Target Organ Toxicology Series

Ophthalmic Toxicology

Target Organ Toxicology Series

Series Editors
A. Wallace Hayes, John A. Thomas, and Donald E. Gardner

Cardiovascular Toxicology, Second Edition
Daniel Acosta, Jr., editor, 576 pp., 1992

Ophthalmic Toxicology
George C. Y. Chiou, editor, 352 pp., 1992

Neurotoxicology
Hugh A. Tilson and Clifford L. Mitchell, editors, 416 pp., 1992

Toxicology of the Lung
Donald E. Gardner, James D. Crapo, and Edward J. Massaro, editors, 540 pp., 1988

Endocrine Toxicology
John A. Thomas, Kenneth S. Korach, and John A. McLachlan, editors, 414 pp., 1985

Immunotoxicology and Immunopharmacology
Jack H. Dean, Michael I. Luster, Albert E. Munson, and Harry Amos, editors, 528 pp., 1985

* **Reproductive Toxicology**
Robert L. Dixon, editor, 368 pp., 1985

Toxicology of the Blood and Bone Marrow
Richard D. Irons, editor, 192 pp., 1985

Toxicology of the Eye, Ear, and Other Special Senses
A. Wallace Hayes, editor, 264 pp., 1985

* **Toxicology of the Immune System**
Jack H. Dean and Albert E. Munson, editors, 528 pp., 1985

Cutaneous Toxicity
Victor A. Drill and Paul Lazar, editors, 288 pp., 1984

Intestinal Toxicology
Carol M. Schiller, editor, 252 pp., 1984

Cardiovascular Toxicology
Ethard W. Van Stee, editor, 400 pp., 1982

---

* Out of print

Target Organ Toxicology Series

Ophthalmic Toxicology

Editor

George C. Y. Chiou, Ph.D.
Professor and Head, Department of Medical Pharmacology and Toxicology
Texas A&M University College of Medicine
College Station, Texas

Raven Press   New York

Raven Press, Ltd., 1185 Avenue of the Americas, New York, New York 10036

Made in the United States of America

Library of Congress Cataloging-in-Publication Data

Ophthalmic toxicology / edited by George C. Y. Chiou.
p. cm. — (Target organ toxicology series.)
Includes bibliographical references and index.
ISBN 0-88167-939-9
1. Ocular toxicology. I. Chiou, George C. Y. II. Series.
[DNLM: 1. Eye—drug effects. 2. Toxicology. WW 525 061]
RE901.T67064 1992
617.71'1—dc20
DNLM/DLC
for Library of Congress 92-16986

9 8 7 6 5 4 3 2 1

To Professor Chen-Yuan Lee, my beloved mentor, an outstanding scholar, a distinguished toxicologist, and an impeccable, unselfish, brave warrior for human welfare.

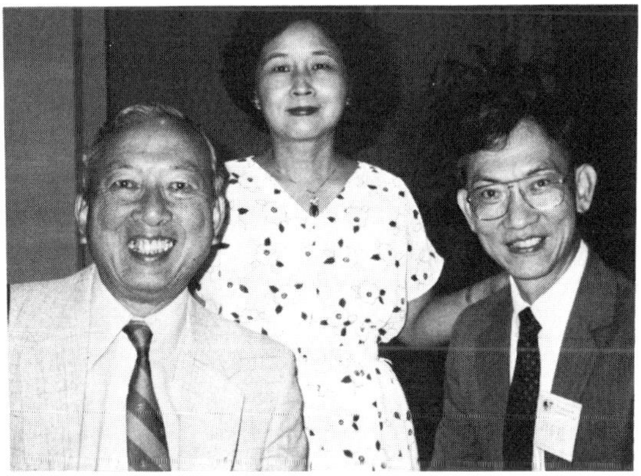

Professor Chen-Yuan Lee, Tricia Chiou, and George Chiou

Contents

Contributing Authors

Jimmy D. Bartlett, O.D. *Department of Optometry, University of Alabama at Birmingham, School of Optometry, Birmingham, Alabama 35294*

Lynn Baxter, B.S. *Department of Medical Pharmacology and Toxicology, Texas A & M University Health Science Center, College Station, Texas 77843*

Elizabeth P. Cannon, Ph.D. *Department of Medical Pharmacology and Toxicology, Texas A & M University Health Science Center, College Station, Texas 77843*

George C. Y. Chiou, Ph.D. *Department of Medical Pharmacology and Toxicology, Institute of Ocular Pharmacology, Texas A & M University Health Science Center, College Station, Texas 77843*

Linda C. Epner, M.D. *Private Practice, Baltimore, Maryland 21225*

Keith Green, Ph.D., D.Sci. *Department of Ophthalmology and Department of Physiology and Endocrinology, Medical College of Georgia, Augusta, Georgia 30912*

David McGuinn, Ph.D. *Department of Medical Pharmacology and Toxicology, Texas A & M University Health Science Center, College Station, Texas 77843*

Nicholas J. Millichamp, D.V.M., Ph.D. *Department of Small Animal Medicine and Surgery, College of Veterinary Medicine, Texas A & M University, College Station, Texas 77843*

Luqi Pei, B.S., M.S. *Department of Medical Pharmacology and Toxicology, Texas A & M University Health Science Center, College Station, Texas 77843*

Ilona Petrikovics, Ph.D. *Department of Medical Pharmacology and Toxicology, Texas A & M University Health Science Center, College Station, Texas 77843*

Brooks H. Rohde, Ph.D. *Department of Medical Pharmacology and Toxicology, Institute of Ocular Pharmacology, Texas A & M University Health Science Center, College Station, Texas 77843*

James L. Way, Ph.D. *Department of Medical Pharmacology and Toxicology, Texas A & M University Health Science Center, College Station, Texas 77843*

Ann Hawkins Zitzer, B.S. *Department of Medical Pharmacology and Toxicology, Texas A & M University Health Science Center, College Station, Texas 77843*

Preface

The uniqueness of this book is the coverage of all aspects of ophthalmic toxicology, including the history and research methods of ophthalmic toxicology: tissue specificity and species differences in ocular responses to chemical injuries, eye toxicities caused by systemic drugs, local agents, air pollutants and occupational hazards, and medical treatment of chemical eye injuries. Although several books are available that cover one or two aspects of the aforementioned areas on an individual basis, none is available that covers all of them in one book as does *Ophthalmic Toxicology*. Therefore, this book will be useful to a broad audience, including researchers, teachers, students, ophthalmologists, optometrists, pharmacists, nurses, and general health-related professionals.

Another unique feature of this book is the concise text that provides an ample number of reference literature. The references provide readers with useful information needed for ordinary purposes or for in-depth information and further investigation of certain aspects of ophthalmic toxicology.

Chapter 1 summarizes the historical perspective of ophthalmic toxicology. Although the history of ophthalmic toxicology originated in 1785 when Withering first noted the visual side effects of foxglove, the explosive development of ophthalmic toxicology is a relatively recent event in medical science.

Chapter 2 concisely reviews the tissue specificity in response to toxic agents. This chapter is designed to assist in the understanding of ocular toxicity caused by systemic and local agents that are presented in later chapters. Although numerous articles are available that discuss the species specificity of anatomy, physiology, and pharmacology, this is the first time that a species specificity of ophthalmic toxicology has been summarized and analyzed.

A good research on ophthalmic toxicology depends very much on reliable animal models. Although the Draize test has been used since 1944 and still is used as the official test method for prediction of clinical toxicities on the eyes in humans, it has inherited numerous problems and disadvantages, as discussed in Chapter 4. For humane reasons, the Draize test should be used as a safety assurance rather than for toxicity testing and only after *in vitro* tests or skin irritation tests show either no irritation or only a mild irritation of the agents. In addition to the skin test, various *in vitro* methods have been developed recently as alternatives to the Draize test (Chapter 5). However, no single *in vitro* method can be used as a complete alternative to the Draize test, as the eye *in vivo* is a very complex structure that is capable of producing a wide variety of responses to toxic insults.

The toxic eye responses caused by representative systemic agents are presented in Chapter 6. The author lists each class of agent with pathogenesis, ocular manifestation, and patient management.

The toxic ocular responses to local contacts are presented in Chapter 7. Unlike systemic agents, tens of thousands of new chemicals are introduced into the world every year, and a large portion of these compounds are toxic to the eyes. Therefore, local agents are treated differently from the systemic drugs by mentioning the ocular toxicity of only a few representative chemicals in each class of agent based on their uses.

Chapter 8 and 9 discuss the ocular toxicity caused by air pollutants and occupational hazards, respectively. Ocular irritations caused by smog and air pollution have become a daily problem for those residents of cities and industrial towns, while ocular toxicities in chemical plants are obvious problems that are experienced by many workers.

The medical treatment of ophthalmic toxicity is presented in Chapter 10. With proper and immediate treatment of ocular toxicity, the result can be happy restoration of eyesight; without it, tragic loss of partial or total eyesight can occur. Therefore, this chapter should be read not only by ophthalmologists, optometrists, nurses and emergency personnel but by general health-related professionals as well.

George C. Y. Chiou

Acknowledgments

It was a delightful experience working with all of the contributors to this book. Completing the chapters on time was not an easy task, and I was grateful to all the contributors who understood my requests and cooperated fully in meeting the deadline. Because of the vast amount of information and the wide range of fields covered in this book, it took almost two years to develop. I am deeply grateful to the secretarial assistance provided by Mrs. Patty Sampson. Without her superb handling of the word processor and her careful proofreading, this book could not have been completed as efficiently and pleasantly as it was.

Target Organ Toxicology Series

Ophthalmic Toxicology

Ophthalmic Toxicology, edited by
George C. Y. Chiou. Raven Press, Ltd.,
New York © 1992.

1

History of Ophthalmic Toxicology

Keith Green

Department of Ophthalmology and Department of Physiology and Endocrinology, Medical College of Georgia, Augusta, Georgia 30912

DEFINITION OF OPHTHALMIC TOXICOLOGY

Despite the occurrence of many events and observations over a period of decades, the science of ocular toxicology, as a recognizably separate discipline from other subspecialties, is of relatively recent origin. The majority of incidents of ocular toxicology, of either single drug effects or of drug interactions, are case reports where the use or addition of a medication has led to an unexpected or unwanted reaction. Very few reports offer the results of a rechallenge with the same drug used by a patient in order to discern whether or not the drug was indeed the cause of the initial reaction. Many of these observations, therefore, are anecdotal in nature. Individually each report may be of relatively little importance, but when a number of similar observations are accumulated they may represent a significant finding. Reactions to drugs or agents may be idiosyncratic or reflect a true, adverse ill effect that is noted in a significant number of individuals exposed to a particular drug or agent.

The expansion of medicine into a scientific and drug-based discipline rather than an empirical and herbal art, in the late 19th and early 20th centuries, gave rise to the development of specific drug products. Following World War II the use of specific, targeted drugs exploded and gave rise to the need to assess these compounds before their exposure to man (1). This progress, in turn, led to the need for an assessment of a single variable against a background of relative constants (2). The veritable explosion of new chemicals and devices requires research protocols in order to determine not only their efficacy, but also any side effects. This has given rise, over the past three or four decades, to the study of mechanisms of drug effects rather than descriptions of responses.

Ocular toxicology consists of two primary systems: One, the study of drugs, devices, or agents given prophylactically in animal trials before their use in man in order to provide some prediction of any potential hazard in human use. Two, the study of the effect of drugs, agents, or drug interactions that have been shown to create adverse effects following their use in, or exposure to, man. The latter include not only ocular effects of systemic drugs but also the systemic effects of ocular drugs (3,4). Such definitions must be viewed relatively conservatively, however, or many substances would be considered toxic. Most drugs or agents, for example, will cause an adverse effect if a sufficiently high concentration is reached. Even oxygen if inhaled at 100% concentration is toxic, and distilled water, if continually ingested, would ultimately lead to problems. The nature and time course of adverse effects depend upon many factors. These include the drug or agent per se, the route of administration or exposure, whether or not a disease or disorder preexists (e.g., the corneal penetration of a drug may be altered during anterior segment or corneal inflammation), age, sex, use or exposure to other drugs or agents, idiosyncrasies, etc. The key is to make careful observations to determine any correlation with drug intake or exposure and identify the variable. One then makes observations that explore the accuracy, or truthfulness, of the observed effects, and their precision or reproducibility. Once a causal relationship has been established, then one can indicate that a toxic effect has occurred (5). It then behooves the investigator to quantitate the observations.

DIVERSITY OF OPHTHALMIC TOXICOLOGY

Given the huge number of prescription drugs (reportedly over 30,000 in the United States alone) and over-the-counter medications (reportedly about 300,000 in the United States) together with all of the various manufactured and natural products to which we are exposed (6), it is not surprising that toxic reactions occur. These occurrences may be due to a single drug, device, or agent or due to an interaction between two or more drugs. There is also an entire ocular toxicology associated with cosmetics that includes safety testing and prognostic ocular toxicology. This area includes mascaras, eyeliners, eye shadows, and eyebrow pencils, as well as devices such as eyelash curlers. There was, and still is, a need for standardization of the observations and an appropriate means of record keeping. These standards have been set by various authorities (e.g., the European Community [7,8], the United States [9], and others) and must be met before approval for human use is permitted. There is still a need for the acceptance of worldwide standards for the labeling of drugs, medications, chemicals, and agents, especially those with the potential for eye damage. Of particular benefit would be worldwide acceptance of standard criteria for ocular toxicity testing. Such standards would allow transference of data from one continent to another, alleviating the need for duplication of effort and expediting the utilization of medications on a wider basis.

OBSERVATIONS OF OPHTHALMIC TOXICOLOGY

Perhaps the earliest observation of ocular toxicity was made in 1785 by Withering (10) who noted that ingestion of foxglove caused confused vision in man, with objects appearing green or yellow. These observations were supported by Carroll (11), who noted similar eye and vision changes after the use of digitalis. Grant (12) has summarized over 100 years of observations on the effects of drugs or agents on the visual system in an elegant synopsis of what is known about substances having toxic effects on the eye. Some observations are dependent upon data from laboratory studies but the majority of observations are case reports.

CLINICAL OBSERVATIONS

Bron (13) drew attention to the remarkable diversity of ocular responses that drugs may cause, some occurring during drug intake, others showing the occurrence of a toxic response after drug withdrawal. Experience has taught us that corticosteroids may cause cataracts and that chloroquine can induce a keratopathy and/ or a retinopathy. These side effects of drugs used for the treatment of nonocular disorders, among others, are well known. Experience has also taught us when it is prudent to monitor for toxic side effects of drugs (13). A variety of tests may be employed to determine whether certain parameters of ocular function fall within normal limits; these include biomicroscopy, intraocular pressure, near and distance visual acuity, visual fields, electroretinography, color vision, dark adaptation, and fluorescein angiography. Changes that may disturb vision include corneal deposits, cataracts, glaucoma, retinal and optic nerve disease, and nystagmus (13).

NEED FOR DOCUMENTATION OF TOXIC RESPONSES

The Physicians Desk Reference (PDR) (14) and Ophthalmic PDR (15) are frequently used as reference sources of drug side effects. Both PDRs contain the same information as supplied on the Food and Drug Administration (FDA)-approved package insert that is made available by the drug manufacturer. The PDR began in 1946 and the Ophthalmic PDR in 1974, indicating an early awareness of the need to provide a resource that listed the possible side effects of various medications. These side effects were recognized as extensions of the observed therapeutic effect with some responses being of an allergic nature (15), and reflected the transition from descriptive to mechanistic medicine. Inorganic materials tend to cause an irritant reaction whose components include hyperemia, edema, increased vascular permeability, and blistering. Organic compounds cause many effects on different tissues, with many of the effects being reversible upon withdrawal of the drug (16). Many observations and descriptions were made dating to the later 1800s and early 1900s for cataracts and other less-evident ocular disorders. As steroids began to be introduced and more widely used to combat either ocular or systemic inflammatory diseases, the secondary side effects of cataracts and elevated intraocular pressure became evident. Other examples of such side effects are the cataract-inducing effects of echothiophate and the occurrence of superficial punctate keratitis, due to surfactants in topical medications, that appear long after the primary disease has disappeared.

One of the major concerns of ocular toxicology research in the mid-1960s was the development of a meaningful and practical test of safety of many manufactured products. These products include drugs, medicines, devices, and agents, in addition to the multitude of chemicals to which the consumer is exposed in the home ranging from household cleaning products to cosmetics. Knowledge of the mechanisms of an injury to the eye caused by direct contact of toxic substances is, in the majority of cases, unknown. Rather, many compounds are known only as an inducer of a response (17). As discussed below, the underlying question concerning the similarity of the response of the widely chosen test model, the rabbit, relative to the effects in man caused by the same agent, is one that remains unanswered.

TOXICITY TESTING

Introduction of the Draize Test

The aim of the study of ocular toxicology is to anticipate and avoid considerable side effects of drugs or agents. This is achieved best through a series of comprehensive tests prior to human use. Testing normally occurs in animals, with the choice of the model system being very important because different species give different responses to the same stimulus. Testing is usually performed by noting the severity of injury to the eye, and the data are used as a guide to determine any labeling of the drug or agent for human use. Because many agents, chemicals, or drugs reach the eye by a topical route, considerable emphasis was placed originally on the assessment of ocular injury or irritation by this route.

The earliest standardized test schedule for determining external ocular toxicity was published in 1944 by Friedenwald et al. (18). This basic grading schedule was upgraded by Draize, Woodard, and Calvery (19) with a system that was modified in 1952 and 1959 (20,21). Standard use of this scheme for testing commercial substances has occurred through its specified use by several different government agencies. The Federal Hazardous Substances Act (22), as detailed in the 1979 Code of Federation Regulations (23), provided the criteria for determining what constitutes "safe" or "hazardous" materials. The Federal Hazardous Substances Act Regulation (1982) is the most recent outline of the protocols to be employed in the United States (24).

No discussion of the history of ocular toxicity would be complete without an exploration of the use of the so-called Draize test and the various other *in vitro* tests that it has generated. It could be said that the other tests would have evolved anyway, and in some cases the technology has been developed because of other needs such as the understanding of physiological processes, but there is little question that the Draize test has acted as a stimulus for the development of many *in vitro* or alternative systems.

The Draize test has been subject to analysis by a number of authors who have addressed the accuracy and reproducibility of the method, the scoring system (25,26), and the comparisons of rabbit data, in which the test is specified, to the human experience. The Draize test scores the effects of drugs or agents, when delivered as 0.1 mg of a solid or 0.1 ml of a liquid into the lower cul-de-sac of the eye. The effects on the cornea, conjunctiva, and iris of rinsed and unrinsed eyes are evaluated at 24, 48, 72 hr, and 4 and 7 days after administration of the test material. Because of the scoring procedures corneal and iris lesions have greater emphasis in the accumulation of "points" for the total score. The corneal scores, because of the multiplication of the different individual subsections, tend to rank very high. The observations required by the testing agencies involve only nonmicroscopic observations of the eye. To assist in the evaluation process a series of color slides is available (27–29). Many authors have stressed greater precision and sensitivity of the test by using different grading systems, the use of slit-lamp biomicroscopy or objective physical measurements of parameters such as corneal thickness (30–34) or corneal epithelial permeability to fluorescein (31,35). Several aspects of this literature have been reviewed earlier (36–39).

The primary objections to the Draize test are those of interlaboratory variation and the accuracy of predicting effects on man. These concerns have been expressed for quite some time, but the level of concern has increased over the past 10 years. Laboratory-to-laboratory variation is expected because the observations required in the Draize test are subjective, although comparisons of unknown samples to known standards often produce similar data. The greater reactivity of the rabbit eye compared to that of man has been one of the major problems with the Draize test. The development of more intense, and prolonged, responses on the rabbit eye compared to man means that the effects are overestimated relative to human responses. Similarly, the use of a large amount, or volume, of test material relative to the smaller amount that humans are estimated to receive on their ocular surface tends to maximize the response of the rabbit eye. The use of other species has been suggested as a means of overcoming this problem.

Modification of the Draize Test

Primate testing, however, although providing more accurate comparisons to man than rabbit (40), has the disadvantages of much greater cost, restricted availability, dangers associated with handling the animals, and the potential for the loss of the animals' sight. Other alternatives (41) suggest that making the rabbit test less severe so as to give results consistent with the known experience is a more practical approach. This is especially true for the lids and conjunctiva of the rabbit that have a much more vigorous reaction than those same tissues in man. The corneal response is almost equal.

Historically, a reduction in dose of applied material and an assessment of reversibility of the response were suggested by the National Research Council Committee of the National Academy of Sciences. This group was asked by the Consumer Product Safety Commission to review the criteria utilized in the Federal Hazardous Substances Act for their ability to predict human ocular responses. As a result of its deliberations, the committee suggested that a smaller dose be used in order to reduce the ocular responses of rabbits to a range more consistent with known responses available from the human experience (42). The committee further suggested that the use of at least two dose levels would provide useful information, and that longer observation times would allow the factoring of reversibility of any response. Testing of a series of substances with different degrees of recognized irritation potential indicated that the Federal Hazardous Substance Act test criteria overrated the irritancy of all the moderate irritants. The National Academy of Sciences test criteria, however, when using a 0.01 ml dose, best predicted the human experience. The latter, of course, are based on anecdotal information, reports to companies from consumers, and occupational incidents, and in many cases form only an incomplete series of reports.

Other Refinements

Subsequent studies, during the intervening years, on the interrelationship between animal experimental data and the human experience after exposure to the same materials has only supported the notion that responses after low-dose applications of materials in rabbits is equivalent to human responses. This result has been substantiated in several studies (41,43–47). It is evident, therefore, that a further modification of the Draize test that incorporates dilute solutions or smaller quantities or volumes of material needs to be accepted by the appropriate authorities to allow more appropriate use of this test for predication of human responses. Smaller numbers of animals have also been advocated for *in vivo* irritancy testing and this has been demonstrated to provide equally adequate data (48).

Replacement of the Draize Test

Several *in vitro* tests have been developed that complement the Draize test and allow initial screening of drugs, chemicals, or agents prior to final testing in an *in vivo* animal model system. *In vitro* tests such as the isolated bovine cornea (49), isolated eyes (50–53), isolated rabbit ileum (54), tissue cultured cells (55–63), chick chorioallantoic membrane (CAM) (64–66), and nonliving systems (67–70) have been employed. Each of these alternative testing methods has drawbacks compared to the response of the *in vivo* eye. The isolated cornea represents but one facet of the ocular response by eliminating the vasoactive and chemotic components of the conjunctival response; tissue cultured cells have no blood supply thus no vascular response can be observed; the CAM offers an elegant alternative for the ocular response but does not include the membranes and connective tissue similar to the cornea and, in addition, an assumption is made concerning a relationship between angiogenesis and inflammation; the totally synthetic system offers no vascular response, although apparently showing clouding similar to the corneal stroma (67–70). Initial testing using these systems has a valuable role in the assessment of potential toxicity of materials that we use or are exposed to either accidentally or deliberately. All roads for the present, however, lead to use of the final *in vivo* assessment as the ultimate test procedure. Further testing of *in vitro* methodologies may yield a system, or a combination of systems, that may predict the behavior of chemicals, drugs, and agents in man.

Can one, with sufficient accuracy, predict the human experience from rabbit or even *in vitro* data? The present evidence, if the correct low dosage test is used in rabbit, is that it is possible to obtain a valid comparison that would reflect human eye behavior. Known experience after exposure to specific chemicals is most often less drastic in man than equivalent exposure in other test species. The experience thus far with entirely *in vitro* test methods appears promising, although it is probably unlikely that a single test will replace the Draize. As Beckley (17) points out, however, we would condemn the placement of known substances into the human eye without first testing it in animal eyes. This does not imply that one treats the test with impunity, but approaches the test in a compassionate and thoughtful manner with use of a lower initial concentration of the material in only a few test cases before proceeding to the test of the full-strength material. The testing in animals follows *in vitro* tests that eliminate harmful irritants.

In 1981, the cosmetics industry took the lead in expanding studies on alternate approaches to assessment of *in vivo* irritancy by establishing the Center for Alternatives to Animal Testing based in the School of Hygiene and Public Health at the Johns Hopkins University Medical Institutions. The aim of this center is to serve as a focal point for the utilization of industry funds for the study of cellular and molecular events occurring with inflammatory processes in cell and tissue culture systems. The results of the studies supported by the center have been published (71–77). In the *in vitro* organic test system a high correlation has been obtained with the *in vivo* Draize test (67,78). Indeed, the high success rate of this test has already caused some cosmetic companies to adopt this method as an *in vitro* alternative for ocular irritancy testing (1). There has been a marked transition over the last 40 years, therefore, from the introduction of the Draize test to a spectrum of alternative tests that allow the use of fewer animals, and in some cases total replacement of animals by other test systems.

DEVELOPMENT OF TECHNIQUES

While there has been an emphasis on the Draize test and its modification or replacement with alternative *in vitro* test systems over the years, there has also been a vast expansion in oculotoxicity methods for tissues other than the cornea. Specifically for the cornea, the use of specular microscopy (with or without simultaneous pachymetry [79]) has allowed the assessment of corneal endothelial changes in the living eye by permitting measurement of cell density and shape. Sophisticated analytical methods exist that allow one to distinguish the various changes in cell morphology that may occur in the endothelium (80).

Similarly, new technologies have allowed assessment of lens changes. Equipment developed to allow slit-image photography of the lens using Scheimpflug's principle has permitted quantitative analysis of lens toxicity (81–86). Evaluations have been made of a whole range of environmental and drug influences upon the development of cataracts in different animal models, allowing a differentiation to be made between drug-induced effects and aging changes (86–88). In addition, more recent analytical techniques such as nuclear magnetic resonance have been used *in vivo* and *in vitro* to examine lens changes (89). *In vitro* examination methods for analyzing changes in lenses after experimental study have also become available. These techniques allow the use of smaller portions of tissue such that thin sections can now be analyzed, instead of whole lenses (90). Use has also been made of chemical structures and known phototoxicity of chemicals in predicting behavior in lenses (91). Other studies on eye tissues such as those in the anterior segment or relative to intraocular pressure control have also profited from the application of new techniques (92,93). Electrophysiological studies of the retina (94,95), combined with morphological studies, have enabled toxicity tests to be performed on a variety of inorganic (96) and organic compounds (97–102). Detailed examinations have also outlined age-related tissue changes (103) as well as the toxicological differences between pigmented and albino animals (104).

The response of an eye to a foreign agent or chemical is determined in part by the longevity of its residence on the corneal surface. Experimentally, however, it has been found that irrigation of eyes is of little benefit if delayed for more than 20 to 30 sec after exposure (105,106). This may be related to the production of prostaglandins and other mediators (such as histamine) in eye tissues following exposure to chemicals or agents that contact the eye. Although the degree of susceptibility of different tissues from different species is highly variable (107,108), there is a common underlying release of prostaglandins in response to a physical or chemical insult. It has been well documented, however, that different species respond in quite different ways to the same stimulus (109); thus, the impact of prostaglandin metabolism differs between species.

In vitro tests have demonstrated a variety of responses, depending upon the type of cells used and the chemical under test. Good correlations or even inverse conditions have been found with different cell systems used in a variety of different techniques (106). The data obtained with surfactants suggest that the mechanism of surfactant irritation to the eye is not straightforward, being complicated by the degree of hydrophobicity of the cornea. Thus, data obtained would be considered as a guide for the test compounds, but not a result that could be slavishly followed. This, and other tests, might be used to exclude certain chemicals, drugs, or agents that would be extremely harmful in the living eye.

Toxicity testing has undergone an evolution during the past 40 years on at least two fronts. In one there has been a shift from anecdotal reports based upon single observations of drug-induced side effects in recipients to a more sophisticated reporting system exemplified in the United States by the National

Registry of Drug-Induced Ocular Side Effects. On the second front, there has been a revolution in the assessment of toxicity from the subjective Draize type of test to ones including the use of quantitative measures of different parameters, whether this be the specular microscope to permit corneal endothelial cell counts to be performed, Scheimpflug photography of the lens with subsequent densitometric analysis, or electroretinographic determinations. Each of these, and other, technological advances has allowed a more precise analysis to be performed on the effects of drugs, whether they be primary or secondary.

Despite these advances, and the publication of drug-induced side effects either from laboratory or from clinical experience, it must be remembered that by far the largest proportion of all the data in ocular toxicology studies (as with all toxicology) is held within the proprietary interests of drug companies. Much of what has been published has come from the public sector when scientists or physicians have had access to materials for testing before or after public release and this data has resulted in publications. Although there has been a considerable increase in the quantity and quality of data that has been published in the area of toxicology, the validation of the data concerning drug-induced side effects or drug-induced ocular toxicology occurs primarily through epidemiological studies. Studies of this type are not only rare but also tremendously expensive; voluntary reporting of side effects and suspected ocular toxicology through a system such as the National Registry of Drug-Induced Ocular Side Effects in the United States is a cost-effective means of partly accomplishing this goal.

PUBLICATIONS

The considerable developments in ocular toxicology over the past few years are exemplified by the appearance of Fraunfelder's book (110) on drug-induced ocular side effects, which discusses probable and possible medication-induced side effects and drug interactions. This burgeoning area of oculotoxicity is replete with possible drug-induced effects. It is the previous reports of drug effects or interactions that may alert the ophthalmologist or other physicians to make the connection between drug use and drug-related effects. This book, in addition to including many references of observations, contains compilations of reports from the National Registry of Drug-Induced Ocular Side Effects, which was organized in 1976 to act as a resource for reports of ocular toxicity (111,112). Data are reported by physicians who suspect adverse reactions secondary to drug therapy. The national registry serves as a focal point for all physicians to report possible cause-and-effect relationships between drugs and unwanted side effects. At the national level, accumulation of data can occur at a vastly enhanced rate compared to what would occur in individual groups of physicians in a common discipline such as in an academic department. When associations are found, they are reported back to the physicians regarding the use and concentration of drugs, or interaction of drugs with each other, so that appropriate adjustments can be made in drug use by patients.

While an earlier book (113), which was the result of a meeting, addressed drug effects on the eye and eye tissues, the focus was more on physiological and pharmacological events, although the responses to excess concentrations (toxicity) was also discussed. Over the past 12 years a series of meetings has been held on drug-induced ocular side effects and ocular toxicology at various locations. The initial meeting (1977) was in Little Rock, Arkansas. This was followed by meetings in Portland, Oregon (1980), Milwaukee, Wisconsin (1982), Augusta, Georgia (1984), Bonn, Germany (1986), Toronto, Canada (1988) and Deidesheim, Germany (1990). Beginning with the Toronto meeting the International Society of Ocular Toxicology was formally founded. The 1992 meeting was held in Sedona, Arizona. The proceedings of the 1986 meeting, which was the fifth international symposium on the subject of ocular toxicology, was published (114) in book form. The Deidesheim meeting proceedings were published in 1990 as an issue of the journal *Lens and Eye Toxicity Research*.

Publications also occur from the registry when sufficient data are available on a particular topic or when a specific drug side effect occurs within the reporting system with a greater than usual frequency. These papers have addressed subjects as diverse as the ocular use of topical phenylephrine at high (115) or low (116) concentrations to the systemic side effects of beta blockers (117,118) and carbonic anhydrase inhibitors (119). Other authors have addressed the side effects of beta blockers (120) and systemic drug interactions with topical glaucoma medications (121), and still others, for example, have addressed drug-induced side effects in Japan (122).

FUTURE AREAS FOR DEVELOPMENT

Although the Draize test has been subject to criticism and modification over the past 40 years, discussions on the use and validity of this test have increased recently. This is, of course, but one aspect of ocular toxicity that excludes examination of what is probably the most susceptible tissue to toxic effects of drugs, namely the lens. The overall view of ocular toxicity, while incorporating the testing of agents and products to which consumers are exposed, must encompass all drugs, chemicals, agents, and devices as well as all eye tissues because no eye tissue is free from the induction of such effects.

In vitro techniques cannot completely replace *in vivo* testing because of their inability to reflect all of the potential manifestations of irritancy. As has been pointed out, however, perhaps a battery of *in vitro* tests, each addressing specific response situations may one day replace the Draize test (106,123). Acceptance of standards for procedures and scoring systems by all regulatory agencies worldwide would certainly be a major achievement, even though the possibility of such unanimity seems remote. Certainly, refinement of the *in vivo* test procedure is required with acceptance by the appropriate agencies of lower doses and fewer animals per test material. Similarly, the use of precedent should be allowable on a larger scale; such a maneuver would limit the need to test yet another material for which the ingredients have been sufficiently tested in the past. The use of *in vitro* techniques to screen materials that have a high irritancy potential would eliminate the need for a number of *in vivo* tests, and eliminate materials that show eye irritancy potential.

Succeeding chapters in this volume address many aspects of ocular toxicology, providing an overview of where this science stands as applied to different tissues of the eye, the methods used to assess toxicity, and the various sources of toxic effects ranging from drugs administered to alleviate a disease to air pollutants. To date, the history of ocular toxicology is brief and somewhat narrowly focused. Recent years have seen an expansion of interests into many diverse areas despite the lack of funding for such approaches by government agencies. An assessment after the next decade will provide a better perspective on whether or not ocular toxicology has assumed a greater role in the marketing of all products, whether designed for systemic or topical use or reaching the eye accidently.

ACKNOWLEDGMENTS

Some of the work reported herein from the author's laboratory was supported in part by National Eye Institute Research Grant EY04558, in part by National Glaucoma Research, a program of the American Health Assistance Foundation, and in part by an Unrestricted Departmental Award from Research to Prevent Blindness, Inc. I thank Brenda Sheppard for her valuable secretarial assistance and Lisa Cheeks and Myra Green for their editorial assistance. I wish to thank Drs. Frederick T. Fraunfelder, Edward M. Jackson, and Malcolm N. Luxenberg for their valuable critiques of this contribution and for their numerous constructive suggestions.

REFERENCES

1. Jackson EM. Animal testing in biomedical research. In: Hockwin O, Green K, Rubin L, eds. *Manual of oculotoxicity testing of drugs*. Stuttgart: G Fischer-Verlag, 1992; 1–8.
2. Jackson EM. Ocular irritancy: the search for acceptable and humane test methods. In: Estrin NF, ed. *The cosmetic industry: scientific and regulatory foundations*. New York: Marcel Dekker, 1984;437–464.
3. Bartlett JD, Jaanus SD. Ocular effects of systemic drugs. In: Bartlett JD, Jaanus SD, eds. *Clinical ocular pharmacology*. Boston: Butterworth's, 1989;801–842.
4. Newcomb RD, Priest ML. Systemic effects of ocular drugs. In: Bartlett JD, Jaanus SD, eds. *Clinical ocular pharmacology*. Boston: Butterworth's, 1989;843–862.
5. Havener W. *Ocular pharmacology*, 5th ed. St. Louis: C.V. Mosby, 1983.
6. Meyer SM, Fraunfelder FT. National registry of drug-induced ocular side effects. In: Hockwin O, ed. *Drug-induced ocular side effects and ocular toxicology*. Basel: Karger, 1987;40–44.
7. Schnieders B. Recommendations concerning toxicity tests on medical products. State of affairs within the European Community. In: Hockwin O, ed. *Drug-induced ocular side effects and ocular toxicology*. Basel: Karger, 1987;1–8.
8. Lehnert T, Ulrich B. Requirements of preclinical examinations. *Lens Eye Toxic Res* 1990;7:207–219.
9. Hackett RB. Nonclinical study requirements for ophthalmic drugs and devices in the United States. *Lens Eye Toxic Res* 1990;7:181–205.
10. Withering W. *An account of the foxglove and some of its medical uses: with practical remarks on dropsy and other diseases*. Birmingham, England: Broomsleigh Press, 1785.
11. Carroll FD. Visual symptoms caused by digitalis. *Am J Ophthalmol* 1945;28:373–376.

12. Grant WM. *Toxicology of the eye*, 2nd ed. Springfield, IL: Charles C. Thomas, 1974.
13. Bron AJ. Mechanisms of ocular toxicity. In: Gorrod JW, ed. *Drug toxicity*. London: Taylor & Francis, 1979;229–253.
14. *Physicians Desk Reference*. Oradell, NJ: Medical Economics, 1990.
15. *Physicians Desk Reference for Ophthalmology*. Oradell, NJ: Medical Economics, 1990.
16. Duke-Elder S. *System of ophthalmology, vol XIV: Injuries*, part 2, Non-mechanical injuries. St. Louis: C.V. Mosby, 1972.
17. Beckley JH. Comparative eye testing: man vs. animal. *Toxicol Appl Pharmacol* 1965;7(suppl):93–101.
18. Friedenwald JS, Hughes WF, Hermann H. Acid-base tolerance of the cornea. *Arch Ophthalmol* 1944;31:279–283.
19. Draize JH, Woodard G. Calvery HO. Methods for the study of irritation and toxicity of substances applied topically to the skin and mucous membranes. *J Pharmacol Exp Ther* 1944;82:377–390.
20. Draize JH, Kelley EA. Toxicity to eye mucosa of certain cosmetic preparations containing surface-active agents. *Proc Sci Sect Toilet Goods Assoc* 1952;17:1–4.
21. Draize JH. Dermal toxicity. In: *Appraisal of the safety of chemicals in foods, drugs and cosmetics*. Austin, TX: Assoc Food and Drug Officials of the United States, 1959;46–59.
22. Consumer Product Safety Commission. *Hazardous substances labeling guide*, Appendix 1. Washington, DC: 1979;29,53.
23. Code of Federal Regulations. *Title 16, part 1500.42*. Washington DC: U.S. Government Printing Office, 1979.
24. Federal Hazardous Substances Act Regulations. *Code of Federal Regulations* 1982;16:part 1500.
25. Weltman AS, Sparber SB, Jurtshuk T. Comparative evaluation and the influence of various factors on eye-irritation scores. *Toxicol Appl Pharmacol* 1965;7:308–319.
26. Baldwin HA, McDonald TO, Beasley CH. Slit-lamp examination of experimental animal eyes. II. Grading scales and photographic evaluation of induced pathological conditions. *J Soc Cosmet Chem* 1973;24:181–195.
27. *Federal Register*. September 17, 1964;29:13009.
28. Focd and Drug Administration. *Illustrated guide for grading eye irritation by hazardous substances*. Washington, DC: U.S. Government Printing Office, 1965.
29. Marzulli FN. New data on eye and skin tests. *Toxicol Appl Pharmacol* 1965;7(suppl):79–85.
30. Burton ABG. A method for the objective assessment of eye irritation. *Food Cosmet Toxicol* 1972;10:209–217.
31. Green K, Bowman KA, Elijah RD, Mermelstein R, Kilpper RW. Dose-effect response of the rabbit eye to cetylpyridinium chloride. *J Toxicol Cutan Ocular Toxicol* 1985;4:13–26.
32. Morgan RL, Sorenson SS, Castles TR. Prediction of ocular irritation by corneal pachymetry. *Food Chem Toxicol* 1987;25:609–613.
33. Kennah HE, Hignet S, Laux PE, Dorko JD, Barrow CS. An objective procedure for quantitating eye irritation based upon changes of corneal thickness. *Fundam Appl Toxicol* 1989;12:258–268.
34. Green K, Crosby VA, Cheeks L. Toxicity of intracameral thymoxamine. *Lens Eye Toxic Res* 1990;7:121–132.
35. Ramselaar JAM, Boot JP, van Haeringen NJ, van Best JA, Oosterhuis JA. Corneal epithelial permeability after instillation of ophthalmic solutions containing local anaesthetics and preservatives. *Curr Eye Res* 1988;7:947–950.
36. McDonald TO, Shadduck JA. Eye irritation. In: Marzulli FN, Maibach HI, eds. *Dermatotoxicology and pharmacology. Advances in modern toxicology, vol 4*. Washington, DC: Hemisphere, 1977;139–191.
37. McDonald TO, Seabaugh V, Shadduck JA, Edelhauser HF. Eye irritation. In: Marzulli FN, Maibach HI, eds. *Dermatotoxicology*, 3rd ed. Washington, DC: Hemisphere, 1987;641–696.
38. McDonald TO, Hiddeman JW, Howe WE, Robertson SM. Ocular safety evaluation: alternatives and the future. In: Marzulli FN, Maibach HI, eds. *Dermatotoxicology*, 3rd ed. Washington, DC: Hemisphere, 1987;697–710.
39. Chan PK, Hayes AW. Principles and methods for acute toxicity and eye irritancy. In: Hayes AW, ed. *Principles and methods of toxicology*. New York: Raven Press, 1988;169–220.
40. Green WR, Sullivan JB, Hehir RM, Scharpf LG, Dickinson AW. *A systematic comparison of chemically induced eye injury in the albino rabbit and rhesus monkey*. New York: Soap and Detergent Association, 1978.
41. Griffith JF, Nixon GA, Bruce RD, Reer PJ, Bannan EA. Dose-response studies with chemical irritants

in the albino rabbit eye as a basis for selecting optimum testing conditions for predicting hazard to the human eye. *Toxicol Appl Pharmacol* 1982;55:501-513.

42. Committee for the Revision of NAS Publication 1138. Dermal and eye toxicity tests. In: *Principles and procedures for evaluating the toxicity of household substances.* Washington, DC: National Academy of Science, 1977;41-54.
43. Freeberg FE, Nixon GA, Reer PJ, et al. Human and rabbit eye responses to chemical insult. *Fundam Appl Toxicol* 1986;7:626-634.
44. Freeberg FE, Griffith JF, Bruce RD, Bay PHS. Correlation of animal test methods with human experience for household products. *J Toxicol Cutan Ocular Toxicol* 1984;1:53-64.
45. Freeberg FE, Hooker DT, Griffith JF. Correlation of animal eye test data with human experience for household products: an update. *J Toxicol Cutan Ocular Toxicol* 1986;5:115-123.
46. Allgood GS. Use of animal eye test data and human experience for determining the ocular irritation potential of shampoos. *J Toxicol Cutan Ocular Toxicol* 1989;8:321-326.
47. Arthur BH, Pennisi SC, DiPasquale LC, et al. Effects of anesthetic pretreatment and low volume dosage on ocular irritancy potential of cosmetics: a collaborative study. *J Toxicol Cutan Ocular Toxicol* 1986;5:215-227.
48. Talsma DM, Leach CL, Hatoum NS, Gibbons RD, Roger JC, Garvin PJ. Reducing the number of rabbits in the Draize eye irritancy test: a statistical analysis of 155 studies conducted over 6 years. *Fundam Appl Toxicol* 1988;10:146-153.
49. Muir CK. Opacity of bovine cornea in vitro induced by surfactants and industrial chemicals compared with ocular irritancy in vivo. *Toxicol Lett* 1985;24:157-162.
50. Price JB, Andrews IJ. The in vitro assessment of eye irritancy using isolated eyes. *Food Chem Toxicol* 1985;23:313-315.
51. Himber J, Andermann G, Erhart M, Leclerc G. Bouzoubaa M. In vitro potential measurement, anaesthetic and antimicrobial effects as indications of beta-blocker toxicity of the cornea. *Methods Find Exp Clin Pharmacol* 1985;7:195-201.
52. Burton ABG, York M, Lawrence RS. The in vitro assessment of severe eye irritants. *Food Cosmet Toxicol* 1981;19:471-480.
53. Maurice D, Singh T. A permeability test for acute corneal toxicity. *Toxicol Lett* 1986;31:125-130.
54. Muir CK. The comparative toxic effects of proprietary antidandruff, adult and baby shampoos on rabbit ileum. *Toxicol Lett* 1983;18:227-230.
55. North-Root H, Yackovich F, Demetrulias J, Gacula M, Heinze JE. Evaluation of an in vitro cell toxicity test using rabbit corneal cells to predict eye irritation potential of surfactants. *Toxicol Lett* 1982;14:207-212.
56. North-Root H, Yackovich F, Demetrulias J, Gacula M, Heinze JE. Prediction of the eye irritation potential of shampoos using the in vitro SIRC cell toxicity test. *Food Chem Toxicol* 1985;23:271-273.
57. Kemp RB, Meredith RW, Gamble S, Frost M. A rapid cell culture technique for assessing the toxicity of detergent-based products in vitro as a possible screen for eye irritancy in vivo. *Cytobios* 1983;36:153-159.
58. Kemp RB, Meredith RW, Gamble SH. Toxicity of commercial products on cells in suspension culture: a possible screen for the Draize eye irritation test. *Food Chem Toxicol* 1985;23:267-270.
59. Bracher M, Faller C, Spengler J, Reinhardt CA. Comparison of in vitro cell toxicity with in vivo eye irritation. *Mol Toxicol* 1987/8;1:561-570.
60. Rink H, Hockwin O. Tissue culture in toxicological research applied to lens epithelial cells. In: Hockwin O, ed. *Drug-induced ocular side effects and ocular toxicology.* Basel: Karger, 1987;368-375.
61. Scaife MC. An in vitro cytotoxicity test to predict the ocular irritation potential of detergents and detergent products. *Food Chem Toxicol* 1985;23:253-258.
62. Simmons SJ, Jumblatt MM, Neufeld AH. Corneal epithelial wound closure in tissue culture: an in vitro model of ocular irritancy. *Toxicol Appl Pharmacol* 1987;88:13-23.
63. Nardone RM, Bradlaw JA. Toxicity testing with *in vitro* systems. 1. Ocular tissue culture. *J Toxicol Cutan Ocular Toxicol* 1983;2:81-98.
64. Luepke NP. Hen's egg chorioallantoic membrane test for irritation potential. *Food Chem Toxicol* 1985;23:287-291.
65. Parish WE. Ability of in vitro (corneal injury—eye organ—and chorioallantoic membrane) tests to represent histopathological features of acute eye inflammation. *Food Chem Toxicol* 1985;23:215-227.

66. Leighton J, Nassaeur J, Tchao R. The chick embryo in toxicology: an alternative to the rabbit eye. *Food Chem Toxicol* 1985;23:293-298.
67. Wallin RF, Hume RD, Jackson EM. The agarose diffusion method for ocular irritancy screening: cosmetic products, part I. *J Toxicol Cutan Ocular Toxicol* 1987;6:239-250.
68. Gordon VC, Kelly CP, Bergman HC. Applications of the Eyetex method. *Toxic in Vitro* 1990;4:314-317.
69. Gordon VC, Bergman HC. Eyetex: an in vitro method for evaluation of ocular irritancy. In: Goldberg AM, ed. *In vitro toxicology: approaches to validation.* New York: Mary Ann Liebert, 1987;293-302.
70. Gordon VC, Bergman HC. External evaluation of the standard Eyetex system in six laboratories to determine intra- and inter-laboratory accuracy and precision. In: Goldberg AM, ed. *Progress in in vitro toxicology.* New York: Mary Ann Liebert, 1988;317-323.
71. Goldberg AM, ed. *Product Safety Evaluation.* New York: Mary Ann Liebert, 1983.
72. Goldberg AM. *Acute toxicity testing: alternative approaches.* New York: Mary Ann Liebert, 1984.
73. Goldberg AM, ed. *In vitro toxicology: a progress report from the Johns Hopkins Center for Alternatives to Animal Testing.* New York: Mary Ann Liebert, 1985.
74. Goldberg AM, ed. *A critical evaluation of alternatives to acute ocular irritation testing.* New York: Mary Ann Liebert, 1987.
75. Goldberg AM, ed. *In vitro toxicology: approaches to validation.* New York: Mary Ann Liebert, 1987.
76. Goldberg AM, ed. *Progress in in vitro toxicology.* New York: Mary Ann Liebert, 1988.
77. Goldberg, AM, ed. *In vitro toxicology: new directions.* New York: Mary Ann Liebert, 1989.
78. Jackson EM, Hume RD, Wallin RF. The agarose diffusion method for ocular irritancy screening: cosmetic products, part II. *J Toxicol Cutan Ocular Toxicol* 1988;7:187-194.
79. Santoul C, Decrouez E, Droit JY, Bonne C. Use of a specular microscope with pachymeter in ocular tolerance studies of eye drops in the rabbit. Evaluation of ocular tolerance of benzalkonium chloride (BAK) in aqueous solution, 0.01% and 0.1%. *Lens Eye Toxic Res* 1990;7:359-369.
80. Edelhauser HF, Ubels J. Models and methods for testing toxicity with tear fluid, cornea, and conjunctiva. In: Hockwin O, Green K, Rubin L, eds. *Manual of oculotoxicity testing of drugs.* Stuttgart: G Fischer-Verlag, 1992; 195-218.
81. Wegener A, Laser H, Hockwin O. Measurement of lens transparency changes in animals. Comparison of the Topcon SL-45 combined with linear microdensitometry and the Zeiss SLC system. In: Hockwin O, ed. *Drug-induced ocular side effects and ocular toxicology.* Basel: Karger, 1987;263-275.
82. Dragomirescu V, Hockwin O, Koch HR, Sasaki K. Development of a new equipment for rotating slit image photography according to Scheimpflug's principle. In: Hockwin O, ed. *Gerontological aspects of eye research.* Basel: Karger, 1978;13:118-130.
83. Eckerskorn U, Hockwin O, Chen TT, Knowles W, Dobbs RE. Contribution of cataract epidemiological studies to the evaluation of cataractogenic risk factors. In: Hockwin O, ed. *Drug-induced ocular side effects and ocular toxicology.* Basel: Karger, 1987;71-78.
84. Lerman S. In vivo methods to evaluate ocular drug efficacy and side effects. In: Hockwin O, ed. *Drug-induced ocular side effects and ocular toxicology.* Basel: Karger, 1987;87-104.
85. Lehnert T, Grosdanoff P, Hockwin O. Assessment of drug-induced oculotoxicity by animal models. In: Hockwin O, ed. *Drug-induced ocular side effects and ocular toxicology.* Basel: Karger, 1987;232-240.
86. Wegener A, Hockwin O. Animal models as a tool to detect the subliminal cocataractogenic potential of drugs. In: Hockwin O, ed. *Drug-induced ocular side effects and ocular toxicology.* Basel: Karger, 1987;250-262.
87. Schmitt C, Schmidt J, Hockwin O. Ocular drug-safety study with the HMG-CoA reductase inhibitor Pravastatin. *Lens Eye Toxic Res* 1990;7:631-641.
88. Kojima M, Hockwin O, Rao GS, Garcia J. Investigations on the presence of 3-hydroxy-3-methylglutaryl coenzyme—a reductase (HMG-CoA-reductase, E.C. 1.1.1.34) in lenses of various animal species. *Lens Eye Toxic Res* 1990;7:605-623.
89. Lerman S. Biophysical methods to monitor lens aging and pre-cataractous changes in vivo. *Lens Eye Toxic Res* 1990;7:243-249.
90. Bours J, Ahrend MHJ, Hockwin O. Crystallin profiles of calf and bovine lens in microsections stained for free sulfhydryl groups and proteins. *Lens Eye Toxic Res* 1990;7:531-545.
91. Roberts JE, Dillon J. Screening for potential in vivo phototoxicity in the lens/retina. *Lens Eye Toxic Res* 1990;7:655-666.
92. Green K. Models and methods for testing toxicity with intraocular pressure. In: Hockwin O, Green

K, Rubin L, eds. *Manual of oculotoxicity testing of drugs.* Stuttgart: G Fischer Verlag, 1992; 243-253.
93. Green K. Models and methods for testing toxicity with aqueous humor, iris and ciliary body. In: Hockwin O, Green K, Rubin L, eds. *Manual of oculotoxicity testing of drugs.* Stuttgart: G Fischer Verlag, 1992;219-242.
94. Brown GC, Eagle RC, Shakin EP, Gruber M, Arbizio VV. Retinal toxicity of intravitreal gentamicin. *Arch Ophthalmol* 1990;108:1740-1744.
95. Blain L, Lachapelle P, Molotchnikoff S. The effect of acute triethylene exposure on electroretinogram components. *Neurotoxicol Teratol* 1990;12:633-636.
96. Paylor R, Peyman GA, Badri S. Effects of intravitreal injection of fluorosilicone oil after vitrectomy in the rabbit eye. *Can J Ophthalmol* 1987;22:251-253.
97. Hennekes R, Janssen K, Muñoz C, Winneke G. Lead-induced ERG alterations in rats at high and low levels of exposure. In: Hockwin O, ed. *Drug-induced ocular side effects and ocular toxicology.* Basel: Karger, 1987;193-199.
98. Zlioba A, Peyman GA, Nikoleit J. Retinal toxicity study of intravitreal carboplatin and iproplatin. *Ann Ophthalmol* 1988;20:71-72.
99. Fiscella R, Peyman GA, Kimura A, Small G. Intravitreal toxicity of cotrimoxazole. *Ophthalmic Surg* 1988;19:44-46.
100. Small GH, Peyman GA, Srinivasan A, Smith RT, Fiscella R. Retinal toxicity of combination antiviral drugs in an animal model. *Can J Ophthalmol* 1987;22:300-303.
101. Baldinger J, Doft BH, Burns SA, Johnson B. Retinal toxicity of amphotericin B in vitrectomised versus non-vitrectomised eyes. *Br J Ophthalmol* 1986;70:657-661.
102. D'Amico DJ, Caspers-Velu L, Libert J, et al. Comparative toxicity of intravitreal aminoglycoside antibiotics. *Am J Ophthalmol* 1985;100:264-275.
103. Weisse I, Loosen H, Peil H. Age-related retinal changes—a comparison between albino and pigmented rabbits. *Lens Eye Toxic Res* 1990;7:717-739.
104. Rubin LF. Albino versus pigmented animals for ocular toxicity testing. *Lens Eye Toxic Res* 1990;7:221-230.
105. Davies RE, Kynoch SR, Liggett MP. Eye irritation tests—an assessment of the maximum delay time for remedial irrigation. *J Soc Cosmet Chem* 1976;27:301-306.
106. Swantson DW. Eye irritancy testing. In: Balls M, Riddell RJ, Worden AN, eds. *Animals and alternatives in toxicity testing.* New York: Academic Press, 1983;337-366.
107. Kulkarni PS, Fleisher L, Srinivasan BD. The synthesis of cyclooxygenase products in ocular tissues of various species. *Curr Eye Res* 1984;3:447-452.
108. Yousufzai SYK, Chen AL, Abdel-Latif AA. Species differences in the effects of prostaglandins on inositol triphosphate accumulation, phosphatidic acid formation, myosin light chain phosphorylation and contraction in iris sphincter of the mammalian eye: interaction with the cyclic AMP system. *J Pharmacol Exp Ther* 1988;247:1064-1072.
109. Bito LZ. Species differences in the responses of the eye to irritation and trauma: a hypothesis of divergence in ocular defense mechanisms, and the choice of experimental animals for eye research. *Exp Eye Res* 1984;39:807-829.
110. Fraunfelder FT. *Drug-induced ocular side effects and drug interactions*, 3rd ed. Philadelphia: Lea & Febiger, 1989.
111. Fraunfelder FT, Meyer SM. The National Registry of Drug-Induced Ocular Side Effects. *J Toxicol Cutan Ocular Toxicol* 1982;1:65-70.
112. Fraunfelder FT. What's new in ocular toxicology? *Sightsaving Rev* 1978;48:53-58.
113. Dikstein S, ed. *Drugs and ocular tissues.* Basel: Karger, 1977.
114. Hockwin O, ed. *Drug-induced ocular side effects and ocular toxicology.* Basel: Karger, 1987.
115. Fraunfelder FT, Scafidi A. Possible adverse effects from topical ocular 10% phenylephrine. *Am J Ophthalmol* 1978;85:447-453.
116. Fraunfelder FT, Meyer SM. Possible cardiovascular effects secondary to topical ophthalmic 2.5% phenylephrine. *Am J Ophthalmol* 1985;99:362-363.
117. Van Buskirk EM. Adverse reactions from timolol administration. *Ophthalmology* 1980;87:447-450.
118. Van Buskirk EM, Fraunfelder FT. Ocular beta-blockers and systemic effects. *Am J Ophthalmol* 1984;98:623-624.
119. Fraunfelder FT, Meyer SM. Recent advances in ocular drug toxicity. In: Hockwin O, ed. *Drug-induced ocular side effects and ocular toxicology.* Basel: Karger, 1987;30-39.

120. Novack GD, Leopold IH. The toxicity of topical ophthalmic beta blockers. *J Toxicol Cutan Ocular Toxicol* 1987;6:283–297.
121. Gerber SL, Cantor LB, Brater DC. Systemic drug interactions with topical glaucoma medications. *Surv Ophthalmol* 1990;35:205–218.
122. Sasaki K, Yamamura T. A review of drug-induced ocular side effects in Japan. In: Hockwin O, ed. *Drug-induced ocular side effects and ocular toxicology*. Basel: Karger, 1987;21–29.
123. Holden C. New focus on replacing animals in the lab. *Science* 1982;215:35–38.

Ophthalmic Toxicology, edited by
George C. Y. Chiou. Raven Press, Ltd.,
New York © 1992.

2

Toxicity in Specific Ocular Tissues

Nicholas J. Millichamp

Department of Small Animal Medicine and Surgery, College of Veterinary Medicine, Texas A & M University, College Station, Texas 77843

Toxins may affect all parts of the eye. Topical substances tend to have more local effects in the eyelids, conjunctiva, and cornea, whereas systemic drugs often have diffuse effects in several parts of the eye. Some drugs have more specific effects on a particular ocular structure. Most of the drugs that cause ocular toxicity cause some degree of visual dysfunction. Many visual disturbances have been reported and are beyond the scope of this review.

This chapter is intended as an introduction to some of the effects of toxins in the eye of humans and animals. This is in no way an attempt at an exhaustive review. For readers who wish to obtain more information either on drugs and effects discussed here, or to determine if other less common drug reactions or toxicities occur with a particular agent, other more exhaustive sources of information are available. In particular the National Registry of Drug-Induced Ocular Side Effects has been incorporated into the comprehensive text by Fraunfelder and Meyer (1). This provides a listing with some indication of significance for every reported ocular side effect in man. This is a valuable source to determine whether a drug has ever caused a particular toxic reaction.

Grant's third edition of *Toxicology of the Eye* (2) remains the most comprehensive source of detailed information on topical and systemic toxic reactions in the eye. This text is very thorough, presenting worldwide literature in a very complete and readable manner.

Throughout this chapter reference is made to ocular structures and some aspects of ocular physiology. The reader is referred to more detailed texts on these subjects for further information (3–12).

EYELIDS

The eyelids can be divided into outer skin and orbicularis layers and inner fibrous connective tissue lined by the palpebral conjunctiva. The connective tissue layer in primates forms a semirigid curved tarsal plate in the upper eyelid that conforms to the shape of the globe. The levator palpebrae superioris muscle and sympathetically innervated Müller's muscle insert into the tarsal plate and effect elevation of the upper lid. The eyelids are variably pigmented in different species. Cilia arise at the margins of the eyelids of upper and/or lower lids associated with modified sweat glands. Glands in the tarsal plate (meibomian glands) contribute to the lipid layer of the tear film. In animals, hair covers the eyelids extending onto the face. In humans, cilia are also located at the eyebrow. Closure of the eyelids is largely caused by contraction of the orbicularis oculi muscle, which encircles the eyelid margins.

The eyelids may be affected by toxins in various ways. Neurological effects on levator palpebrae superioris muscle or sympathetically innervated muscle of the upper lid results in ptosis, whereas contraction of these muscles will retract the upper lid. Blepharospasm is a nonspecific response of the eyelids to any painful or irritating stimulus, including conjunctival or corneal irritation or injury, or deeper injury or inflammation in the uvea. Drugs that cause corneal epithelial injury, uveitis, or elevated intraocular pressure and cause a painful sensation in the eye will cause blepharospasm.

Ptosis and Lid Retraction

Drooping of the upper eyelid is seen with several systemic agents. Ptosis or blepharoplegia is a common feature of **venomous snakebite**, being caused by most types of snake venom but especially that of **elapid** and some **viperids**. **Snake venoms** act like **curariform** drugs to reduce muscle end-plate potentials and prevent action potentials spreading into the muscle. Depolarizing neuromuscular blocking drugs like **succinylcholine** also cause lid drooping (13). The venom of the **black widow spider** also may cause ptosis, along with eyelid edema (14). **Botulinus toxin** causes ptosis by inhibiting acetylcholine release at the muscle ending (13).

Tetraethylammonium, a ganglion blocking agent, causes ptosis. **Guanethidine**, a sympatholytic drug used to reduce lid retraction reduces tone in the sympathetically innervated upper eyelid muscle fibers, causing ptosis. **Mephenesin** is a muscle relaxant that causes ptosis. The metal-chelating agent **penicillamine** has caused toxicity that has often presented with ptosis (2).

Sedatives and related drugs including **barbiturates, primidone**, and **alcohol** often cause ptosis (1,2). **Vincristine** causes ptosis in patients by inducing a neuropathy of peripheral motor nerves (15).

Retraction of the upper eyelid occurs with drugs that stimulate the sympathetic innervation of the upper eyelid, including **phenylephrine**, **amphetamine**, and **cocaine** (2).

Blepharitis

Inflammation of the eyelids has been described with numerous topical drugs including the antivirals **vidarabine**, **idoxuridine**, and **trifluridine**, and ophthalmic drug preservatives (**benzalkonium**, **thimerosal**). Reactions to most topically applied ophthalmic preparations as well as numerous systemic drugs appear to have been reported on occasion as a cause of blepharoconjunctivitis (1).

Alopecia and Poliosis

Grant (2) and Fraunfelder and Meyer (1) list various drugs that have caused hair loss or depigmentation of the eyelashes or eyebrows. Most notable in causing alopecia are **actinomycin D, triparanol, thallium**, and **vitamin A** (2).

Poliosis has been reported to occur with **corticosteroids, chloroquine, hydroxychloroquine, amodiaquine**, and **triparanol** (1,2).

LACRIMAL SYSTEM

Many substances cause increased lacrimation and are discussed under corneal and conjunctival irritation. Decreased lacrimation occurs as a side effect of many human drugs (1), and may occur due to pharmacological blockage of secretion in the lacrimal gland. A component of this innervation is from the parasympathetic system. Parasympatholytic drugs, including **atropine**, and **scopolamine**, reduce tearing in this manner.

Other compounds have been reported to be toxic to the lacrimal gland in animals and potentially capable of causing clinical keratoconjunctivitis sicca. Drugs toxic to the canine lacrimal gland include **phenazopyridine, sulfadiazine**, and **salicylazosulfapyridine** (16–18). **Phenazopyridine** causes necrosis and fibrosis of lacrimal gland acini (17).

CORNEA AND CONJUNCTIVA

The cornea comprises the anterior 1/4 to 1/16 of the outer fibrous tunic of the eye (depending upon the species), and functions as the major refractive surface of the eye. The cornea is made up of four main layers, excluding the precorneal tear film. The outer epithelium is several cells thick, with columnar germinal cells resting on a basement membrane. The cells become nonkeratinized, stratified squamous as they are displaced superficially and eventually lost into the tear film. The stroma, which lies beneath the epithelial basement membrane comprises 90% of the total corneal thickness. This layer is made up of layers of corneal lamellae that span the entire corneal surface. The lamellae comprise regularly arranged bundles of collagen fibrils maintained evenly spaced by a proteoglycan ground substance. The water content of the cornea is maintained at 78%. Few keratocytes (specialized fibroblasts) are found in the corneal stroma. Noncollagenous protein, lipids, and glycoproteins comprise the rest of the biochemical makeup of the cornea.

At the inner face of the stroma is a highly elastic layer, Descemet's membrane, which is the basement membrane of the posterior endothelium of the cornea; it apposes the anterior chamber. The endothelial layer is one cell in thickness and has the important function of maintaining corneal hydration and detumescence by pumping water that has leaked into the stroma back into the anterior chamber. This leak pump mechanism is an active process that provides for corneal nutrition from the aqueous humor while maintaining normal stromal hydration. Normal stromal hydration ensures that the collagen fibrils maintain regular spacing, an important feature in maintaining corneal transparency and preventing the development of corneal edema. Focal loss of either the corneal epithelium and to an even greater extent the corneal endothelium results in edema accumulation in the corneal stroma and epithelial layers. Polymorphonuclear leukocytes (PMNs), which may reach the site of epithelial injury, have significant potential to slow epithelial wound healing.

Erosions of the corneal epithelium are healed by rapid sliding of adjacent cells into the defect followed by mitosis of the basal germinal cells to thicken the epithelial layer. Epithelial cells will attach to undamaged basement membrane. If the basement membrane is also damaged (corneal ulcer) epithelial attachment may take several weeks to be complete, pending reformation of an underlying basement membrane.

Stromal lacerations initially fill with fibrin and PMNs attracted to the site of injury to provide phagocytosis of infectious agents that may be present. Keratocytes become activated and produce new collagen into the area of the fibrin clot. Neovascularization of the stroma with granulation tissue production occurs in cases of severe stromal injury. Epithelial cells cover the area of the defect and stromal scarring is eventually remodeled over many months. In some instances PMNs, corneal breakdown products, or toxins may cause rapid dissolution of the stromal collagen and ground substance, which may result in ulceration to Descemet's membrane or perforation of the cornea.

The conjunctiva is a thin mucous membrane that extends from the limbus of the eye to the margin of the eyelids. The conjunctiva, which covers the anterior portion of the sclera, is the bulbar conjunctiva. It is reflected at the conjunctival fornix to line the inner surface of the eyelids as the palpebral conjunctiva and to cover the third eyelid in species where this structure is found. The space bounded by the conjunctival and corneal surfaces is the conjunctival sac. The conjunctiva is divided histologically into two layers: a superficial layer of stratified columnar epithelium, which is continuous with the stratified squamous epithelium of the cornea, and a deeper substantia propria. The palpebral conjunctival epithelium contains goblet cells, which are particularly numerous at the fornices and over the base of the anterior surface of the third eyelid. The conjunctival epithelium is variably pigmented in different species particularly near the limbus.

The substantia propria has a superficial glandular layer and a deeper layer of loose fibrous tissue. Two layers of lymphatics are present—one at the depth of the superficial blood vessels and the other in the deep fibrous layer. Lymph follicles are especially numerous in the bulbar conjunctiva of the third eyelid and fornices. The blood supply of the conjunctiva is derived from the anterior ciliary arteries, and the vascular arcades of the eyelids. The conjunctiva and cornea is innervated by the trigeminal nerve.

Corneal and Conjunctival Chemical Burns

Chemical burns to the cornea are due to either acids or alkalis. Acids that may be involved include **sulfuric** and **sulfurous acids, hydrochloric acid, hydrofluoric acid, chromic acid, nitric acid, sulfur dioxide,** and **silver nitrate**. Acids cause coagulation and precipitation of proteins. This occurs in both the epithelium and stroma; however, precipitation of protein in the more superficial layers tends to prevent acid from reaching deeper layers of the cornea and thus the severity of at least weak acid burns is not usually as great as alkali burns where no such superficial protection occurs. With strong acids the protective effect may not be particularly significant and the eye may sustain severe injury. Acids coagulate the epithelial cells and cause contraction (shrinkage) of stromal collagen fibrils. Proteoglycan matrix is precipitated by acids (19).

In mild acid burns the initial changes are turbidity and dulling of the conjunctival surface, possibly with corneal epithelial erosion. The conjunctiva becomes hyperemic and petechial hemorrhages may be seen. With stronger acids the cornea and conjunctiva immediately become opaque (usually white). Necrotic epithelium is lost within a few days, but will regenerate rapidly in mild cases. In severe cases the stroma may be clear or becomes thinner and a descemetocele may develop or the cornea may perforate. Healing is by neovascularization with extensive scarring in severe cases (2).

Alkalis that may burn the cornea and conjunctiva include **hydroxides of sodium, ammonium, calcium, magnesium,** and **potassium**. Several other hydroxide-containing substances are known to cause ocular damage (2). Most severe injury occurs with alkalis at pH over 12 (20). Variations in the severity of corneal injury appear to correlate with the differences in the epithelial damaging potential of the various alkalis (2).

Alkalis cause fatty acid saponification and dissociation in cell membranes. This causes cell destruction allowing penetration of the epithelial layer. In the stroma the alkali causes swelling of the collagen fibrils, either directly or after hydrolyzation of proteoglycans and render the stromal collagen more susceptible to enzymes (particularly collagenase). Collagenases are produced by PMNs (21) that enter the cornea in response to high molecular weight substances and collagen breakdown products, which act as PMN chemoattractants (22). Collagenase further degrades collagen, causing a melting appearance to the stroma. Plasmin from damaged epithelial cells and fibroblasts (23) may additionally retard epithelial healing and potentiate a cascade of events resulting in further collagen and stromal breakdown (10).

Corneal Epithelial Defects and Erosions

Minor defects or erosions in the corneal epithelium, which may heal rapidly, have been described after exposure to several groups of toxins. These are reviewed extensively by Grant (2). Epithelial erosions may occur secondary to impaired sensory innervation of the cornea (neurotropic keratitis). This may occur in **acid** and **alkali burns**, or with exposure to **carbon** or **hydrogen disulfide**.

Elapid venoms cause excessive lacrimation, conjunctival hyperemia, and corneal edema, and may damage the epithelium, causing erosions (24). In severe cases ulceration, perforation, and uveitis occur (25,26).

Solvents cause irritation and pain and loss of epithelium, which in most cases will regenerate again rapidly (2).

Surfactants are used as surgical preoperative antiseptic agents and topically applied ophthalmic drops as preservatives. **Benzalkonium chloride** is a cationic surfactant commonly used to increase the penetration of certain drugs into the eye. **Dodecyl sodium sulfate** and **soaps** are examples of anionic surfactants, and **Tween** is a nonionic surfactant. Cationic surfactants are in general more injurious to the conjunctiva and cornea than anionic or nonionic types, although the concentration applied to the eye is a more important determinant of the severity of injury. Surfactants cause conjunctival hyperemia, corneal opacification, and epithelial edema, with occasional epithelial erosions.

Chloroacetophenone is a component of a solvent spray tear gas used for self-defense. This agent causes extensive lacrimation, and epithelial erosions or loss with stromal edema. Epithelial lesions usually heal rapidly (27). Numerous other related agents that cause excessive lacrimation and epithelial damage have been described by Grant (2). These agents at low concentrations cause marked stimulation of the trigeminal nerve endings in the cornea, and only at higher concentration cause epithelial damage.

Local anesthetics such as **lidocaine, proparacaine**, and **butacaine** cause epithelial damage and retard epithelial healing. These drugs should not be used therapeutically where ocular pain is present (28).

Epithelial injury occurs with many substances applied topically to the eyes. **Hydrogen sulfide** gas and **sulfur** dust causes conjunctival hyperemia and epithelial cell loss, which may be due to the inhibition of cytochrome oxidase in the epithelium. **Surfactants** such as **benzalkonium chloride** cause slight damage to epithelial cells and have been used to promote drug penetration into the eye (29). **Vinblastine** applied topically to the human cornea causes a punctate epithelial keratopathy and erosions (30). Low concentrations of **mustard gas** applied topically to the rabbit eye cause epithelial edema and conjunctival hyperemia several hours after topical application. Longer contact with the irritant can result in stromal ulceration (31). **Nitrogen mustard** has similar although more rapid effects on the conjunctiva and corneal epithelium when applied topically in experimental animals or with exposure in humans. Additionally acute ocular irritation occurs in the anterior uvea (32,33). **Allyl alcohol** causes conjunctival hyperemia and chemosis and reversible corneal opacification due to epithelial damage and edema (34). **Colchicine** causes stromal edema and will reduce the rate of epithelialization of epithelial defects (2,35). Other agents that have been found to be toxic to the corneal epithelium include **emetine, dimethyl sulfoxide diisopropylamine in various dyes, and formaldehyde** in various concentrations (2).

Conjunctivitis and keratitis have been described with many drugs given systemically. These include **phenylbutazone**, **sulfonamides** (2), **cytarabine** (36), **methotrexate** (37), **ß-blockers** (1), and **phenazopyridine** (16).

Follicular conjunctivitis may occur with topical use of several ophthalmic drugs, including **idoxuridine, vidarabine, pilocarpine,** and **atropine** (38).

The corneal endothelium may be damaged by air or intraocular irrigating solutions used for cataract surgery (39). Certain preservatives (**benzalkonium chloride**) may be very destructive when applied to the corneal endothelium (40). Damage may occur from certain photosensitizing agents. In cattle, **phenothiazine** causes photosensitization and corneal endothelial damage resulting in severe corneal edema (41). **Dichloroethane**, a solvent, is selectively toxic to the canine corneal endothelium, either after parenteral administration or inhalation. Endothelial cells become swollen and detach from the endothelium and later attempt to cover the defect by sliding from adjacent undamaged areas (42).

Deposits in the corneal epithelium, which appear as fine gray granules (cornea verticillata), have been described in humans with several systemic drugs, including **clofazimine, amiodarone, chloroquine,** and **triparanol. Chlorpromazine** causes fine deposits both deep in the stroma and in the epithelium with chronic use as well as conjunctival pigmentation (1,2). **Epinephrine** used topically causes fine multifocal pigmented deposits in the conjunctiva and sometimes the corneal stroma if the epithelial surface is damaged. The deposits are oxidized epinephrine (43).

Corneal Lipidosis

Amphiphilic cationic substances cause lipid deposition in the cornea in several species. In man **chloroquine** and **amiodarone** cause whorl- or streak-like lipid deposits in the epithelium (2). Topical applications of **amiodarone** to rats results in cytoplasmic lipid inclusions in all corneal layers (44–47). Corneal lipidosis has also been caused in rats by **chlorphentermine**, **iprindole**, **tamoxifen**, and **chloroquine** (47).

Corneal Mucopolysaccharidosis

Glycosaminoglycans (GAGS) may accumulate in keratocytes and the endothelium and basal layers of the epithelium of rats treated with the dicationic amphiphilic drug **tilorone** (47).

ANTERIOR UVEA

The anterior uvea comprises the iris and ciliary body. The iris comprises an anterior stroma of collagen fibers, melanocytes, and fibroblasts. The anterior border is made up of fibroblasts and melanocytes. The posterior aspects of the iris is made up of two epithelial layers; the anterior forms the myoepithelial-type dilator muscle and continues as the anterior pigmented epithelium of the ciliary body. The posterior pigmented layer of iris epithelium continues into the ciliary body as the nonpigmented layer of ciliary epithelium. The iris also has a smooth iridal sphincter muscle near the margin of the pupil in the stroma. The ciliary body extends posteriorly from the iris base to the retina. The most anterior aspect of the ciliary body forms the iridocorneal angle, the site of most aqueous humor drainage from the eye. The ciliary body comprises the ciliary muscle, which inserts into the region of the iridocorneal angle, and the ciliary processes, which project inward from the ciliary body toward the lens. The ciliary processes are histologically divided into a highly vascular collagenous stroma, which is separated from the posterior chamber by the two layers of ciliary epithelium. The ciliary epithelium is the cell layer responsible for active secretion of aqueous humor. The zonule fibers that support the lens arise from between adjacent ciliary processes.

Acute Ocular Irritative Response and Uveitis

The most significant ocular pathological responses of the uvea are the acute ocular irritative response and uveitis (inflammation of the uvea). The ocular irritative response consists of miosis, disruption of the blood-aqueous barrier, and changes in the intraocular pressure of the eye in response to various noxious substances, trauma, radiation, or paracentesis of the anterior chamber. The mechanisms whereby the ocular irritative responses develop and their variation in different species are discussed in the chapter by Millichamp, "Species Specificity."

Numerous toxic substances can potentially cause disruption of the blood-aqueous barrier. In several species irritation of the cornea with compounds such as **nitrogen mustards** will cause breakdown of the blood-aqueous barrier and miosis. Clinically, treatment with **miotics** may cause dilatation of iris blood vessels, pigment dispersion in the aqueous, and occasionally iritis (2). Several related substances including **organophosphates** (irreversible acetylcholinesterase inhibitors) have similar effects. There appears to be little specificity as to which substances that cause ocular surface irritation will also affect the ocular barriers. Variations are more closely tied to the species being tested.

Iris Cysts

Cysts of the pupillary margin occur in patients treated for long periods with **miotics**, including **pilocarpine**, demecarium, and echothiophate (29).

Hippus

Rapid, small oscillations in pupil size have been reported as a side effect of barbiturate usage and toxicity (1).

LENS

The lens of the eye is a clear spheroidal structure, composed of an inner, embryologically older nucleus surrounded by a cortex. The whole structure is enclosed by the lens capsule. The anterior lens capsule is lined as far as the lens equator by a single layer of epithelial cells, the continued division of which results in the deposition of successive layers of anucleate lens fibers around the outside of the cortex like the layers of an onion. Consequently the lens increases in size throughout life. The main biochemical components of the lens are protein and water. The protein fractions are both soluble and insoluble, the latter increasing in proportion to the former with age or in the development of cataract. The lens is suspended behind the iris by zonular fibers that arise from the ciliary body and insert onto the lens capsule circumferentially at the lens equator. Lens protein turnover is limited within the lens fibers, most of the metabolic and synthetic activity of the lens taking place in the anterior epithelium (9,10).

Nuclear Sclerosis

Aging changes in animals referred to as nuclear sclerosis involve a change in the refractive properties of the nucleus. These have also been seen as a reversible change in experimental species, including dogs and rabbits but not man, systemically administered **dimethylsulfoxide** (48,49).

Cataract

Cataract is the most common and significant abnormality of the lens. A cataract is defined as any opacity or loss of transparency, partial or complete, of the lens. The metabolic causes of cataracts have been reviewed elsewhere (50). Changes in lens proteins during cataract formation are similar to those seen in aging. These include tryptophan oxidation, deamination, development of lens pigmentation, increase in fluorescence, formation of disulfide bonds, cross linking, increase in insoluble protein, glycation, and formation of high molecular weight aggregates (10). The appearance of cataracts varies considerably between species and differences in the metabolism of the lens in different species may account for particular sensitivity of one species to toxic cataract development over another.

Numerous topical and systemic drugs have been reported causing cataracts in man and animals. Complete lists are available in Grant (2) and Fraunfelder and Meyer (1). The various toxic agents that cause cataracts have been thoroughly reviewed in a systematic manner by Harding and Crabbe (50). This section lists some of the better known toxic causes of cataracts.

Many photosensitizing agents have been described as causes of cataracts (2). Light (including sunlight and ultraviolet light [UVL]) although often cited as causes of cataracts are probably not able to cause cataracts alone without some photosensitizing agent (50). **8–Methoxypsoralen** (methoxsalen) causes anterior cortical cataracts in mice and guinea pigs with UVL exposure (51,52). Other agents that may cause cataracts associated with photosensitization in various species include **nafoxidine, hematoporphyrin, 1,4-bis-(phenylisopropyl)-piperazine**, and **bleomycin (antineoplastic and antibiotic)** (2).

Various drugs produce cataracts that resemble those caused by ionizing radiation. These cataracts often affect the actively mitotic cells at the lens equator, thus forming equatorial cataracts in the early stages (2). **4-(p-Dimethylaminostyryl) quinoline** produces such cataracts in mice (53). Systemic **iodoacetate** causes posterior polar cataracts in rabbits when given systemically or by intracameral injection (54). Other agents that have produced cataracts resembling radiation damage include **nitrogen mustard** (2). Various antimitotic and antineoplastic drugs cause cataracts in man and animals that resemble radiation cataracts. **Busulfan** affects lens epithelial nucleic acid and reduces mitosis and causes cataracts in rats and humans (55,56). ***p*-Chlorophenylalanine**, an antimetabolite, may cause cataracts in rats by reducing entry of amino acids into the aqueous or lens (57,58). **Triethylenemelamine** (tretamine) causes cataracts when administered systemically to mice (53). **Myleran** causes cataracts in rats, presumably by preventing division of lens epithelial cells (59).

Cataracts may result from interference with protein synthesis and metabolism and interference with enzyme systems in the lens. **Naphthalene** and related compounds produce cataracts in rabbits and rats and possibly humans. The drug was used as an antiseptic and anthelminthic. Cataracts are seen with systemic but not intraocular administration (2). Both albino and pigmented rabbits are equally affected, whereas pigmented rats are more likely to be affected than albinos due to enzyme differences between the strains. Cataracts can develop to maturity in 2 weeks in rabbits fed naphthalene. Breakdown of the blood-aqueous barrier in rabbits apparently enhances development of cataracts (60). Naphthalene is probably metabolized to toxic products, in particular **1-2-naphthoquinone**, that reach the eye and cause changes in lens electrolytes (reduced potassium, increased sodium and chloride, and reduced gluthathione and amino acids), all of which have been associated with cataract development (61). **Methionine sulfoxime** interferes with protein synthesis and causes cataracts in rats fed a low protein diet (62). **Mimosine**, a plant extract that affects protein metabolism and enzyme activity, causes various ocular changes when fed to rats, including cataracts, which appears to be a primary effect (63). Lens vacuolation and epithelial hyperplasia also occur in cattle fed a diet of **Leucaena leucocephala**, due to its high mimosine content (64). **2,4-Dinitrophenol** was used orally for weight reduction in humans and cataracts were seen as a common complication. Cataracts have variously been described in some experimental animals (2). The drug uncouples oxidative phosphorylation, which might be expected to increase the lens consumption of oxygen, although this is not the case with incubated lenses *in vitro* (65). Other mechanisms suggested include a reduction of lens glutathione, although this is not particularly specific and occurs in most cataract formation (66). Both the anterior capsule and anterior and posterior cortices around the lens sutures were initially involved with progressing to a complete intumescent cataract (50).

Galactose can cause cataracts when given in high doses to experimental animals (2). In humans with hereditary galactosemia and in macropods (kangaroos, wallabies, etc.) the enzyme galactose 1-phosphate-uridyltransferase and galactokinase are usually absent. Galactose and galactose-1-phosphate saturate the lens and are converted to galactitol, or dulcitol, which accumulates in lens cells. Cows milk (high in lactose and galactose) will cause cataracts in these species. Accumulated sugars in the lens (as in diabetes) cause cataracts by exerting an osmotic effect, drawing water into the lens and causing hydropic degeneration. Additionally protein synthesis and lens enzyme systems may be affected and contribute to cataract development (50). A similar type of sugar cataract is caused by **xylose** toxicity in weanling rats, with accumulation of sorbitol in the lens cells (67). **Arabinose** produces cataracts similar to those caused by galactose and xylose (2). **Alloxan** causes cataracts in rabbits and rats, and although it also causes diabetes mellitus, which could contribute to cataract development, it may have a direct antimitotic effect on the lens epithelial cells (68,69). Cataracts develop in rats within 2 weeks of a single injection of **streptozotocin**, which destroys pancreatic ß-cells and causes diabetes (70). Interestingly, cataract development in this case can be reduced by aldose reductase inhibitors, suggesting that the streptozotocin cataracts are secondary to the diabetes induced by the drug (71,72). Oral hypoglycemic drugs such as **carbutamide**, **tolbutamide**, and **chlorpropamide** have induced cataracts in rats (73).

Chronic dosing with topical or systemic **corticosteroids** have on several occasions resulted in posterior subcapsular cataracts in humans (74). The same does not always appear to occur in experimental animals (2), although cataracts possibly induced by corticosteroids have been reported in adult rabbits and neonatal mice (75). Various mechanisms have been suggested for corticosteroid cataracts including elevation of glucose in the plasma and aqueous, increased cation permeability, inhibition of glucose-6-phosphate dehydrogenase, inhibition of RNA synthesis, loss of lens adenosine triphosphate (ATP), and covalent binding of steroid to lens proteins. It is suggested that steroid cataract could have a multifactorial etiology (50). **Clomiphene** used as a hormonal treatment has produced cataracts in rats (76).

Triparanol and **diazocholesterol** block the conversion of desmosterol to cholesterol by inhibiting the enzyme desmosterol reductase. Cataracts have been reported in various species including man, dog, and rat. Affected lenses accumulate abnormally high concentrations of desmosterol, which presumably is associated with the changes of permeability and with sodium and water accumulation in the lens. Opacities are seen initially in the anterior and posterior subcapsular regions, followed by cortical clouding progressing to total opacification (77,78).

Various drugs may cause cataracts by producing damaging free radicals in the eye. **Diquat** causes initially posterior subcapsular cataracts which, progress to involve the nucleus and later entire lens in the rat (79). Glutathione concentrations are unaffected, but the production of diquat free radical might have a damaging effect on the lens by conversion to superoxide radicals (80). However, superoxide can usually be destroyed by several substances present in the lens (including glutathione and ascorbate) and therefore the concept of superoxide damage in diquat toxicity is still unresolved (50). **Hydrogen peroxide** has been found in high concentrations in the aqueous of humans with senile nuclear cataract. Since nuclear proteins become oxidized with aging it has been suggested that increased concentrations of hydrogen peroxide might be etiologic in causing these aging changes (81). Hydrogen peroxide, which reduces lens superoxide dismutase making the lens more prone to damage from free radicals formed in response to sunlight (UVL), might be involved in causing these changes. **Aminotriazole** causes cataracts in the rabbit, possibly by reducing lens catalase concentrations, and increasing local hydrogen peroxide concentrations (82,83).

Miotic anticholinesterase drugs (usually used in man for glaucoma therapy) including **demecarium bromide**, and **phospholine iodide** have caused cataracts in man and monkeys (84,85). Cataracts in man begin as anterior subcapsular vacuoles and progress to involve the nucleus and posterior cortex and ultimately the entire lens. *In vitro* studies of rabbit lenses show a fall in potassium and a rise of sodium and water concentration in the lens (86,87). **Epinephrine** given in large doses causes transient lens opacities in rodents (88), although these may be more related to a decrease in blinking, and corneal exposure with subsequent lens dehydration. Cataracts have similarly been produced in rodents with **opiates, phenelzine** combined with **serotonin** (2,89).

Hygromycin B, an anthelminthic, has caused cataracts in sows when fed in the diet. Lesions are posterior subcapsular cataracts with lens fiber swelling, with cortical vacuolation and degeneration (90–92). **Disophenol** when used in puppies may cause transient lens opacities (93,94). **Rafoxanide** induces equatorial cataracts and papilledema in dogs (95,96). Reversible lens opacities have been seen in dogs administered the systemic antihypertensive agents **diazoxide** (97) and **dichloroacetate** (98).

Thallium, a heavy metal, causes cataracts in experimental animals. The metal is concentrated in lenses *in vitro* (2).

Chlorphentermine is an amphiphilic catatonic drug that causes subcapsular lens opacities in rats by upsetting lipid metabolism (99,100).

Cyanate has caused posterior subcapsular cataracts in dogs and in humans treated for sickle-cell anemia (101,102). Raised aqueous concentrations of **urea** have been suggested as the cause of cataracts occasionally seen in uremic patients due to **ammonium cyanate** carbamylation of lens proteins (50).

Boron hydride disulfide causes cataracts in mice possibly by inactivating **Na-adenosine triphosphatase (ATPase)** and reducing water pumping across the anterior lens epithelium, resulting in increased lens hydration (103).

Selenium causes nuclear and later cortical cataracts in rats possibly by depressing lens glutathione, catalase, and superoxide dismutase, which normally provide protection against free radical damage (104–106). **Sulfaethoxy-pyridazine, an antimicrobial drug, has caused cataracts in dogs and rats (2).**

Trinitrotoluene (TNT) causes equatorial cataracts in humans chronically exposed to its dust or vapor (2).

Verapamil, a calcium blocker, has occasionally been reported to cause cataracts in dogs when given at toxic doses (2).

The metal chelator **dithizone** causes equatorial cataracts in rats (2), and may cause cataracts in dogs along with severe fundus pathology (107,108). Cataracts may also occur with the chelators **deferoxamine** and **pyrithione** (109). Since these agents cause severe inflammatory changes elsewhere in the eye the cataracts are likely to be secondary occurrences (2).

Lens Deposits

Lamellated inclusions and vacuoles formed in the lens epithelium appear as lens opacities in the anterior and posterior cortex in rats fed amphiphilic cationic agents **chloroquine, chlorphentermine**, or **iprindole** (99).

Deposits (presumably of the particular toxin) may occur beneath the anterior lens capsule with systemic toxicity from several **metals** and chronic use of **chlorpromazine** and possibly **thiothixene** (2).

INTRAOCULAR PRESSURE AND GLAUCOMA

The intraocular pressure (IOP) is maintained within normal limits by an equal rate of secretion and ultrafiltration of aqueous from the ciliary processes and outflow of aqueous via the iridocorneal angle (comprising particularly the trabecular meshwork) and uveoscleral pathway (across the iris and ciliary body into the suprachoroidal space). Drugs may affect the production or drainage of aqueous by systemic peripheral or central effects on the cardiovascular system (for instance by increasing or lowering the intraarterial or intravenous pressure which is directly reflected in alterations of IOP), or by affecting central control of IOP. Outflow from the anterior chamber via the trabecular meshwork is facilitated by contraction of the ciliary muscle. Drugs may reduce this effect.

Reduction in intraocular pressure is a desired effect of many topical and systemic drugs, including **carbonic anhydrase inhibitors, miotics** (parasympathomimetic drugs), **adrenergics, ß-blockers**, and **osmotic agents**. Since these are used clinically in the treatment of glaucoma in man and animals, these drugs rarely lower intraocular pressure to such an extent that it affects ocular function or results in ocular pathology. For this reason lowering of intraocular pressure is not considered a toxic reaction in the eye. Numerous drugs have the potential to reduce IOP and are listed in Grant (2) and Fraunfelder and Meyer (1).

Elevation of IOP is, however, a significant toxic effect of some drugs that may be used in clinical therapy and is therefore a toxic reaction. Glaucoma may arise as a primary disease or secondary to other ocular pathology such as uveitis, lens luxation, neoplasia, or drug effects in the eye. Obviously there may be interaction between these etiologies—for instance a drug that causes breakdown of the blood-aqueous barrier (BAB), cellular infiltrate into the eye, could result in reduced aqueous outflow due to inflammatory debris clogging the trabecular meshwork and thus cause a secondary rise of IOP. In rabbits use of drugs that cause disruption of the blood-aqueous barrier (**nitrogen mustard, acids, alkalis**) may cause a rise of IOP associated with disruption of the BAB and changes in the blood flow within the eye. Conversely in some situations drugs used to treat uveitis might potentiate a rise in IOP; this occurs in man with **atropine**. In dogs with acute uveitis, inflammatory debris may obstruct the trabecular meshwork and elevate IOP. Use of a nonsteroidal anti-inflammatory drug **flurbiprofen** reduces prostaglandin (PG) production in the eye and further elevates IOP (110). This probably occurs because PGs act as a safety valve in ocular inflammation to increase uveoscleral outflow to compensate for any reduction in iridocorneal outflow.

Parasympatholytic drugs such as **atropine, homatropine, scopolamine, cyclopentolate**, and **tropicamide** paralyze the ciliary muscle and may in some species (certainly man, dog, cat, and horse) increase IOP. Elevated IOP occurs in humans with open-angle glaucoma and can precipitate angle closure in individuals with narrow angles (111). Several mechanisms may be involved, including the formation of peripheral anterior synechiae in noninflamed eyes as the base of the iris is dilated into the angle region, and reduced outflow through the ciliary muscle due to paralysis of the ciliary muscle.

Corticosteroids may cause glaucoma in man when used either systemically or topically. A genetic predisposition is seen in man in sensitivity to corticosteroid-induced glaucoma (112). Corticosteroids have been suggested as affecting intraocular pressure by various mechanisms. The most frequently cited cause of glaucoma is that corticosteroids increase the amounts of glycosaminoglycans (GAG) in the trabecular meshwork possibly by limiting degradation of GAG by lysosomal enzymes. Lysosome membranes are stabilized by corticosteroids. Other possible pathogenetic mechanisms include corticosteroid reduction of phagocytosis by the trabecular meshwork and accumulation of debris (cells) in the meshwork, which blocks flow (10,113). Corticosteroids have been shown *in vitro* to reduce prostaglandin production by trabecular meshwork cells. If PGs are acting to fine-tune IOP in the eye through the uveoscleral outflow pathway, a reduction of PG in the eye might cause reduced uveoscleral outflow and, thus, a rise in IOP (114).

In other species it has been more difficult to demonstrate any effect of corticosteroids on IOP. In rabbits prolonged therapy with high-enough doses to cause systemic toxicity do transiently elevate IOP (2). In cats IOP elevation has been reported with topically applied **dexamethasone** (115). The tricyclic antidepressant **amitriptyline** has caused angle-closure glaucoma at high doses (116). The H_2-blockers **cimetidine** and **ranitidine** cause elevation of IOP when injected into the cerebral ventricles of rabbits, suggesting an action via the CNS regulatory mechanisms for IOP (117).

Acetazolamide reduces intraocular pressure by reducing aqueous secretion, due to its action as a carbonic anhydrase inhibitor (CAI). Cases have been reported in man, however, where the IOP was increased, associated with swelling of the lens and transient myopia (111). Despite the normal effect of the CAI-type drug in reducing IOP, swallowing of the anterior chamber induced by lens swelling might be a significant precipitating factor in narrow-angle glaucoma in man.

Several agents including the vasodilator **tolazoline,** and sympathomimetics **epinephrine, ephedrine,** and **amphetamine** dilate the pupil and thus might potentiate angle-closure glaucoma in susceptible individuals. Subconjunctival injections of vasodilators are more likely to produce IOP increases than systemic administration (1,2,111).

Parasympathomimetic drugs such as **pilocarpine**, **carbachol**, and **demecarium** although indicated for treating open-angle glaucoma, may cause dilatation of iridal vessels and swelling of the iris and ciliary body, and the increased curvature of the lens may displace the iris anteriorly, reducing the depth of the anterior chamber and narrowing the angle. In humans predisposed to narrow-angle glaucoma this may precipitate angle closure. Additionally, the miotic pupil induced by these drugs may limit aqueous flow from the posterior to the anterior chamber and cause pupil block with iris bombe, thus further narrowing the angle (2,111).

Viscoelastic substances injected into the eye during intraocular surgery to protect the corneal endothelium and facilitate intraocular lens implantation have been associated with a significant rise in IOP after surgery in humans and dogs. Presumably these agents, which are viscous, interfere with aqueous outflow through the angle (118). Several other examples of fine particulate matter causing elevation of the IOP have been cited (2).

RETINA AND CHOROID

The retina is a multilayered structure that lines the posterior segment of the eye. During embryonic development the optic cup, an evagination of neuroectoderm from the diencephalon, forms inner and outer layers. The cells of the inner layer undergo division and differentiation into the perikarya of the neural retina, whereas the outer layer becomes the retinal pigment epithelium (RPE). The neural retina (hereafter referred to as retina) and RPE become apposed, although a potential intraretinal or subretinal space remains as a site for retinal detachment later in life (119).

Ten layers of RPE and retina are recognized. The RPE is a single layer of cuboidal cells. The folded basal surface of each cell lies on Bruch's membrane, adjacent to the vascular choroid, which provides a blood supply to the outer retina. In some species (such as the guinea pig) most of the retinal nutrition comes from this source. The apical surface of each cell forms elongated processes that extend between the outer segments of the photoreceptors of the retina. The RPE is variably pigmented depending upon the species, the position in the retina, and, in some animals, the age.

The photoreceptors compose the outermost layer of the neural retina. Two main photoreceptor types are recognized—the rods and cones. The proportions of these cell types vary between species and at different geographic locations in the posterior segment. Rod outer segments (ROS) are tubular in shape. The plasma membrane encloses a stack of membrane-bound discs, each held separate from the next and the plasma membrane by a cytoskeletal array of filaments. Cone outer segments are generally shorter than those of rods, and have a more conical shape. The cone plasma membrane forms membranous lamellae by continuous infolding throughout the outer segment. The cytoplasm of the outer and inner segments is continuous through a connecting cilium.

An interphotoreceptor matrix (IPM) fills the potential subretinal space between the RPE cells, photoreceptor outer segments, and glia of the neurosensory retina. The IPM is biochemically composed of carbohydrates (glycosaminoglycans and sialic acid-containing molecules) mostly linked to glycoproteins. The IPM functions may include transfer of retinoids between the photoreceptors and RPE (via the interphotoreceptor retinol-binding protein [IBRP]), maintenance of retinal attachment to the RPE, and support of retinal development and maturation via trophic factors in the IPM (119).

The inner segments of the photoreceptors are highly metabolically active, containing numerous mitochondria. The perikarya of the photoreceptor cells lie in the outer nuclear layer, comprising from 5 to 12 nuclear layers in the peripheral and central retina, which again varies with species. Axons of the photoreceptors terminate in rod spherules and cone pedicles, which synapse with bipolar and horizontal cells in the outer plexiform layer (OPL) (120).

Nuclei of the bipolar, horizontal, amacrine, and retinal glial (Müller) cells are located in the inner nuclear layer (INL).

The ganglion cell layer comprises mainly ganglion cells, of which as many as 23 different morphological types may occur in the cat retina. The ganglion cell processes project into the nerve fiber layer, the fibers of which radiate toward the optic nerve papilla and leave the eye through the lamina cribrosa of the sclera (121).

The internal limiting membrane is formed by flat expansions of the Müller cells at the vitreal surface.

The blood supply to the retina comes from two sources. The choroidal circulation provides oxygen and other nutrients to the outer part of the retina, including the photoreceptors. The retinal pigment epithelium controls the flow of nutrients and metabolites into and out of the neurosensory retina. In man, the central artery of the retina forms the ophthalmic artery, which crosses the subarachnoid space and penetrates the optic nerve ventrally and enters the retina with the nerve. In dogs, approximately 20 retinal arteries branch from the short posterior ciliary arteries at the optic disc and supply blood to the inner retinal layers. Choroidal vessels are fenestrated and therefore contribute little to the blood-retinal barrier. Retinal vessels are nonfenestrated and along with tight junctions between RPE cells provide a blood-retinal barrier to limit the size of molecules that can gain access to the neurosensory retina (8).

The choroid in several domestic species is modified anteriorly by the presence of a tapetum lucidum. This is cellular in carnivores (cat, dog, ferret) and fibrous in herbivores (cattle, horse). The tapetum as seen ophthalmoscopically varies in color and surface area depending upon the species, the breed or strain, age, and extent of pigmentation elsewhere in the skin and eye. In carnivores the tapetal cells are packed with elongated rods of modified melanin granules and vary in the concentrations of trace elements or other constituents. The presence of a tapetum and its interspecies variations may affect the response of the retina in tapetal species to various toxins (8).

Toxicity may occur at various sites in the retina and choroid. Drugs that affect the cardiovascular system elsewhere in the body may affect the retinal or choroidal circulations. The retinal pigment epithelium may be the primary site of a toxin's actions, possibly determined by the presence or absence of pigment in this layer to which the toxin may bind and become concentrated. Within the retina itself the photoreceptors, ganglion cells or other neurons, synaptic junctions, or glial cells may be the primary targets of toxins.

Tapetal Color Change and Choroidal Edema

Changes in the appearance or color of the tapetum have been described in dogs due to either the action of systemic vasodilator or drugs with toxic effects in the tapetum itself, the retina, RPE, or underlying choroid. Many of the effects reflect choroidal edema, necrosis, or degeneration of the tapetum and choroid. **Vasodilating agents** produce reversible color changes along a horizontal meridian of the canine tapetum superior to the optic nerve, without histological abnormalities. This site corresponds to the position of the long posterior retinal arteries and may simply be an optical effect due to distortion of retinal and choroidal blood vessels (95). **Trans-11-amino-10,11-dihydro-5-(3-dimethylaminopropyl)-5,10 epoxy-5-H-dibenzo [a,d] cycloheptene** causes reduced visual acuity and tapetal color reduction, apparently due to tapetal necrosis and resorption in the beagle (95). Another compound has been described that causes pigmentation of the RPE in dogs over the normally nonpigmented tapetal area (95). **Ethambutol** and other **ethylenediamenes** also discolor the tapetum of dogs and possibly cats, causing a fluffy-white appearance (95). The changes, which are reversible after discontinuing drug treatment, may be due to altered refraction by the tapetal cell rodlets, which lose osmophilia and longitudinal orientation in the cell and become swollen. The color changes may reflect a loss in zinc content of the tapetal cells (2,122). Tapetal discoloration also occurs with the zinc chelator **diphenylthiocarbazone** (**dithizone**) toxicity in dogs due to retinal, choroidal, and tapetal edema associated with necrosis and degeneration of the choroid and tapetum (107,108,123). Another chelating agent, **pyrithione** also causes tapetal necrosis and choroidal, tapetal, and retinal edema (108,124,125). It would be reasonable to assume that the tapetal damage from these drugs in dogs is due to zinc chelation, since that metal occurs in high concentration in the tapetal cells. However, both **pyrithione** and **zinc pyridinethione** (which does not cause chelation and has a high zinc concentration) also causes severe tapetal edema, degeneration, retinal edema, and detachment in dogs and tapetal atrophy in cats (126). These changes seem specific for species with a tapetum since no retinal changes are seen in primates, rats, or rabbits, or in beagles with an inherited absence of a tapetum (2). Additionally, **ethambutol**, which is also a chelating agent, causes far less severe effects in tapetal species. It has been suggested that some of the severe toxic effects on the tapetum of agents such as zinc pyrithione, and dithizone may be partly due to zinc chelation (like ethambutol effects) and partly due to reaction with sulfydryl groups necessary for tapetal metabolic processes (126).

Retinal Edema

Retinal edema may arise from breakdown of the blood-retinal barrier (BRB), or from edema in the optic nerve. This comprises the tight junctions between adjacent endothelial cells of retinal blood vessels and between retinal pigment epithelial cells (the choroidal vessels are fenestrated and thus are not a barrier to quite large molecules). These two barriers are respectively the inner and outer blood retinal barriers. Disruption of either may result in protein and water loss into the retinal extracellular space, seen clinically as retinal edema. In man and other primates with a macula, the latter is often the site of edema (macular edema), especially in the outer plexiform or inner nuclear layers. In some instances the edema may be seen as clear cystic spaces in the macula (cystoid macular edema) (127).

Naphthalene causes edema of the retina in rabbits. Small doses cause deposition of calcium oxalate crystals in the retina and vitreous. Larger doses produce the appearance of small circular white lesions, initially in the periphery of the fundus. The edema eventually causes splitting of the retinal layers and detachment above and below the medullary rays (95,128,129).

Intracarotid injections of **triaziquone (Treminon)** in rabbits, used to achieve high ocular concentrations, will cause initial retinal edema either in sharply delineated spots or diffuse cloudiness throughout the fundus, and later retinal degeneration and pigment dispersion (130).

Dithizone, a metal chelator, causes retinal edema in rabbits and dogs. Edema in dogs occurs in the retina and tapetum. The changes in the rabbit fundus are less than in the dog, which may in part be due to the lower concentration of zinc in the tapetum of the rabbit (107,108,123,131,132).

Fluoride has been reported to cause retinal edema when given intravenously to rabbits (133,134). This does not appear to be a significant problem in humans receiving high doses of fluoride for osteoporosis (2).

Glutamate causes massive retinal edema in neonatal mice until 10 days after birth associated with damage to ganglion cells and cells in the inner nuclear layer (135,136).

Sheep and cattle grazing *Helichrysum argyrosphaerum* may develop retinal edema associated with optic nerve edema and hemorrhage, photoreceptor degeneration, and blindness (137).

Iminodipropionitrile causes various ocular lesions in different species. In rats, systemic administration causes retinal edema associated with endothelial proliferation and microaneurysm formation in retinal vessels (138–140).

Methanol causes nerve fiber layer edema in humans, monkeys and primates associated with the major toxic action of methanol in the eye—papilledema (141–143).

Iodopyracet, a radiopaque contrast medium, has occasionally caused retinal edema in humans after intracarotid injection (144). Retinal or macular edema is a reported side effect of several radiographic contrast media.

Retinal edema may occur after intravitreal injection of various substances including **streptomycin** (145).

Macular and retinal edema may occur in cases of severe **quinine** toxicity in humans (146). Cystoid macula edema (CME) may develop in aphakic eyes. It is suggested that surgical inflammation involves production of prostaglandins, which disrupt the perifoveal capillary endothelial cells, and breakdown of the perifoveal BRB. This may be exacerbated by free radicals released in the eye in response to ultraviolet light reaching the macula in the absence of the lens (127). Epinephrine use for glaucoma has been associated with aphakic CME, possibly by causing prostaglandin production (147). Transient CME occurs in humans treated with nicotinic acid used to reduce serum lipid levels (148). The antiestrogen **tamoxifen** used to treat breast cancer has caused CME with prolonged high doses (149).

Retinal and macular edema has also been described as a side effect of many drugs including carbonic anhydrase inhibitors, corticosteroids, tranquilizers, diuretics, and amebicides (1).

Retinal Detachment

The normal retina adheres to the apical processes of the retinal pigment epithelium due to various adhesive forces, mechanical properties of the photoreceptor outer segments, and the presence of an interphotoreceptor matrix in the subretinal space (150). The majority of retinal detachments in man arise from peripheral retinal tearing and vitreous flow into the subretinal space (rhegmatogenous detachments). Detachments may also arise from traction of fibrous strands in the vitreous, or serous exudate from the retina or choroid associated with disruption of the blood-retinal barriers, which enters the subretinal space pushing the retina from the underlying pigment epithelium. Most retinal detachments caused by toxins in animals are exudative. Such detachments may be seen with several of the agents described as causing retinal or choroidal edema or tapetal changes.

Retinal detachment associated with retinal folds and subretinal transudate is seen in cats poisoned with **ethylene glycol** (antifreeze) (151). **Iodate** causes toxic effects on the RPE and disrupts the BRB, which may present as serous detachment in various experimental animals and man (2). Serous retinal detachments have been rarely reported associated with several systemic drugs in man including **corticosteroids** and **penicillamine** (1). **Dithizone** may cause bullous retinal detachments in dogs (108).

Topical use of various miotics for glaucoma, including **pilocarpine, demecarium bromide**, and **echothiophate**, has been suggested as a cause of retinal detachment, and although circumstantial evidence suggests that this may be the case, examination of available evidence does not confirm the hypothesis that the occurrence of detachments is more than coincidental (29,152).

Premature newborn humans and experimental animals exposed to high **oxygen** concentrations during late stages of retinal development respond with initial cessation of peripheral retinal vascularization, followed by the formation of peripheral retinal neovascularization and fibrotic bands in the vitreous. Retinal detachment occurs associated with traction of fibrotic bands on the peripheral retina and subretinal exudate formation (153,154). Oxygen toxicity (pure oxygen) in adult dogs has appeared as choroidal and retinal exudative detachment (155).

Retinal Hemorrhage

Retinal hemorrhage is a commonly reported feature of retinal toxicosis in man, less so in animals. It has been suggested that this is because humans more frequently undergo ocular examination (2), although it could also reflect the greater incidence of retinovascular disease in man (and thus some peculiarities of the human retinal vasculature) as compared with domestic or laboratory species in which it is rarely seen. Hemorrhage may result from toxin-induced retinal vasculitis, plasma hyperviscosity, hypertension, neovascularization, or coagulopathies.

Dicumarol, warfarin, and other anticoagulant drugs may occasionally cause retinal hemorrhage by reducing blood clotting mechanisms (2). **Viper** and **rattlesnake** bites have caused retinal hemorrhages (156,157). These venoms contain anticoagulant factors (158). Retinal hemorrhage has occasionally been reported in animals administered **alloxan** to induce diabetes mellitus. Changes at most are comparable to the background retinopathy described in man without vascular proliferative changes (2). **Carbon disulfide** is a volatile liquid that may cause formation of retinal microaneurysms and hemorrhage without retinal neovascularization (159). **Chloramphenicol** administration in children has resulted in hemorrhage of the optic papilla associated with optic neuritis (160). Plasma hyperviscosity induced by intravenous **dextrans** in monkeys has caused retinal hemorrhages (161).

Dithizone, pyrithione, and **zinc pyrithione** cause retinal hemorrhage in dogs associated with severe exudative changes in the posterior segment and choroidal degeneration (107,108,126).

Retinal hemorrhages in the retinal nerve fiber layer are seen in some aphakic patients with **epinephrine**-induced cystoid macular edema (162). **Systemic lead** or **phosphorus** toxicity may result in retinal hemorrhages, either associated with optic neuritis or due to vasculitis, sclerosis, or degeneration of retinal vessels (2,163). Occasional case reports of retinal hemorrhage have been described in humans or animals administered **aspirin, benzene, dapsone, diquat, ethambutol, hexachlorophene, methyl bromide,** or **radiopaque x-ray media** (2).

Retinal Vessel Abnormalities

Toxins may cause various changes in retinal blood vessels, most notably narrowing, which may occur acutely due to undefined mechanisms, or occur secondary to retinal or optic atrophy due to reduced demand in the degenerate tissue for nutrients. This appears to be the reason for retinal vessels narrowing with a considerable number of toxins (see retinal degeneration). **Quinine** and some of its derivatives cause acute narrowing of retinal arterioles. These changes occur later than the acute and reversible blindness that occurs with quinine toxicity and thus probably do not contrast to the loss of visual acuity (146). **Ergotamine** has also been associated with visual deficits and retinal arteriole narrowing in humans that persisted after other funduscopic and visual signs improved (164). **Oxygen** causes retinal vasoconstriction in adult humans (165). Various anesthetic agents including **barbiturates** also cause retinal vasoconstriction (1).

Occlusion of central retinal arteries or veins has been described in many reports of women taking **oral contraceptives**, although as pointed out by Grant (2) there is no evidence that vascular occlusions occurred more frequently in these patients than the general population (2,166). Thrombosis may occur in retinal vessels in humans treated with pheylpropanolamine hydrochloride (167).

Carbon dioxide, amyl nitrate, and hypoxia cause vasodilation of retinal blood vessels.

Engorgement of retinal vessels may be seen in **methanol toxicosis** (2).

Retinal Pigment Epithelium

The retinal pigment epithelium (RPE) serves an important function both in providing a means for nutrition and waste removal (phagocytosis of the photoreceptor outer segments) in the outer layers of the retina. It also forms an integral part of the outer blood-retinal barrier. Toxins that damage the RPE often have functional and morphological effects on the neural retina. Several groups of compounds have been found to have toxic effects that may involve the RPE, most notably the quinolines and phenothiazines (168). Changes in the RPE are clinically manifest as pigmentary retinopathy with either a decrease or increase of pigmentation.

Primary toxic effects on the RPE appearing as RPE degeneration with secondary effects on the neural retinal have been reported with several agents. **Sodium iodate** given intravenously causes selective damage to the RPE with swelling of the cells, with later degeneration of the photoreceptors and pigment migration and proliferation (169–171). Electrophysiological data in sheep demonstrate that the earliest functional changes are in the RPE (171). **Sodium azide** does not specifically damage the RPE cells although it does change the standing potential across the retina (attributable to RPE) (172). This effect can be abolished by sodium iodate (173). Aminophenoxyalkanes cause retinal degeneration in several species (**aminophenoxyalkanes** in cats and rabbits [174,175], **diaminodiphenoxyheptane** in monkeys, cats, and dogs [174,176,177], and **diaminodiphenoxyheptane [168]). These appear clinically as pigmentary retinopathies. The RPE cells become swollen and proliferate, causing retinal distortion and then photoreceptor outer segment loss. RPE over the tapetal fundus undergoes reactionary pigmentation. Urethane** damages the RPE in rats possibly by effects on RPE mitochondria (178,179). **Oxalate metabolized from methoxyflurane** results in deposition of oxalate crystals in the RPE (180). The RPE atrophies or undergoes peripheral proliferation and hyperpigmentation in response to intravitreal **iron** damage to retinal photoreceptors (181). **Systemic lead** toxicity in rabbits results in RPE cell swelling due to accumulation of phagosomes and lipofuscin (182). ***N*-Methyl-*N*-nitrosourea** causes swelling of RPE cells with pigment dispersion and later degeneration of photoreceptors, seen clinically as a pigmentary retinopathy in hamsters (183).

Chloroquine in high doses causes retinopathy in man. The main lesion appears to be in the photoreceptors and ganglion cells (184–186). The drug is concentrated in melanin-containing RPE cells, which may provide a reservoir for release of the drug into and toxic effects on the retinal neurons (187). RPE changes consist of variable depigmentation and hyperpigmentation (macular "bull's-eye" lesion) (168), hyperplasia, and migration of pigment into the retina (188). In other species similar pigmentary changes occur in RPE cells (95). **Amopyroquin** causes pigment proliferation from the RPE in beagles (189). **Hydroxychloroquine** and **diiodohydroxyquin** have similar effects on the RPE (168). **Quinine** causes blindness and changes in the electroretinogram (ERG) c-wave and electro-oculogram (EOG) during the acute phases of toxicity, which suggests that the RPE may be primarily affected (190,191).

Phenothiazines are also concentrated in RPE melanin and persist in RPE cells for long periods of time (192). Overdosage with **thioridazine** causes a pigmentary retinopathy with visual loss in man. Irreversible black pigmentary stippling is seen throughout the posterior fundus, which may progress to RPE atrophy and patchy depigmentation (168,193). **Piperidylchlorophenothiazine** selectively damages rods, resulting in excessive accumulation of outer segment lamellar debris and inclusions in the RPE, which appears as a pigmentary retinopathy in humans and cats (194–196). **Dithizone** toxicity in dogs may result in RPE hypertrophy, which gives the tapetum a granular appearance (95). **Sparsomycin causes primary clumping of RPE pigment with degeneration of adjacent photoreceptors (197). Intravitreal cephaloridine causes photoreceptor degeneration and degeneration of the RPE (198). Amphilphilic cationic compounds** cause the formation of membrane-bound crystalloid or lamellar inclusions in the RPE and ganglion cells in rats (199). **Fenthione** causes retinal degeneration in rats associated with swelling and disorganization of RPE cells (200).

Photoreceptor Degeneration

Degeneration of the retinal rods and cones may occur from primary action of a toxin on the cells, damage to the RPE or choroid and outer blood-retinal barrier with secondary photoreceptor degeneration, or following extensive damage and degeneration in the inner retinal layers.

Piperidylchlorophenothiazine (NP-207) causes retinal toxicity in man and cats although not in several other species (2). The drug accumulates in the melanin of the choroid. In man, NP-207 affects dim light vision and later visual acuity (201). Its effects may be partially reversible. Electrophysiological studies identify the site of toxicity as the photoreceptor layer (202). The ophthalmoscopic appearance in the cat is of a pigmentary retinopathy that develops after 4 to 6 weeks of treatment, spreading as a horizontal band from the area centralis (95). Pigmentary changes deep in the retina also occur in man. In both species the drug causes disruption of the rod outer segments and may activate photoreceptor shedding. The excess membranous lipid material engulfed by the RPE produces the clinical appearance of pigmentation. NP-207 acts on the ellipsoids of the rods and probably inhibits oxidative phosphorylation by inhibiting flavine nucleotides (196,203,204).

Ammeline, a herbicide, causes degeneration of photoreceptors secondary to histological degeneration of the RPE. **Aramite**, a plant pesticide, causes electroretinographic signs of photoreceptor damage in mice. **Benzoic acid** causes exudative retinal detachment and degeneration of rods and cones (2).

"Bright blindness" is seen in sheep fed bracken fern (*Pteridium aquilinum*). Tapetal hyperreflectivity is seen due to thinning of the overlying retina. Degeneration initially affects the rods and cones, the outer segments of which become fragmented and vesicular, and later the nuclear layers (205,206). The plant *Stypandra imbricata* or blindgrass causes degeneration of photoreceptors and optic neuritis in sheep that graze it. Similar lesions are seen in rats fed blindgrass (207,208).

Several cardiac glycosides, including **digitalis** and **digoxin**, have been shown to have toxic effects in the eye. The most commonly reported are central and paracentral scotomas, reduced visual acuity, and color vision deficits. These are reversible when the drug is discontinued and may be associated with a reduction of the ERG amplitude. This suggests that the toxic effects are probably at the level of the outer retina. No histological degeneration of the photoreceptors has been reported (2).

Colchicine, an antimitotic agent, causes photoreceptor degeneration and blocks axonal transport in rats when administered intravitreally.

Ethylenimine, an alkylating agent and a related compound **4,4′-diaminodiphenylmethane**, causes specific atrophy of rods and cones in cats, but not in man or other species tested (209).

Sodium fluroescein and **hematoporphyrin** have been reported to act as photosensitizing agents in albino mice and pigmented rabbits, causing photoreceptor damage (2).

Vitamin A causes retinal damage in rats with signs of mitochondrial damage evident both in the photoreceptors and RPE (210).

Sodium fluoride causes outer segment disorganization and loss following changes in the RPE in rabbits given high doses of the drug intravenously (133,211).

Hexachlorophene causes photoreceptor outer segment disorganization and degeneration, and optic atrophy and retinal hemorrhage. Photoreceptor degeneration appears to be distinct from changes in the optic nerve and ganglion cells (212).

Sodium iodate causes photoreceptor degeneration secondary to damage to the RPE and blood-retinal barrier (171).

Iodoacetate causes rapid and selective toxicity on the photoreceptors when administered by intravenous or intraarterial injection. Rods are more sensitive to iodoacetate than cones. Within a few hours of injection swelling of mitochondria in the rod inner segments is seen, with rapid progression of photoreceptor and RPE disorganization and degeneration (213,214). **Bromoacetate** causes a similar retinal degeneration in rabbits (215).

***N*-methyl-*N*-nitrosourea**, a carcinogenic agent, causes retinal degeneration (RPE and photoreceptors) in the hamster when given intravenously (183).

Quinine appears to have several effects in the retina at the level of the photoreceptors, RPE, ganglion cells, and optic nerve fibers. In reviewing the literature Grant (2) concluded that electrophysiological data points to early toxicity in the RPE and photoreceptors with later changes in the optic nerve, ganglion cells, and inner retinal vasculature.

Quinoline and its derivatives have caused retinal degeneration and optic nerve atrophy in several species (1,2).

Sodium azide causes changes in the ERG that point to the RPE as the primary site of damage. Photoreceptors can be shown to undergo degeneration, which is probably secondary to RPE degeneration (216).

Sucrose causes specific degeneration of the rods and cones that does not affect the RPE or inner retinal neurons. Retinal vascular changes are reminiscent of background retinopathy in man (217).

Urethane administered parenterally to pigmented rats causes photoreceptor degeneration and growth of new vessels into the retinal pigment epithelium (218).

Guanosine 3′,5′-cyclic monophosphate (cyclic GMP) has been shown to be toxic to photoreceptors, causing disorganization and breakup of outer segments in retinas *in vitro* (219). This is believed to be involved in the pathogenesis of certain inherited photoreceptor degenerations in rodents, dogs, and cats (220).

Tunicamycin causes photoreceptor-specific degeneration by suppressing the renewal mechanisms of the photoreceptor outer segments (221).

Vincristine, an antineoplastic agent, causes photoreceptor inner segment degeneration when injected into the vitreous in rats (222), whereas in a human who became night blind after vincristine therapy, the normal a-wave and abnormally small b-wave suggested that the drug might cause a neurotransmission defect in the outer plexiform layer (223).

Vitamin A inhibits the alcohol dehydrogenase systems of the photoreceptors and RPE with disruption of mitochondrial membranes in the photoreceptor inner segments (210).

Ganglion Cells and Inner Retina

Ganglion cells can be damaged by toxins that exert their effects directly on these proximal retinal neurons, through damage to the optic nerve into which they project and by toxic effects on the other retinal neurons and glia or retinal pigment epithelium. In many cases it is difficult to separate these actions and determine that the ganglion cell is the primary target of a toxin. Other cells in the inner retina (bipolar, horizontal, or amacrine cells) may be affected, particularly by neurotransmitter-like substances.

Doxorubicin causes neurofilament accumulation in the cell body and central axon of ganglion cells and then loss of ganglion cells in the rat retina possibly by inhibiting slow axoplasmic flow, causing axon swelling and death (224).

Arsanilic acid causes degeneration of the ganglion cells in humans (2). In pigs this compound causes blindness due to optic nerve atrophy without any evident retinal lesions (225). Ducks fed **Ammi majus** seeds develop vacuolation and degeneration of the ganglion cells (226). ***Dryopteris felix mas*** toxicity causes blindness in cattle fed upon the plant. Histology reveals the main lesion to be ganglion cell and optic nerve fiber degeneration (227). Similar findings occur in **chloramphenicol** toxicity causing optic atrophy and ganglion cell loss (160,228). **Carbon dioxide** toxicity in man may cause degeneration of ganglion cells and associated blindness. Dogs are very sensitive to the effects of quinine and cinchona derivatives. The drug selectively causes degeneration of retinal ganglion cells and subsequent optic atrophy. Ophthalmoscopically, cinchona toxicity causes retinal arteriolar vasoconstriction and pallor of the optic disc (95).

Carbon disulfide appears to cause primary damage to the ganglion cells with associated retrobulbar optic neuritis (2). In rats it causes acute ganglion cell degeneration (229).

***L*-Cysteine** is selectively toxic to ganglion cells and amacrine cells in the rat retina (230,231).

Glutamate is a neurotransmitter in the retina. At toxic doses it causes very specific degeneration of ganglion cells in rat neonates with destruction of the inner retinal layers by 17 days of age. The glial cells and inner nuclear layer later degenerate (215,232).

Trimethyltin causes most degeneration in the inner retinal layers with pyknosis seen in the inner and outer nuclear layers and swelling of the photoreceptor inner segments (233).

Locoweed (*Astragalus mollissimus*) causes vacuolation of ganglion and bipolar cells in cattle and sheep (234) by suppressing the enzyme α-mannosidase. Oligosaccharides accumulate in and affect the function of ganglion cells and neurons in the central nervous system (CNS) (235).

Methanol poisoning in man presents typically with blindness due to optic atrophy. In acute cases optic nerve edema is seen. Histologically in advanced cases optic and ganglion cell atrophy is detected, although these are not seen in acute cases. In monkeys the earliest signs of methanol toxicity are optic nerve edema. Ganglion cell degeneration occurs secondary to restricted axoplasmic flow because of swollen optic nerve oligodendroglia (2).

Quinine toxicity results in vacuolation of ganglion cells and associated optic atrophy (as well as outer retinal degeneration and later vascular attenuation) (2).

Orthochromic granules are seen in the ganglion cells of rats treated with **chloroquine** apart from its toxic effects of the RPE and photoreceptors (236).

As in other sites in the retina and cornea **amphiphilic cationic compounds** may cause accumulation of lipids in ganglion cells (199).

Kainic acid causes pyknosis of amacrine cells and edema in the inner plexiform layer possibly by causing persistent depolarization of the neurons (237).

Retinal Lipidosis

Lipid deposits in the retina occur with **cationic amphiphilic drugs** such as **chlorphentermine, triparanol,** and **1-chloroamitriptyline** administered to rats. These cause no significant pathology and are only diagnosed by ultrastructural examination of the RPE, ganglion cells, Müller cells, and neurons of the inner nuclear layer (238,239). Retinal lipidosis occurs in several other species treated long term with **chloroquine** (239).

OPTIC NERVE

The ganglion cell's central axons pass into the nerve fiber layer of the retina and converge to a point just below and medial to the posterior pole of the eye to form the optic nerve at the optic disc or papilla.

The optic nerve may be considered to consist of three portions: (a) ocular, the part seen within the eye and composed of retina, choroidal, and scleral portions; (b) orbital, which extends from the lamina cribrosa of the sclera to the optic foramen; and (c) intracranial, which passes from the optic foramen to the optic chiasm.

The optic nerve is formed by ganglion cell axons, glia (astrocytes and microglia), collagenous setae arising from the ensheathing pia mater, blood vessels, and in the retrobulbar part of the nerve myelin.

The site in the sclera where the nerve fibers leave the eye is the lamina cribrosa, a sieve-like arrangement of scleral collagen through which fascicles of nerve fibers and ensheathing glia pass.

In dogs the entire optic nerve, extending up into the peripapillary area of the retina, may be myelinated. In man, cats, and horses, the nerve becomes myelinated after it exits through the lamina cribrosa.

The orbital and intracranial portions of the optic nerve are invested by the outer dura mater, subarachnoid, and pia mater.

The blood supply to the optic nerve is from the internal ophthalmic artery in domestic species, whereas the blood supply to the choroid and retina is derived from the external maxillary artery via the external ophthalmic artery and long and short posterior ciliary arteries. In primates, by contrast, both the anterior and posterior segment are supplied by the internal carotid artery via the internal ophthalmic artery. The central retinal artery in primates penetrates the dura mater and crosses the subarachnoid space to form the central retinal artery. In animals the long posterior ciliary arteries, giving rise to cilioretinal arteries, pierce the globe around the periphery of the optic nerve.

Toxic influences on the nerve may be a reflection of processes occurring in the retina and particularly the ganglion cells or CNS disease. Specific toxic disorders may be caused by demyelinating drugs. The most common lesions caused by drug toxicity are optic neuritis (often loosely referred to as optic neuropathy) and (often as a consequence) optic atrophy. The optic nerve may become inflamed in association with chorioretinitis or meningoencephalitis and undergo atrophy secondary to retinal (or chorioretinal) degeneration.

Optic Neuritis, Neuropathy, and Atrophy

Optic neuritis may be seen within the eye or occur in any part of the nerve as far back as the chiasm. Lesions behind the eye are referred to as retrobulbar optic neuritis. In man this involves, in particular, ganglion cell fibers from the papillomacular bundle. Optic neuritis may result in various disturbances of vision, although a central scotoma, complete loss of vision, and color deficiencies are commonly reported.

Hexachlorophene causes signs of intraocular or retrobulbar optic neuritis in man (2). In rats there is demyelination and degeneration of axons of the optic nerve and pathways, associated with severe lesions in the white matter of the brain. Optic nerve destruction precedes ganglion cell loss.

Arsanilic acid and its derivatives, including **acetarsone**, cause optic neuritis and atrophy in humans and pigs. The damage to the nerve causes sudden blindness (225).

Poisoning with *Dryopteris felix mas*, the active ingredient of which is **felicin**, causes retrobulbar neuropathy in man, cattle, and dogs. In man ophthalmoscopic signs of optic neuritis have been described progressing to optic atrophy. In dogs and rabbits, histologic evidence of ganglion cell death and axon degeneration is seen without signs of neuronal inflammation, although endovasculitis and perivasculitis is described (2). In cattle, hemorrhages and edema are seen at the optic disc and optic atrophy ensues. Histologically, axons persist in areas devoid of myelin, suggesting that medullary sheaths and oligodendrocytes may be more susceptible to the toxin due to their high lipid content (227). In sheep and goats grazed on *Stypandra glauca* (blindgrass), similar optic neuropathy affects the intracranial and intracanalicular portions of the nerve (208). *Stypandra imbricata* consumed by sheep, goats, or rats causes blindness due to vacuolation of optic nerve myelin, degeneration of the axons, and gliosis. The orbital and intracranial nerves in the rats were considerably swollen (207). *Helichrysum argyrosphaerum* causes almost identical lesions in cattle (137).

Carbon disulfide may cause retrobulbar neuritis and atrophy in man and experimentally in rabbits and mice ganglion cell, and optic nerve fiber degeneration is seen (2).

Chronic thallium toxicosis causes optic neuritis and atrophy with relative sparing of the outer retina (240).

Chloramphenicol has caused optic neuritis and atrophy in children treated for cystic fibrosis (160). Atrophy of ganglion cells in the macular region and optic nerve fibers is seen histologically (228).

Clioquinol, an antiamebic drug, exerts a very specific toxic effect on the long tracts of the spinal cord and the optic nerves. The disease has been seen in humans and reproduced in dogs and cats. Degeneration of the nerve may extend from the ganglion cells to the lateral geniculate synapse (241-244).

Cyanides in near-lethal doses will cause retrobulbar optic atrophy in rats, possibly associated with a paucity of capillaries at this site, which would render the tissue more susceptible to the acidotic effects of cyanide (245,246).

Dinitrobenzene and related compounds are believed (based on the signs of central scotomas and color deficiencies) to cause retrobulbar neuropathy in man (1,2).

Disulfiram has caused several cases of bilateral optic neuritis in humans (2). **Penicillamine** has caused several cases of optic neuritis in man (2). Several **monoamine oxidase inhibitors (isoniazid, octamoxin, pheniprazine)** have caused cases of optic neuritis and atrophy in man (2,247). **Plasmocid**, an 8-aminoquinoline, has caused optic neuritis and atrophy in humans, cats, dogs, and rabbits (2).

Lead toxicity in man has caused optic neuropathy. Optic atrophy may result from increased intracranial pressure (affecting the pressure around the optic nerve via the subarachnoid) or as a direct toxic effect of lead on the optic nerve. Papilledema is a consistent feature due to raised intracranial pressure (2).

The antitubercular drug **ethambutol** specifically causes chiasmal retrobulbar neuritis in monkeys and rats (248,249), and based upon clinical findings also in humans. In rabbits the drug causes demyelination of the optic nerve (250).

Ethylene glycol when ingested causes acidosis, and clinical signs suggestive of retrobulbar neuropathy have been described in man (251,252).

Glutamate administered to rats or mice during the first 10 postnatal days causes specific ganglion cell degeneration that progresses to optic atrophy (136,253,254).

In **methanol** toxicity in humans an early change appears to be demyelinization of the retrolaminar portion of the optic nerve (255). Later findings are of optic nerve atrophy and ganglion cell death. Clinically patients initially have evidence of retinal and optic nerve edema, from which they may recover or progress to optic atrophy and blindness (256).

Optic Nerve Edema

In dogs oral **rafoxanide** causes edema and vacuolation of the optic nerve and chiasm. Edema of the optic disc may be due to edema in the ocular and retrobulbar portion of the nerve as well as raised intracranial pressure due to edema of the white matter of the brain (257). **Hexachlorophene** used to treat liver fluke causes transient edema of the optic nerve in sheep between 24 and 72 hr of administration, followed by irreversible loss of the pupillary light reflexes. Affected animals have hydrocephalus and optic nerve edema and vacuolation progressing to gliosis (95).

Optic neuritis and atrophy has been described along with peripapillary edema, and retinal hemorrhages associated with impaired central vision in children treated for several weeks with high doses of **chloramphenicol**. Many cases proceed to optic atrophy. Degenerative changes are confined to ganglion cells and optic nerve.

EXTRAOCULAR MUSCLES

Paralysis of extraocular muscles (EOM) may arise in some toxicities. Signs include strabismus, restricted eye movement, diplopia, and, occasionally, complete external ophthalmoplegia. Toxicity may be due to local action of toxins at the muscle end plate or associated with central nervous system toxicity.

EOM weakness has been described with various animal venoms and plant toxins, including **elapid snake venoms, *Amanita* mushrooms, scorpion venom, botulinus toxin, *d*-tubocurarine**, and ***Gelsemium sempervirens***.

Partial paralysis of EOM may occur in humans some days after receiving **spinal anesthetics** (144).

Primidone, an anticonvulsant, causes occasional cases of ophthalmoplegia, mainly in association with phenytoin (2).

EOM paralysis usually assumed to be due to the CNS effects of the toxin have been reported with **carbamazepine, arsphenamine, barbiturates, lead** (which is unusual in that it may also cause local signs of pathology in the EOM), and **nalidixic acid** (44).

Neurotoxicity with effects on EOM have been described with various antibiotics including furmethanol and streptomycin.

Toxins that have caused total EOM paralysis include **amitriptyline**.

Pamaquine, an 8-aminoquinoline antimalarial, has caused damage to the EOM nuclei in dogs and possible sympathetic effects that appear as divergent strabismus, mild enophthalmos, and miosis (258). **Plasmocid**, another 8-aminoquinoline antimalarial, causes selective injury to the third, fourth, and sixth nerve nuclei, thus affecting extraocular muscle function (2).

Thallium poisoning causes a polyneuropathy that presents with strabismus, ptosis, and paralysis of the extraocular muscles. Degeneration of nerve fibers of the extraocular muscles has been reported (259).

Trichloroethylene causes neuritis affecting cranial nerves resulting in EOM palsy (260,261). Grant (2) points out that this toxicity is probably associated with decomposition products of trichloroethylene (especially dichloracetylene), which might be the toxic principle.

Vincristine can cause a neuropathy that may involve nerves innervating EOM, causing EOM paralysis (262).

Nystagmus has occurred with several toxins. The site of action is usually not the eye but the CNS (1,2).

ORBIT

The most commonly reported toxic orbital abnormality is exophthalmos (1,2). This has been reported commonly as a side effect of various **corticosteroids** in man (263,264).

Lithium, used as an anti-manic depressive therapy in man, causes thyroid dysfunction and an associated exophthalmos (265). **Methyl cyanide** injected into rabbits causes thyroid hyperplasia and exophthalmos (266).

Vitamin A toxicity has caused exophthalmos in dogs and guinea pigs when administered in high doses. In the guinea pig, malformation of the orbit has been shown to be the cause of exophthalmos (267,268).

Aminocaproic acid injected intravenously in cats causes contraction of sympathetically innervated muscle in the orbital cone, resulting in mild exophthalmos (269).

OCULAR TERATOGENESIS

The normal development of the eye may be affected in the uterus by a variety of toxins. The most common ocular malformations reported are varying degrees of microphthalmia to anophthalmia, colobomatous defects, and vitreoretinal dysplasia.

Selenium toxicity in sheep during early embryonic development causes microphthalmia with cysts and normal-sized eyes with microcornea or in which the cornea and iris are missing, with ectopia lentis or aphakia. Other structures may have colobomas. The failure of sclera to form enables the forming vitreous to flow into adjacent mesectodermal tissue to form cysts (270).

Maternal ingestion of the plant *Veratrum californicum* by sheep on the 14th day of gestation produces cyclopia in the offspring. Various alkaloids, **cyclopamine**, **veratrosine**, **jervine**, **cycloposine**, **pseudojervine**, and **isorubijervine**, have been found to be the toxic agents. In severe cases bones of the upper jaw and cranium were distorted with fusion of the cerebral hemispheres, hydrocephalus, cyclopia, and anophthalmia (271-275).

Vitamin A causes various ocular malformations that have included lens and retinal defects, microphthalmia, and colobomas in rabbits, rats, and chickens (2). In hamsters and guinea pigs abnormal growth of the orbital bones may result in abnormally shallow orbits and exophthalmos.

Apholate, an alkylating agent used as an insect chemosterilant, may cause anophthalmia and defective development of cranial and facial bones with absence of the orbital cavities in sheep (276).

Griseofulvin administered to cats in the first half of gestation causes anophthalmia, cyclopia, and optic nerve aplasia in the kittens (277).

Anticoagulants such as **warfarin** taken by humans during pregnancy have caused microphthalmia or abnormally large eyes, optic atrophy, and lens opacities (278).

Chlorambucil, an antineoplastic drug, causes retinal dysplasia in mice, rats, and monkeys, and lens and optic nerve malformations in mice (279,280). **Vinblastine** has produced anophthalmia, microphthalmia, and other developmental defects in hamsters (281). **Cyclophosphamide** used in several species has caused congenital malformation of the nasolacrimal ducts (282–284). **Alloxan**, has caused teratogenic defects of the lens and iris in mice. **Busulfan** has caused congenital malformations in humans (2).

Felicin, the toxic principle of *Dryopteris felix mas*, has caused microphthalmia, anophthalmia, and dysplastic development of the retina and optic nerves when administered to mice (2).

Salicylate produces anophthalmia, microphthalmia, and apparent exophthalmia in rats (285).

Azathioprine causes ocular malformations, including defects in the lens in rabbits (286).

The antioxidant food additive **butylated hydroxytoluene** causes anophthalmia in rats (287).

2,4-Dichlorophenyl-*p*-nitrophenyl ether causes hypoplasia of the harderian gland. The eyes may be normal in size or larger than usual. The enophthalmos due to absence of the harderian gland may resemble microphthalmia (288).

Idoxuridine causes retinal dysplasia and defects in the iris and ciliary body when administered to rabbits (289).

The alkaloid **caffeine** has caused lens abnormalities in developing rat lenses (290).

Corticosteriods applied topically to the eyes of pregnant mice have caused congenital abnormalities in the offspring (291).

Isotretinoin causes ocular teratogenesis in man—defects ranging from microphthalmia to abnormal development of central projections of the visual pathway (292,293).

Trypan blue, an anionic dye, causes anophthalmia and microphthalmia in rats (294).

Lysergic acid diethylamide (LSD) has produced lens epithelial abnormalities similar to those caused by radiation in mice (295) and multiple ocular anomalies in man (296,297).

1-Methyl-3-nitro-1-nitrosoguanidine causes dysgenesis of the anterior segment, hypoplasia of the iris stroma, and ectopia of the ciliary body in rabbits (298).

Abnormal facial development with shortening of the palpebral fissure has been described in humans with fetal alcohol syndrome (299). Attempts to reproduce a model of the human syndrome in mice has demonstrated that **ethanol** causes microphthalmia (300).

Nickel carbonyl has caused anophthalmia and microphthalmia in rats exposed to it in early gestation.

Acute **quinine** toxicity associated with high doses taken during pregnancy has caused optic nerve hypoplasia in humans (301).

Tetracycline has resulted in corneal and lens discoloration in fetuses of mice and rabbits when fed to the dams during gestation, although this cannot be considered a malformation (2).

Thalidomide causes various ocular malformations in humans and some defects have been duplicated in rabbits. Abnormal development of extraocular muscles is commonly reported (302). Other abnormalities include microphthalmia and colobomas of the iris, choroid, retina, and lenticular and retinal dysplasia (303,304).

Ocular teratogenic effects in various animal species have also been described with **cyclizine**, an antihistamine, and **colchicine** (2).

REFERENCES

1. Fraunfelder FT, Meyer SM. *Drug-induced ocular side effects and drug interactions*, 3rd ed. Philadelphia: Lea & Febiger, 1989.
2. Grant WM. *Toxicology of the eye*, 3rd ed. Springfield: Charles C. Thomas, 1986.
3. Prince JH. *Comparative anatomy of the eye*. Springfield: Charles C. Thomas, 1956.
4. Hogan MJ, Alvarado JA, Weddell JE. *Histology of the human eye*. Philadelphia: W.B. Saunders, 1971.
5. Walls GL. *The vertebrate eye and its adaptive radiation*. Bloomfield Hills, MI: Cranbrook Institute of Science, 1942.
6. Duke-Elder S. The eye in evolution. In: *System of ophthalmology, Vol 1*. St. Louis: C.V. Mosby, 1958.
7. Prince JH, Diesem CD, Eglitis I, Ruskell GL. *Anatomy and histology of the eye and orbit in domestic animals*. Springfield: Charles C. Thomas, 1960.
8. Samuelson DA. Ophthalmic anatomy and embryology. In: Gelatt KN, ed. *Veterinary ophthalmology*, 2nd ed. Philadelphia: Lea & Febiger, 1991;3–123.
9. Davson H. *Physiology of the eye*, 5th ed. New York: Pergamon Press, 1990.
10. Berman ER. *Biochemistry of the eye*, New York: Plenum Press, 1991.
11. Ozanics V, Jakobiec FA. Prenatal development of the eye and its adnexa. In: Duane TD, Jaeger EA, eds. *Biomedical foundations of ophthalmology*, Vol 1. Philadelphia: Harper & Row, 1986;9–86.
12. Wilkie DA, Wyman M. Comparative anatomy and physiology of the mammalian eye. In: Hobson DW, ed. *Dermal and ocular toxicology: fundamentals and methods*. 1991;433–491.
13. *The pharmacological basis of therapeutics*, 8th ed. New York: Pergamon Press, 1990.
14. Edwards JJ, Anderson RL, Wood JR. Loxoscelism of the eyelids. *Arch Ophthalmol* 1980;98:1997–2000.
15. Sandler SG, Tobin W, Henderson ES. Vincristine-induced neuropathy. *Neurology* 1969;19:367–374.
16. Bryan GM, Slatter DH. Keratoconjunctivitis sicca induced by phenazopyridine in dogs. *Arch Ophthalmol* 1973;90:310–311.
17. Slatter DH. Keratoconjunctivitis sicca in the dog produced by oral phenazopyridine hydrochloride. *J Small Anim Pract* 1973;14:749–771.
18. Kaswan RL, Salisbury MA. A new perspective on canine keratoconjunctivitis sicca: treatment with ophthalmic cyclosporine. *Vet Clin North Am [Small Anim Pract]* 1990;20:583–613.
19. Friedenwald JS, Hughes WF, Herrmann H. Acid burns of the eye. *Arch Ophthalmol* 1946;35:98–108.
20. Grant WM, Kern HL. Action of alkalies on the corneal stroma. *Arch Ophthalmol* 1955;54:931–939.
21. Kao WW-Y, Ebert J, Kao CW-C, Covington H, Cintron C. Development of monoclonal antibodies recognizing collagenase from rabbit PMN: the presence of this enzyme in ulcerating corneas. *Curr Eye Res* 1986;5:801–815.
22. Elgebaly SA, Downes RT, Bohr M, Forouhar F, O'Rourke J, Kreutzer DL. Inflammatory mediators in alkali-burned corneas: preliminary characterization. *Curr Eye Res* 1987;6:1263–1274.
23. Berman M, Leary R, Gage J. Evidence for a role of the plasminogen activator-plasmin system in corneal ulceration. *Invest Ophthalmol Vis Sci* 1980;19:1204–1221.
24. Brown CJ. Ocular envenomization by the West African spitting cobra. *Ann Ophthalmol* 1980;12:868–870.
25. Payne Y, Warrell DA. Effects of venom in eye from spitting cobra. *Arch Ophthalmol* 1976;94:1803.

26. Warrell DA, Ormerod LD. Snake venom ophthalmia and blindness caused by the spitting cobra (Naja nigricollis) in Nigeria. *Am J Trop Med Hyg* 1976;25:525–529.
27. MacLeod IF. Chemical mace: ocular effects in rabbits and monkeys. *J Forensic Sci* 1969;14:34–47.
28. Smelser G, Ozanics V. Effect of local anesthetics on cell division and migration following thermal burns of the cornea. *Arch Ophthalmol* 1945;34:271–277.
29. Havener WH. *Ocular pharmacology*, 5th ed. St. Louis: C.V. Mosby, 1983.
30. McLendon BF, Bron AJ. Corneal toxicity from vinblastine solution. *Br J Ophthalmol* 1978;62:97–99.
31. Kinsey VE, Grant WM. Determination of the rate of disappearance of mustard gas and mustard intermediates in the corneal tissue. *J Clin Invest* 1946;25:776–779.
32. Mann I, Pirie A, Pullinger BD. An experimental and clinical study of the reaction of the anterior segment of the eye to chemical injury, with special reference to chemical warfare agents. *Br J Ophthalmol* 1948;13(suppl):1–171.
33. Jampol LM, Axelrod A, Tessler H. Pathways of the eye's response to topical nitrogen mustard. *Invest Ophthalmol Vis Sci* 1976;15:486–489.
34. Carpenter CP, Smyth HF. Chemical burns of the rabbit cornea. *Am J Ophthalmol* 1946;29:1363–1374.
35. Gipson IK, Westcott MJ, Brooksby NG. Effects of cytochalasins B and D and colchicine on migration of the corneal epithelium. *Invest Ophthalmol Vis Sci* 1982;22:633–642.
36. Kaufman HE, Capella JA, et al. Corneal toxicity of cytosine arabinoside. *Arch Ophthalmol* 1964;72:535–540.
37. Fraunfelder FT, Meyer SM. Ocular toxicity of antineoplastic agents. *Ophthalmology* 1983;90:1–3.
38. Wilson FM II. Adverse external ocular effects of topical ophthalmic medications. *Surv Ophthalmol* 1979;24:57.
39. Waltman SR, Carroll D, Schimmelpfennig W, Okun E. Intraocular irrigation solutions for clinical vitrectomy. *Ophthalmic Surg* 1975;6:90.
40. Maurice D, Perlman M. Permanent destruction of the corneal endothelium in rabbits. *Invest Ophthalmol* 1977;16:646.
41. Whitman LK, Filmer DB. A photosensitized keratitis in young cattle following the use of phenothiazine as an anthelmintic. *Aust Vet J* 1974;23:336–340.
42. Kuwabara T, Quevedo AT, Cogan DG. An experimental study of dichloroethane poisoning. *Arch Ophthalmol* 1968;79:321–330.
43. Reinecke RD, Kuwabara T. Corneal deposits secondary to topical epinephrine. *Arch Ophthalmol* 1963;70:170–172.
44. Bockhardt H, Drenckhahn D, Lullmann-Rauch R. Amiodarone-induced lipidosis-like alterations in ocular tissues in rats. *Graefes Arch Ophthalmol* 1978;207:91–96.
45. Bockhardt H, Drenckhahn D, Lullmann-Rauch R. Amiodarone-induced lipidosis-like alterations in ocular tissues of rats. *Graefes Arch Clin Exp Ophthalmol* 1978;207:91–96.
46. Drenckhahn D, Jacobi B, Lullmann-Rauch R. Corneal lipidosis in rats treated with amphiphilic cationic drugs. *Arzneimittelforschung* 1983;33:827–831.
47. Lullmann-Rauch R. Lipidosis and mucopolysaccharidosis of the cornea due to cationic amphiphilic drugs, rat. In: Jones TC, Mohr U, Hunt RD, eds. *Eye and ear*. Berlin: Springer-Verlag, 1991;25–29.
48. Rubin LF. Toxicity of dimethyl sulfoxide, alone and in combination. *Ann NY Acad Sci* 1975;243:98–103.
49. Wood DC, Wirth NV. Changes in rabbit lenses following DMSO therapy. *Ophthalmologica* 1969;158:488–493.
50. Harding JJ, Crabbe MJC. The lens: development, proteins, metabolism and cataract. In: Davson H, ed. *The eye*, Vol 1B, 3rd ed. Orlando, FL: Academic Press, 1984;207–492.
51. Cloud TM, Hakim R, Griffin AC. Photosensitization of the eye with methoxsalen. I. Acute effects. *Arch Ophthalmol* 1960;64:346–351.
52. Cloud TM, Hakim R, Griffin AC. Photosensitization of the eye with methoxsalen. II. Chronic effects. *Arch Ophthalmol* 1961;66:689–693.
53. Christenberry KW, Conklin JW, et al. Induction of cataracts in mice by 4-(p-dimethylaminostyryl) quinoline. *Arch Ophthalmol* 1963;70:250–252.
54. Cibis PA. Ocular lesions produced by iodoacetate. *Arch Ophthalmol* 1957;57:509–519.
55. Grimes P, Von Sallmann L, Frichette A. Influence of Myleran on cell proliferation in the lens epithelium. *Invest Ophthalmol* 1965;3:566–576.
56. Hamming NA, Apple DJ, Goldberg MF. Histopathology and ultrastructure of busulfan-induced cataract. *Graefes Arch Ophthalmol* 1976;200:139–147.

57. Gralla EJ, Rubin L. Ocular studies with parachlorophenylalanine in rats and monkeys. *Arch Ophthalmol* 1970;83:734-740.
58. Rowe VD, Zigler S, Andersen AE, Sidbury JB, Guroff G. Some characteristics of the p-chlorophenylalanine-induced cataract. *Exp Eye Res* 1973;17:245-250.
59. Grimes P, Von Sallmann L. Interference with cell proliferation and induction of polyploidy in rat lens epithelium during prolonged myleran treatment. *Exp Cell Res* 1966;42:265-273.
60. Hockwin O, Okamoto T, et al. Genesis of cataracts: cumulative effects of subliminal noxious influences. *Ann Ophthalmol* 1969;1:321-325.
61. van Heyningen R. Naphthalene cataract in rats and rabbits: a resume. *Exp Eye Res* 1979;28:435-439.
62. Bagchi K. The effects of methionine sulphoximine induced by methionine deficiency on the crystalline lens of albino rats. *Indian J Med Res* 1959;47:437-447.
63. Von Sallmann L, Grimes P, Collins E. Mimosine cataract. *Am J Ophthalmol* 1959;47:107-117.
64. Holmes JHC, Humphrey JD, Walton EA, O'Shea JD. Cataracts, goiter and infertility in cattle grazed on an exclusive diet of *Leucaena leucocephala*. *Aust Vet J* 1981;57:257-261.
65. Kleifeld O, Hockwin O. The effect of dinitrophenol (DNP), ethylenediamine tetra-acetic acid, diamox and butazolidin on the metabolism of the lens. *Graefes Arch Ophthalmol* 1956;158:54-63.
66. Miyata A. Studies on the experimental dinitrophenol cataract. *Acta Soc Ophthalmol Jpn* 1968;72:2307-2324.
67. van Heyningen R. Xylose cataract: a comparison between the weanling and the older rat. *Exp Eye Res* 1969;8:379-385.
68. Bernat R, Bombicki K. Changes in the concentration of glutathione, ascorbic acid, and sulfhydryl amino acids in experimental cataracts. *Acta Physiol Pol* 1968;19:205-215.
69. Patterson JW, Patterson ME, Kinsey VE, Reddy DVN. Lens assays on diabetic and galactosemic rats receiving diets that modify cataract development. *Invest Ophthalmol* 1965;4:98-103.
70. Von Sallmann L, Grimes P. Eye changes in streptozotocin diabetes in rats. *Am J Ophthalmol* 1971;71(1-part 2):312-319.
71. Arison RN, Ciaccio EL, Glitzer MS, Cassaro JA, Pruss MP. Light and electron microscopy of lesions in rats rendered diabetic with streptozotocin. *Diabetes* 1967;16:51-56.
72. Poulsom R, Boot Hanford RP, Heath H. Some effects of aldose reductase inhibition upon the eyes of long-term streptozotocin-diabetic rats. *Curr Eye Res* 1982;2:351-355.
73. Wright HN. Corneal and lenticular opacities in eyes of rats following long-term administration of sulfonylurea derivatives. *Diabetes* 1963;12:550-554.
74. Black RL, Oglesby RB, Von Sallmann L, Bunim JJ. Posterior subcapsular cataracts induced by corticosteroids in patients in rheumatoid arthritis. *JAMA* 1960;174:166-171.
75. Render JA, Carlton WW. Induced cataracts, lens, rat. In: Jones TC, Mohr U, Hunt RD, eds. *Eye and ear.* Heidelberg, Berlin: Springer-Verlag, 1991;63-70.
76. Newberne JW, Kuhn WL, Elsea JR. Toxicologic studies on clomiphene. *Toxicol Appl Ophthalmol* 1966;9:44-56.
77. Kirby TJ. Cataracts produced by triparanol. *Trans Am Ophthalmol Soc* 1967;65:493-543.
78. Mizuno G, Ellison E, et al. Lipids of the triparanol cataract in the rat. *Ophthalmic Res* 1974;6:206-215.
79. Pirie A, Rees JR, Holmberg NJ. Diquat cataract in the rat. *Biochem J* 1969;89:114.
80. Stancliffe TC, Pirie A. Production of superoxide radicals in reactions of the herbicide diquat. *Fed Eur Biochem Soc Lett* 1971;17:297-299.
81. Spector A, Garner WH. Hydrogen peroxide and human cataract. *Cesk Oftalmol* 1981;33:673-681.
82. Bhuyan KC, Bhuyan DK, Katzin HM. Amizol-induced cataract and inhibition of lens catalase in rabbit. *Ophthalmic Res* 1973;5:236-247.
83. Bhuyan KC, Bhuyan DK. Regulation of hydrogen peroxide in aqueous humors. *Biochem Biophys Acta* 1978;542:28-38.
84. Axelsson U. Cataracts following the use of long-acting cholinesterase inhibitors in glaucoma. *Proc Eur Soc Study Drug Toxic* 1971;12:199-203.
85. Kaufman PL, Axelsson U, Barany EH. Induction of subcapsular cataracts in cynomolgus monkeys by echothiophate. *Arch Ophthalmol* 1977;95;499-504.
86. Michon J Jr, Kinoshita JH. Experimental miotic cataract. I. *Arch Ophthalmol* 1968;79:79-86.
87. Michon J Jr, Kinoshita JH. Experimental miotic cataract. II. *Arch Ophthalmol* 1968;79:611-616.
88. Scullica L, Bisantis C, Pezzi PP. Effects of epinephrine on the mitotic activity of the lens epithelium. *Bol Oculist* 1968;47:561-567.

89. Fraunfelder FT, Burns RP. Effect of lid closure in drug-induced experimental cataracts. *Arch Ophthalmol* 1966;76:599-601.
90. Sanford SE, Dukes TW. Acquired bilateral cortical cataracts in mature sows. *J Am Vet Med Assoc* 1979;173:852-853.
91. Sanford SE, Dukes TW, Creighton MO, Trevithick JR. Cortical cataracts induced by hygromycin B in swine. *Am J Vet Res* 1981;42:1534-1537.
92. Creighton MO, Trevithick JR, Sanford SE, Dukes TW. Modelling cortical cataractogenesis. IV. Induction by hygromycin B in vivo (swine) and in vitro (rat lens). *Exp Eye Res* 1982;34:467-476.
93. Martin CL, Christmas R, Leipold HW. Formation of temporary cataracts in dogs given a disophenol preparation. *J Am Vet Med Assoc* 1972;161:294-300.
94. Martin CL, Chambreau T. Cataract production in experimentally orphaned puppies fed a commercial replacement for bitch's milk. *J Am Anim Hosp Assoc* 1982;18:115-119.
95. Rubin LF. *Atlas of veterinary ophthalmoscopy*. Philadelphia: Lea & Febiger, 1974.
96. Brown WR, Rubin L, Hite M, Zwickey RE. Experimental papilledema in the dog induced by a salicylanilide. *Toxicol Appl Pharmacol* 1971;21:532-541.
97. Schiavo DM, Field WE, Vymetol FJ. Cataracts in Beagle dogs given diazoxide. *Diabetes* 1975;24:1041.
98. Stacpoole PW, Moore GW, Kornhauser DM. Toxicity of chronic dichloracetate. *N Engl J Med* 1979;300-372.
99. Drenckhahn D, Lullmann-Rauch R. Lens opacities associated with lipidosis-like ultrastructural alterations in rats treated with chloroquine, chlorphentermine, or iprindole. *Exp Eye Res* 1977;24:621-632.
100. Lullmann-Rauch R. Retinal lipidosis in albino rats treated with chlorphentermine and with tricyclic antidepressants. *Acta Neuropathol* 1976;35:55-67.
101. Kern HL, Bellhorn RW, Peterson CM. Sodium cyanate induced ocular lesions in the beagle. *J Pharmacol Exp Ther* 1977;200:10-16.
102. Nicholson DH, Harkness DR, Benson WE, Peterson CM. Cyanate induced cataracts in patients with sickle cell hemoglobinopathies. *Arch Ophthalmol* 1976;94:927-930.
103. Fukui HN, Iwata S, Epstein DL, Merola LO. Cataractogenic effects of a boron hydride disulfide compound. *Invest Ophthalmol* 1977;16:654-657.
104. Bhuyan KC, Bhuyan DK, Podos SM. Cataract induced by selenium in the rat. I. Effect on the lenticular protein and thiols. *IRCS Med Sci* 1981;9:194-195.
105 Bhuyan KC, Bhuyan DK, Podos DM. Selenium-induced cataract; biochemical mechanisms. In: Spallholz JE, Martin JL, Ganther HE, eds. *Proceedings of the 2nd international symposium on selenium in biological medicine*. Westport: 1981;403-412.
106. Bunce GE, Hess JL. Biochemical changes associated with selenite-induced cataract in the rat. *Exp Eye Res* 1981;33:504-514.
107. Budinger JM. Diphenylthiocarbazone blindness in dogs. *Arch Ophthalmol* 1961;71:304-310.
108. Delahunt CS, Stebbins RB, Anderson J, Bailey J. The cause of blindness in dogs given hydroxypyridinethione. *Toxicol Appl Pharmacol* 1962;4:286-291.
109. Bruckner R, Hess R, Keberle H, Pericin C, Tripod J. Tierexperimentelle pathologische Linsenveranderungen nach langdauernder verabreichung hoher dosen von desferal hely. *Acta Physiol Pharmacol* 1967;25:62-77.
110. Millichamp NJ, Dziezyc, JD. Control of the ocular irritative response in the dog: a comparison of flunixin meglumine and flurbiprofen. *Am J Vet Res* 1991;52:1452-1455.
111. Mandelkorn RM, Zimmerman TJ. Effects of nonsteroidal drugs on glaucoma. In: Ritch R, Shields BM, Krupin T, eds. *The glaucomas*. St. Louis: C.V. Mosby, 1989;1169-1184.
112. Armaly MF. Inheritance of dexamethasone hypertension and glaucoma. *Arch Ophthalmol* 1967;77:747.
113. Bill A. The drainage of aqueous humor. *Invest Ophthalmol Vis Sci* 1975;14:1.
114. Weinreb RN, Mitchell MD, Polansky JR. Prostaglandin production by human trabecular cells: in vitro inhibition by dexamethasone. *Invest Ophthalmol Vis Sci* 1983;24:1541-1545.
115. Zhan GL, Miranda OC, Bito LZ. Steroid-induced ocular hypertension in cats. *Invest Ophthalmol Vis Sci* 1989;30:445.
116. Steele CM, O'Duffy J, Brown SS. Clinical effects and treatment of imipramine and amitriptyline poisoning in children. *Br Med J* 1967;3:663.
117. Trzeciakowski JP. Review: central control of intraocular pressure. *J Ocul Pharmacol* 1987;3:367-377.

118. Binkhorst CG. Inflammation and intraocular pressure after the use of Healon in intraocular lens surgery. *Am Intra-Ocul Implant Soc J* 1980;6:340.
119. Hewitt AT, Adler R. Retinal pigment epithelium and interphotoreceptor matrix: structure and specialized functions. In: Ryan SJ, Ogden TE, eds. *Retina*, vol 1. St. Louis: C.V. Mosby, 1989;57-64.
120. Dowling JE. *The retina: an approachable part of the brain.* Cambridge, MA and London, England: The Belknap Press of Harvard University Press, 1987.
121. Blanks JC. Morphology of the retina. In: Ryan SJ, Ogden TE, eds. *Retina*, vol 1. St. Louis: C.V. Mosby, 1989;37-52.
122. Vogul A, Kaiser J. Ethambutol induced transient change and reconstitution (in vivo) of the tapetum lucidum color in the dog. *Exp Mol Pathol* 1963;2(suppl):136-149.
123. Weitzel G, Strecker FJ. Zinc in the tapetum lucidum. *Z Physiol Chem Hoppe-Seyler's* 1954;296:19-30.
124. Moe RA, Kirpan J, Linegar CR. Toxicology of hydroxypyridinethione. *Toxicol Appl Pharamacol* 1960;2:156-170.
125. Snyder FH, Buehler EF, Winek CL. Safety evaluation of zinc 2-pyridinethiol 1-oxide in a shampoo formulation. *Toxicol Appl Pharmacol* 1965;7:425-437.
126. Cloyd GG, Wyman M. Ocular toxicity studies with zinc pyridinethione. *Toxicol Appl Pharmacol* 1978;45:771-782.
127. Jampol LM. Macular edema. In: Ryan SJ, Schachat AP, Murphy RP, et al., eds. *Retina*, vol 2. St. Louis: C.V. Mosby, 1989;81-88.
128. Pirie A. Pathology in the eye of the naphthalene-fed rabbit. *Exp Eye Res* 1968;7:354-357.
129. Adams DR. The nature of the ocular lesions produced experimentally by naphthalene. *Br J Ophthalmol* 1930;14:49-60.
130. Apponi G, Tieri O, Rinaldi E. The retinotoxic action of Trenimon. *Acta Ophthalmol* 1964;42:64-67.
131. Butturini U, Grignolo A, Baronchelli A. "Diabetes" from dithizone: metabolic, ocular and histologic aspects. *G Clin Med* 1953;34:1253-1347.
132. Babel J, Ziv B. The action of dithizone on the retina of the rabbit. *Experientia* 1957;13:122-123.
133. Sorsby A, Harding R. Experimental degeneration of the retina. *Br J Ophthalmol* 1960;44:213-224.
134. Sorsby A, Harding R. Oxidizing agents as potentiators of the retinotoxic action of sodium fluoride, sodium iodate and sodium iodoacetate. *Nature* 1966;210:997-998.
135. Cohen AI. An electron microscopic study of the modification by monosodium glutamate of the retinas of normal and "rodless" mice. *Am J Anat* 1967;120:319.
136. Olney JW. Glutamate-induced retinal degeneration in neonatal mice. *J Neuropathol Exp Neurol* 1969;28:455-474.
137. Basson PA, Kellerman TS. Blindness and encephalopathy caused by *Helichrysum argyrosphaerum DC. (Compositae)* in sheep and cattle. *Onderstepoort J Vet Res* 1975;42:135-147.
138. Paterson RA. The effect of hydroxyethyl-substituted rutosides on the B,B-iminodipropionitrile-induced retinopathy in the rat. *Br J Exp Pathol* 1968;49:283-287.
139. Selye H. Prevention by thyroxine of the ocular changes normally produced by B,B-iminodipropionitrile (IDNP). *Am J Ophthalmol* 1957;44:763-765.
140. Wang MK, Heath H. Effect of B,B-iminodipropionitrile and related compounds on the electroretinogram and the retinal vascular system of the rat. *Exp Eye Res* 1968;7:56-61.
141. Potts AM, Praglin J, Farkas I. Studies on the visual toxicity of methanol. *Am J Ophthalmol* 1955;40:76-83.
142. Gilger AP, Potts AM, Farkas IS. Studies on the visual toxicity of methanol. *Am J Ophthalmol* 1956;42:244-251.
143. Gilger AP, Farkas IS, Potts AM. Studies on visual toxicity of methanol. *Am J Ophthalmol* 1959;48:153-160.
144. Walsh FB, Hoyt WF. *Clinical neuro-ophthalmology*, 3rd ed. Baltimore: Williams & Wilkins, 1969.
145. Gardiner PA, Michaelson IC. Intravitreous streptomycin: its toxicity and diffusion. *Br J Ophthalmol* 1948;32:449-456.
146. Brinton GS, Norton EWD, et al. Ocular quinine toxicity. *Am J Ophthalmol* 1980;90:403-410.
147. Thomas JV, Gragoudas ES, Blair NP, Lapus JV. Correlation of epinephrine use and macular edema in aphakic glaucomatous eyes. *Arch Ophthalmol* 1978;96:625-628.
148. Gass JDM. Nicotinic acid maculopathy. *Am J Ophthalmol* 1973;76:500-510.
149. Kaiser-Kupfer MI, Lippman ME. Tamoxifen retinopathy. *Cancer Treat Rev* 1978;62:315-320.
150. Marmor MF. Mechanisms of normal retinal adhesion. In: Ryan SJ, ed. *Retina*, vol 3. St. Louis: C.V. Mosby, 1989;71-87.

151. Barclay SM, Riis RC. Retinal detachment and reattachment associated with ethylene glycol intoxication in a cat. *J Am Anim Hosp Assoc* 1979;15:719-724.
152. Beasley H, Fraunfelder FT. Retinal detachments and topical ocular miotics. *Am Acad Ophthalmol* 1979;86:95-98.
153. Garner A, Ashton N, Tripathi R, Kohner EM, Bulpitt CJ, Dollery CT. Pathogenesis of hypertensive retinopathy: an experimental study in the monkey. *Br J Ophthalmol* 1975;59:3-44.
154. Foos RY. Chronic retinopathy of prematurity. *Ophthalmology* 1985;92:563-574.
155. Beeler CC, Newton NL, et al. Retinal detachment in adult dogs resulting from oxygen toxicity. *Arch Ophthalmol* 1964;71:665-670.
156. Guttman-Friedmann A. Blindness after snakebite. *Br J Ophthalmol* 1956;40:57-59.
157. McLane J. Retinal hemorrhage in case of rattlesnake bite. *J Fla Med Assoc* 1943;30:22-25.
158. Mebs D. Pharmacology of reptilian venoms. In: Gans C, ed. *Biology of the reptilia, Vol 8: Physiology B*. London, New York: Academic Press, 1978;437-530.
159. Hotta R, Goto S. A fluorescein angiographic study on microangiopathia sulfocarbonica. *Acta Soc Ophthalmol Jpn* 1970;74:1463-1467.
160. Kittell V, Cornelius C. Optic nerve injury by chloramphenicol. *Klin Monatsbl Augenheilkd* 1969;155:83-87.
161. Maurolf FA, Mesher JH. Experimental hyperviscosity retinopathy. *Ann Ophthalmol* 1973;5:205-209.
162. Kolker AE, Becker B. Epinephrine maculopathy. *Arch Ophthalmol* 1968;79:552-562.
163. Lobeck E. On knowledge of retinal changes in chronic lead poisoning. *Graefes Arch Ophthalmol* 1936;135;165-168.
164. Mindel JS, Rubenstein AE, Franklin B. Ocular ergotamine tartrate toxicity during treatment of Vacor-induced orthostatic hypotension. *Am J Ophthalmol* 1981;92:492-496.
165. Anderson B Jr. Ocular effects of changes in oxygen and carbon dioxide tension. *Trans Am Ophthalmol Soc* 1968;66:423-474.
166. Swartz M. Other diseases: drug toxicity and metabolic and nutritional conditions. In: Ryan SJ, Schachat AP, Murphy RP, et al., eds. *Retina*, vol 2. St. Louis: C.V. Mosby, 1989;737-748.
167. Gilmer G, Swartz M, Teske M, Crandall AS. Over-the-counter phenylpropanolamine: a possible cause of central retinal vein occlusion. *Arch Ophthalmol* 1986;104:642.
168. Zinn KM, Marmor MF. Toxicology of the human retinal pigment epithelium. In: Zinn KM, Marmor MF, eds. *The retinal pigment epithelium*. Cambridge, MA: Harvard University Press, 1979;395-412.
169. Noell WK. The effect of iodoacetate on the vertebrate retina. *J Cell Comp Physiol* 1951;37:283-307.
170. Noell WK. Experimentally induced toxic effects on structure and function of visual cells and pigment epithelium. *Am J Ophthalmol* 1953;36:103-116.
171. Nilsson SEG, Knave B, Persson HE. Changes in ultrastructure and function of the sheep pigment epithelium and retina induced by sodium iodate. II. Early effects. *Acta Ophthalmol* 1977;55:1007-1026.
172. Noell WK. Azide sensitive potential difference across the eye bulb. *Am J Physiol* 1952;170:217.
173. Graymore CN. *Biochemistry of the eye*. London, New York: Academic Press, 1970.
174. Ashton N. Degeneration of the retina due to 1,5-bis(p-aminophenoxy) pentane dihydrochloride. *J Pathol Bacteriol* 1957;74:103-112.
175. Sorsby A, Nakajima A. Experimental degeneration of the retina. IV. Diaminodiphenoxy alkanes as inducing agents. *Br J Ophthalmol* 1958;42:563-570.
176. Edge ND, Mason DFJ, Wien R, Ashton N. The pharmacological effects of certain diaminodiphenoxy alkanes. *Nature* 1956;178:806-807.
177. Orzalesi N, Grignolo A, Calabria GA, Castellazzo RA. A study on fine structure and the rhodopsin cycle of the rabbit retina in experimental degeneration induced by diaminodiphenoxypentane. *Exp Eye Res* 1967;6(4):376-382.
178. Bellhorn RW, Bellhorn MS, Friedman AJ, Henkind P. Urethane-induced retinopathy in pigmented rats. *Invest Ophthalmol Vis Sci* 1973;12:65-76.
179. Amemiya T. Electron microscopic study of the retina of rats repeatedly treated with urethane. *Ophthalmol Jap* 1968;72:293-298.
180. Bullock JD, Albert DM, Skinner CW, Miller WH, Galla JH. Calcium oxalate retinopathy associated with generalized oxalosis. X-ray diffraction and electron microscopic studies of crystal deposits. *Invest Ophthalmol* 1974;13:256-265.
181. Barber AN, Catsulis C, Cangelosi RJ. Studies on experimental retinitis light and electron microscopy. *Br J Ophthalmol* 1971;55:91-105.

182. Brown DVL. Reaction of the rabbit retinal pigment epithelium to systemic lead poisoning. *Trans Am Ophthalmol Soc* 1975;72:404–447.
183. Herrold KM. Pigmentary degeneration of the retina induced by *N*-methyl-*N*-nitrosourea. *Arch Ophthalmol* 1967;78:650–653.
184. Abraham R, Hendy RJ. Irreversible lysosomal damage induced by chloroquine in the retinae of pigmented and albino rats. *Exp Mol Pathol* 1970;12:185–200.
185. Ramsey MS, Fine BS. Chloroquine toxicity in the human eye. *Am J Ophthalmol* 1972;73:229–235.
186. Rosenthal AR, Kolb H, Bergsma D, Huxsoll D, Hopkins JL. Chloroquine retinopathy in the rhesus monkey. *Invest Ophthalmol Vis Sci* 1978;17:1158–1175.
187. Bernstein H, Zvaifler N, et al. The ocular deposition of chloroquine. *Invest Ophthalmol* 1963;2:384–391.
188. Berstein HN, Ginsberg J. The pathology of chloroquine retinopathy. *Arch Ophthalmol* 1964;71:238–245.
189. Kurtz SM, Kaump DH, Schardein JL, Roll DE, Reutner TF, Fisken RA. The effect of long-term administration of amopyroquin, a 4-aminoquinoline compound, on the retina of pigmented and nonpigmented laboratory animals. *Invest Ophthalmol* 1967;6:420.
190. Hommer K. The effects of quinine, chloroquine, iodoacetate and chlorodiazepoxide on the ERG of the isolated rabbit retina. *Graefes Arch Ophthalmol* 1968;175:111–120.
191. Cibis GW, Burian HM, Blodi FC. Electroretinogram changes in acute quinine poisoning. *Arch Ophthalmol* 1973;90:307–309.
192. Ullberg S, Linquist NG, Sjostrand SE. Accumulation of chorioretinotoxic drugs in the foetal eye. *Nature* 1970;227:1257–1258.
193. Davidorf FH. Thioridazine pigmentary retinopathy. *Arch Ophthalmol* 1973;90:251–255.
194. Goar EF, Fletcher MC. Toxic chorioretinopathy following the use of NP 207. *Am J Ophthalmol* 1956;44:603–608.
195. Burian HM, Fletcher MC. Visual functions in patients with retinal pigmentary degeneration following the use of NP 207. *Arch Ophthalmol* 1958;60:612–629.
196. Cerletti A, Meier-Ruge W. Toxicological studies on phenothiazine induced retinopathy. *Proc Eur Soc Study Drug Toxic* 1968;9:170–188.
197. McFarlane JR, Yanoff M, Sheie HG. Toxic retinopathy following sparsomycin therapy. *Arch Ophthalmol* 1966;76:532–540.
198. Vlchek JK, Peyman GA. Cephaloridine-induced retinopathy by intravitreal infection: an ultrastructural study. *Ann Ophthalmol* 1975;7:903–914.
199. Drenckhahn D, Lullmann-Rauch R. Drug-induced retinal lipidosis: differential susceptibilities of pigment epithelium and neuroretina toward several amphiphilic cation drugs. *Exp Mol Pathol* 1978;28:360–371.
200. Imai H, Miyamata M, Uga S, Ishikawa S. Retinal degeneration in rats exposed to an organophosphate pesticide (Fenthion). *Environ Res* 1983;30:453.
201. Verrey F. Pigmentary degeneration of the retina of drug origin. *Ophthalmologica* 1956;131:296–303.
202. Bornschein H, Hoyer J, et al. Animal experimental study with a substance harmful to the visual system (NP 207). *Graefes Arch Clin Exp Ophthalmol* 1974;190:13–25.
203. Meier-Ruge W, Cerletti A. On the experimental pathology of phenothiazine retinopathy. *Ophthalmologica* 1966;151:512–533.
204. Meier-Ruge W, Kalberer F, Cerletti A. Microhistoautoradiographic investigations of the distribution of tritium-labeled phenothiazine derivatives in the eye. *Experientia* 1966;22:153–155.
205. Barnett KC, Watson WA. Bright blindness in sheep. *Res Vet Sci* 1970;11:289.
206. Barnett KC, Blakemore WF, Mason J. Bracken retinopathy in sheep. *Trans Ophthalmol Soc U K* 1972;92:741–744.
207. Huxtable CR, Dorling PR, Slatter DH. Myelin oedema, optic neuropathy and retinopathy in experimental *Stypandra imbricata* toxicosis. *Neuropathol Appl Neurobiol* 1980;6:221–232.
208. Main DC, Slatter DH, Huxtable CR. *Stypandra imbricata* ("blind grass") toxicoses in goats and sheep—clinical and pathologic findings in 4 field cases. *Aust Vet J* 1981;57(3):132–135.
209. von Canstatt BS, Hofmann HT, et al. Disturbances of the cat retina by poisoning with perorally or percutaneously administered chemicals. *Verh Dtsch Ges Pathol* 1966:50:429–435.
210. Amemiya T. Cytochemical and electron microscopic examination of the retina of rats with hypervitaminosis A. *Acta Soc Ophthalmol Jpn* 1967;71:2236–2251.
211. Vanysek J, Anton M, et al. Some metabolic disturbances of the retina due to the effect of natrium fluoride. *Ophthalmologica Addit Ad* 1969;158:684–690.

212. Rose AL, Wen GY, Cammer W. Hexachlorophene retinopathy in suckling rats. *J Neurol Sci* 1981;52:163-178.
213. Grignolo A. Rhodopsin cycle and fine structure of rabbit retina in experimental degeneration induced by retinotoxic agents. *Exp Eye Res* 1969;8:254.
214. Reading HW, Sorsby A. Retinal toxicity and tissue-SH levels. *Biochem Pharmacol* 1966;15:1389-1393.
215. Lucas DR, Newhouse JP, Davery JB. Experimental degeneration of the retina. *Br J Ophthalmol* 1957;41:313-316.
216. Hansson HA. Selective effects of metabolic inhibitors on retinal cultures. *Exp Eye Res* 1966;5:335-354.
217. Cohen AM, Michaelson IC, Yanko L. Retinopathy in rats with disturbed carbohydrate metabolism following a high sucrose diet. *Am J Ophthalmol* 1972;73:863-875.
218. Bellhorn RW, Bellhorn W, Friedman AH. Urethane-induced retinopathy in pigmented rats. *Invest Ophthalmol* 1973;12:65-76.
219. Ulshafer RJ, Garcia CA, Hollyfield JG. Elevated levels of cGMP destroy rod photoreceptors in the human retina. *Invest Ophthalmol Vis Sci* 1980;38.
220. Aguirre GD, Farber DB, Lolley RN, et al. Retinal degenerations in the dog. III. Abnormal cyclic nucleotide metabolism in rod-cone dysplasia. *Exp Eye Res* 1982;35:625-642.
221. Fliesler SJ, Rapp LM, Hollyfield JG. Photoreceptor-specific degeneration caused by tunicamycin. *Nature* 1984;311:575-577.
222. Hansson HA. Retinal changes induced by treatment with vincristine and vinblastine. *Doc Ophthalmol* 1972;31:65-88.
223. Ripps H, Carr RE, et al. Functional abnormalities in vincristine-induced night blindness. *Invest Ophthalmol Vis Sci* 1984;25:787-794.
224. Parhad IM, Giffin JW, Clark AW, Koves JF. Doxorubicin intoxication: neuro-filamentous axonal changes with subacute neuronal death. *J Neuropathol Exp Neurol* 1984;43:188-200.
225. Witzel DA, Smith EL, et al. Arsanilic acid-induced blindness in swine. *Am J Vet Res* 1976;37:521-524.
226. Barishak YR, Beemer AM, et al. Histology of the retina and choroid in ducklings photosensitized by feeding *Ammi majus seeds. Ophthalmic Res* 1976;8:169-178.
227. Rosen ES, Edgar JT, Smith JLS. Male fern retro-bulbar neuropathy in cattle. *J Small Anim Pract* 1970;10:619-625.
228. Cogan DG, Truman JT, Smith TR. Optic neuropathy, chloramphenicol and infantile genetic agranulocytosis. *Invest Ophthalmol* 1973;12:534-537.
229. Ide T. Histopathological studies on retina, optic nerve and arachnoidal membrane of mouse exposed to carbon disulfide poisoning. *Acta Soc Ophthalmol Jpn* 1958;62A:85-108.
230. Pederson OO, Karlsen RL. The toxic effect of *L*-cysteine on the rat retina. *Invest Ophthalmol Vis Sci* 1980;19:886-892.
231. Karlsen RL, Pederson OO. A morphological study of the acute toxicity of *L*-cysteine on the retina of young rats. *Exp Eye Res* 1982;34:65-69.
232. Sisk DR, Kuwabara T. Histological changes in the inner retina of albino rats following intravitreal injection of monosodium *L*-glutamate. *Graefes Arch Clin Exp Ophthalmol* 1985;223:250-258.
233. Bouldin TW, Goines ND, Krigman NR. Trimethyltin retinopathy. Relationship of subcellular response to neuronal subspecialization. *J Neuropathol Exp Neurol* 1984;43:162-174.
234. Van Kampen KR, James LF. Sequential development of the lesions in locoweed poisoning. *Clin Toxicol* 1972;5:575-580.
235. Dorling PR, Huxtable CR, Vogel P. Lysosomal storage in *Swainsona* spp. toxicosis, an induced mannosidosis. *Neuropathol Appl Neurobiol* 1978;4:285-295.
236. Thompson SW, Chloroquine toxicity in the rat. *Vet Pathol* 1975;12:71.
237. Lecoll S, Croft JL, Albert DM. Kainic acid induces mitoses in mature retinal neurones in rats. *Exp Eye Res* 1980;30:731-738.
238. Lullmann H, Lullmann-Rauch R, Wassermann O. Lipidosis induced by amphiphilic cationic drugs. *Biochem Pharmacol* 1978;27:1103-1108.
239. Lullmann-Rauch R. Lipidosis of the retina due to cationic amphiphilic drugs, rat. In: Jones TC, Mohr U, Hunt RD, eds. *Eye and ear*. Berlin: Springer Verlag, 1991;87-92.
240. Manschot WA. Ophthalmic pathological findings in a case of thallium poisoning. *Ophthalmologica Addit Ad* 1969;158:348-349.

241. Committee on drugs: blindness and neuropathy from diiodohydroxyquin-like drugs. *Pediatrics* 1974;54:378-379.
242. Tateishi J, Kuroda S, et al. Experimental myelo-optic neuropathy induced by clioquinol. *Acta Neuropathol* 1973;24:304-320.
243. Worden AN, Heywood R, et al. Clioquinol toxicity in the dog. *Toxicology* 1978;9:227-238.
244. Krinke G, Schaumburg HH, et al. Clioquinol and 2,5-hexanedione induce different types of distal axonopathy in the dog. *Acta Neuropathol* 1979;47:213-221.
245. Lessell S. Experimental cyanide optic neuropathy. *Arch Ophthalmol* 1971;86:194-204.
246. Lessell S, Kuwabara T. Fine structure of experimental cyanide optic neuropathy. *Invest Ophthalmol Vis Sci* 1974;13:748-756.
247. Levy J, Michel-Ber E. Difficulties and complications caused in man by monoamine oxidase (MAO) inhibitors, with special reference to their specific and secondary pharmacological effects. *Proc Eur Soc Study Drug Toxic* 1968;9:189-245.
248. Schmidt IG, Schmidt LH. Studies of the neurotoxicity of ethambutol and its racemate for the rhesus monkey. *J Neuropathol Exp Neurol* 1966;25:40-67.
249. Lessell S. Histopathology of experimental ethambutol intoxication. *Invest Ophthalmol Vis Sci* 1976;15:765-769.
250. Matsuoka Y, Mukoyama M, Sobue I. Histopathological study of experimental ethambutol neuropathy. *Clin Neurol* 1972;12:453-459.
251. Beasley VR, Buck WB. Acute ethylene glycol toxicosis: a review. *Vet Hum Toxicol* 1980;22:255-263.
252. Berger JR, Ayyar DR. Neurological complications of ethylene glycol intoxication. *Arch Neurol* 1981;38:724-726.
253. Freedman JK, Potts AM. Repression of glutaminase I in the rat retina by administration of sodium-L-glutamate. *Invest Ophthalmol* 1963;2:252-258.
254. Hansson HA. Ultrastructural studies on the long term effects of sodium glutamate on the rat retina. *Virchows Arch (B)* 1970;6:1-11.
255. Sharpe JA, Hostovsky M, et al. Methanol optic neuropathy: a histopathological study. *Neurology* 1982;32:1093-1100.
256. Benton CD Jr, Calhoun FP Jr. The ocular effects of methyl alcohol poisoning: report of a catastrophe involving 320 persons. *Am J Ophthalmol* 1953;36:1677-1685.
257. Brown WR, Rubin L, Hite M, Zwickey RE. Experimental papilledema induced by a salicylanilide. *Toxicol Appl Pharmacol* 1971;27:532-541.
258. Schmidt IG, Schmidt LH. Neurotoxicity of the 8-aminoquinolines. *J Neuropathol Exp Neurol* 1948;7:368-398.
259. Cavanagh JB, Fuller NH, et al. The effects of the thallium salts, with particular reference to the nervous system changes. *Q J Med* 1974;43:293-319.
260. Buxton PH, Hayward M. Polyneuritis cranialis associated with industrial trichloroethylene poisoning. *J Neurol Neurosurg Psychiatry* 1967;30:511-518.
261. Feldman RG, Mayer RM, Taub A. Evidence for peripheral neurotoxic effect of trichloroethylene. *Neurology* 1970;20:599-606.
262. Albert DM, Wong V, Henderson ES. Ocular complications of vincristine therapy. *Arch Ophthalmol* 1967;78:709-713.
263. Slansky HH, Kolbert G, Gartner S. Exophthalmos induced by corticosteroids. *Arch Ophthalmol* 1967;77:579-581.
264. Hiroz CA, Assimacopoulos T, et al. Ophthalmologic side effects of lithium. *Encephale* 1981;7:123-128.
265. Segal RL, Rosenblatt S, Eliasoph I. Endocrine exophthalmos during lithium therapy of manic-depressive disease. *N Engl J Med* 1973;289:136-138.
266. Marine D, Rosen SH, Cipra A. Further studies on the exophthalmos in rabbits, produced by methyl cyanide. *Proc Soc Exp Biol Med* 1933;30:649-651.
267. Maddock CL, Wolbach SB, Maddock S. Hypervitaminosis A in the dog. *J Nutr* 1949;39:117.
268. Robens JF. Teratogenic effects of hypervitaminosis A in the hamster and in the guinea pig. *Toxicol Appl Pharmacol* 1970;16:88-99.
269. Cummings JR, Welter AN. Cardiovascular studies on aminocaproic acid. *Toxicol Appl Pharmacol* 1966;9:57-69.
270. Miller TR, Gelatt KN. Food animal ophthalmology. In: Gelatt KN, ed. *Veterinary ophthalmology*, 2nd ed. Philadelphia: Lea & Febiger, 1991;611-655.

271. Babbott FL, Binns W, Ingalls TH. Field studies of cyclopian malformations in sheep. *Arch Environ Health* 1962;5:109-113.
272. Mulvihill JJ. Congenital and genetic disease in domestic animals. *Science* 1972;176:132-137.
273. Binns W, et al. A congenital cyclopian-type malformation in lambs induced by material ingestation of a range plant, *Veratrum californicum*. *Am J Vet Res* 1963;24:1164.
274. Keeler RF, Binns W. Teratogenic compounds of V. californicum. *Can Vet J* 1966;44:819.
275. Binns W, et al. Chronologic evaluation of teratogenicity in sheep fed *Veratrum californicum*. *J Am Vet Med Assoc* 1965;147:839.
276. Younger RL. Probable induction of congenital anomalies in a lamb by apholate. *Am J Vet Res* 1965;26:991.
277. Scott FW. Teratogenesis in cats associated with griseofulvin therapy. *Teratology* 1975;11:79.
278. Shaul WL, Hall JG. Multiple congenital anomalies associated with oral anticoagulants. *Am J Obstet Gynecol* 1977;127:191-198.
279. Calvert A, Gabriel Robez O. Eye defects induced by chlorambucil in the mouse. *C R Soc Biol* 1974;168:1115-1118.
280. Rugh R, Skaredoff L. Radiation and radiomimetic chlorambucil and the fetal retina. *Arch Ophthalmol* 1965;74:382-393.
281. Ferm VH. Congenital malformations in hamster embryos after treatment with vinblastine and vincristine. *Science* 1963;141:126.
282. Calvert A, Gabriel RO. Eye defects induced by chlorambucil in the mouse. *C R Soc Biol* 1974;168:1115-1118.
283. Singh S, et al. Eye anomalies induced by cyclophosphamide in rat fetuses. *Acta Anat* 1976;94:490-496.
284. Stuhltrager U. Cyclophosphamide-induced developmental disturbances of the nasolacrimal ducts in the mouse. *Folio Ophthalmol* 1982;7:207-211.
285. Goldman AS, Yakovac WC. Salicylate intoxication and congenital anomalies. *Arch Environ Health* 1964;8:648-656.
286. Tuchmann-Duplessis H, Mercier-Parot L. Dissociation of antitumor and teratogenic properties of a purine antimetabolite, azathioprine. *C R Soc Biol* 1965;159:2290-2294.
287. Johnson AR. A re-examination of the possible teratogenic effects of butylated gydroxytoluene (BHT). *Food Cosmet Toxicol* 1965;3:371-375.
288. Gray LEJ, Kavlock RJ, et al. Prenatal exposure to the herbicide 2,4-dichlorophenyl-p-nitrophenyl ether destroys the rodent Harderian gland. *Science* 1982;215:293-294.
289. Itoi M, Gefter JW, et al. Teratogenicities of ophthalmic drugs. *Arch Ophthalmol* 1975;93:46-51.
290. Pitel M, Lerman L. Further studies on the effects of intrauterine vasoconstrictors on the fetal rat lens. *Am J Ophthalmol* 1964;58:464-470.
291. Ballard PD, Hearney EF, et al. Comparative teratogenicity of selected glucocorticoids applied ocularly in mice. *Teratology* 1977;16:175-180.
292. Benke PJ. The isotretinoin teratogen syndrome. *JAMA* 1984;251:3267-3269.
293. Hill RM. Isotretinoin teratogenicity. *Lancet* 1984;1:1465.
294. Beck F, Lloyd JB. The preparation and teratogenic properties of pure trypan blue and its common contaminants. *J Embryol Exp Morph* 1963;11:175-184.
295. Hanaway JK. Lysergic acid diethylamide: effects on the developing mouse lens. *Science* 1969;164:574-575.
296. Apple DJ, Bennett TO. Multiple systemic and ocular malformations associated with maternal LSD usage. *Arch Ophthalmol* 1974;92:301-303.
297. Chan CC, Fishman M, Egbert PR. Multiple ocular anomalies associated with maternal LSD ingestion. *Arch Ophthalmol* 1978;96:282-284.
298. Alfieri G, Alfieri-Rolla G. Ocular alterations in the newborn rabbit after treatment of the mother during gestation with *N*-methyl-*N*-nitro-*N*-nitrosoguanidine. *Arch Rass Ital Ottal* 1973;3:247-256.
299. Miller M, Israel J, Cuttone J. Fetal alcohol syndrome. *J Pediatr Ophthalmol Strabismus* 1981;18:6-15.
300. Cook CS, Nowotny AZ, Sulik KK. Fetal alcohol syndrome: eye malformation in a mouse model. *Arch Ophthalmol* 1987;105:1576-1581.
301. McKinna AJ. Quinine induced hypoplasia of the optic nerve. *Can J Ophthalmol* 1966;1:261-266.
302. Laszczyk WA, et al. Changes in the visual system of rabbit fetuses after thalidomide administration. *Ophthalmic Res* 1976;8:146-151.
303. Cullen JF. Teratogenic agents and thalidomide. *Trans Ophthalmol Soc UK* 1966;86:101-113.
304. Cullen JF. Clinical anophthalmos in a thalidomide child. *J Pediatr Ophthalmol* 1966;3:10-14.

Ophthalmic Toxicology, edited by
George C. Y. Chiou. Raven Press, Ltd.,
New York © 1992.

3

Species Specificity

Factors Affecting the Interpretation of Species Differences in Toxic Responses of Ocular Tissues

Nicholas J. Millichamp

Department of Small Animal Medicine and Surgery, College of Veterinary Medicine, Texas A & M University, College Station, Texas 77843

The manner in which the eye responds to chemicals, radiation, and other toxic insults is influenced by many factors, some of which are described elsewhere in this book. Variations in morphology, physiology, biochemistry, and pharmacology of the eye in different species of animal may have a significant effect on the reaction of the eye to injury or toxins. Even within a particular species, differences in age and degree of ocular pigmentation may affect the eye's response to, and recovery or repair from, noxious substances. The area of the eye in which most differences are seen and about which most is known is the anterior uvea and the response of the iris sphincter muscle and blood-aqueous barrier to toxic substances. For this reason the anterior uvea will receive most attention.

Both humans and animals are affected by a number of inherited ocular diseases. Since many of these may mimic the response of the eye to toxic substances it is important that the toxicologist be aware of which inherited eye diseases occur in the species being used in any study. It is important that both human and veterinary ophthalmologists are able to differentiate between toxic reactions in the eye and inherited diseases, since this will profoundly influence the course any planned therapy will take.

Additionally most of the species used in ocular toxicity testing are prone to various infectious ocular diseases. Although these are beyond the scope of this chapter details may be found in veterinary ophthalmologic texts (1,2). Certain species have been used to develop models of infectious and metabolic ocular diseases (3).

This chapter examines some of the considerations that affect species specificity in ocular toxic reactions. Most of the reported toxic reactions of the eyes in animals have been the result of experimental studies, whereas in man the preponderance of toxic reactions are noted as accidental occurrences or the side effects of drugs in use for other purposes. It is usually difficult to make meaningful direct comparisons between species in the reaction to a particular toxin due to differences in experimental protocols, routes of administration, dose of drug, and duration of the study. Rarely is information available about the pharmacokinetics of absorption, distribution, biotransformation, and excretion of drugs in the eye of even one test species, let alone controlled comparative studies in several species. Thus, in many instances we are unable to say that a particular species significantly differs in the type of ocular response to a toxin when compared to another species. There are few examples of well-controlled studies between particular species or strains to demonstrate differences in toxic effects. The varying susceptibilities of different strains of mice to light-induced retinal damage is one example (4).

The species of animal that are most commonly used in toxicological and pharmacological studies and thus are most frequently compared to man are the rabbit, rat, cat, dog, and monkey. Little is known of toxic reactions in the eye of other domestic species.

A detailed review of comparative ocular anatomy, histology, physiology, biochemistry, and pharmacology is beyond the scope of this chapter. The reader is referred to appropriate publications in the reference list that cover these aspects in some depth (2,5-10). Aspects of comparative anatomy and physiology relevant to toxicological studies has recently been reviewed (11). Other aspects of spontaneous or experimental ocular disease in laboratory animals have been reviewed elsewhere (12,13).

EYELIDS

The eyelids can be divided into two layers—an outer layer of skin and muscle and an inner layer of fibrous connective tissue lined by the palpebral conjunctiva. The skin is variably pigmented and has hair follicles and associated sebaceous and sweat glands. The fibrous layer of the upper eyelid is especially well developed into a tarsal plate in primates; however, this is poorly developed in other laboratory and domestic species. The perimarginal tarsal plate in all species contains modified sebaceous tarsal or meibomian glands that contribute lipid to the tear film. Several muscles are present in the lids. The orbicularis muscle encircles the margin and closes the lids. The upper lid is elevated primarily by the levator palpebrae superioris muscle with a contribution from the deeper, sympathetically innervated Müller's muscle.

Cilia arising at the lid margins are present in most species but are absent in the cat and only found on the upper eyelid of the dog and horse.

The shape of the palpebral fissure varies among species, being almond shaped in carnivores and man, and more circular in rodents, rabbits, and some subhuman primates. The lids are pigmented in most species, although not in albinos, which may affect the response of the eyelids to toxins.

There are relatively few specific conditions affecting the eyelid that may mimic toxic effects in different species. Drooping of the upper eyelid (ptosis) is reported in man in response to several systemic drugs and toxins (14,15), and may develop with advancing age in man and occasionally in dogs. In dogs the ptotic upper eyelid cilia may contact and irritate the cornea (trichiasis). Ptosis of the upper eyelid may be seen in man, cat, and dog as part of Horner's syndrome due to denervation of the sympathetic innervation to the upper eyelid. Sagging of the lower eyelid (ectropion), which may become more marked with age, may be seen in certain canine breeds.

The presence of the third eyelid in laboratory species has been considered a factor that would affect the ocular response to drugs compared to primates by trapping test substances in the conjunctival fornix. Studies in monkeys and rabbits in which the nictitans was removed from the latter do not suggest this to be a significant factor in the differential response to irritants (16), although entrapment may be more of a factor when using viscous formulations of drugs (17).

LACRIMAL SYSTEM

The precorneal tear film is secreted by a variety of glands in the eyelids and orbital region in all laboratory and domestic species and man. The lipid portion of tears is secreted by meibomian glands in the fibrous tarsal region of the upper and lower lid, the mucous portion by goblet cells in the conjunctiva. These components of the tear film appear to differ little between species. The major portion of the tear film is made up of an aqueous component that maintains wetting and lubrication of the lids, cornea, and conjunctiva, provides nutrition to and removes waste products from the corneal epithelium and anterior corneal stroma, and provides specific and nonspecific defense mechanisms against infectious disease. This serous portion of the tear film is secreted by the lacrimal gland in most species and by various auxiliary glands in several species. In man and other primates only a lacrimal gland is present; in dogs and cats a lacrimal and nictitating membrane occurs. In mice a harderian gland is found in addition to the lacrimal gland; in rats there are three lacrimal glands, the intra- and extraorbital glands and a harderian gland, and in rabbits, lacrimal, nictitans, and harderian glands occur. Tear volumes produced vary between the species. In man 15 μl of tears are produced in 5 min with the stimulus of a Schirmer tear test strip. In dogs the same volume is produced in 1 min (11). The tear film turnover rate in rabbits is approximately half that in man despite the presence of three lacrimal glands (18,19).

Tears are lost from the ocular surface by evaporation and drainage through the nasolacrimal system. The contact time of tears at the ocular surface may be affected by the rate of production, extent of evaporation, which may be greater in species like rabbits that have protruding eyes and blink infrequently, and the rate of drainage. Drainage may be influenced by the rate of blinking, by the lacrimal pump action of the eyelids, and the presence of one or two lacrimal puncta (rabbits and pigs have only one punctum, rodents, carnivores, and primates have two). Tear film pH is similar in laboratory species and man, averaging 7.5; however, the pH of the rabbit tear film at 8.2 falls well outside the 6.6 to 7.8 considered the nonirritating range in man (11,19).

Dog and man are species in which a deficiency of the aqueous portion of the tears (keratoconjunctivitis sicca; KCS) occur with some frequency. In dogs the disease may be an autoimmune disorder and there are particular breeds and families that are more predisposed than others. This may interfere with drug toxicity studies since several drugs including phenazopyridine and sulfonamides can result in KCS due to toxic effects on the lacrimal gland (20).

In rats viral sialodacryoadenitis is a common disease. Clinical signs may vary and include exophthalmos, epiphora, and blood staining of the tears and nares, keratoconjunctivitis, iritis, chorioretinitis, and retinal degeneration. These may be confusing in toxicological studies where similar ocular toxic responses are seen. The disease appears at 6 to 12 months of age (21-23).

CONJUNCTIVA AND CORNEA

Despite reported differences in the response of various species to surface irritants, there is no evidence to suggest that these are due to differences in the anatomy or morphology of the conjunctiva or cornea. The relevance of differences in the size, thickness, and curvature of the cornea in different species in responses to surface irritants has not been demonstrated (11). Similarly, although presumably any differences must reflect interspecies variation in conjunctival and corneal innervation, no comparative studies of the nerve supply or the neuropharmacology exist. It is likely that factors that affect the uveal response of the eye to irritation in various species (see below) may also play some as yet undefined part in variable response of the ocular surface. Comparative studies are needed in particular to determine the ability of the corneal epithelium to resist surface acting toxins and to examine healing rates of the corneal surface in different species. The corneal endothelium by contrast does vary in its reparative capacity. Endothelial healing capacity is greatest in young animals and in rabbits and to a lesser extent in dogs (24).

The cornea varies in thickness in different species as does the number of cell layers in the epithelium. One might speculate that this could affect the resistance of the eye of some species to certain epithelial-damaging toxins or caustic substances, although this is unproven. It has been suggested that the rabbit, which has a thin layer of epithelial cells, would be more sensitive to topically applied irritants since these would penetrate the epithelium more readily than in species such as the cat or dog with thicker layers of epithelial cells (25). However, any differences in sensitivity might lie in pharmacological differences in the cornea or conjunctiva or differences in the density of nerve endings in the epithelium in different species.

Several studies have attempted to compare the sensitivity of the cornea and conjunctiva to ocular irritants (gases, surfactants, or detergents). In one early study it was concluded that corneal sensitivity declines in the following order: bovine, man, rabbit, dog, and cat (26). Various studies have found that in comparisons of rabbits, monkeys, and man that the rabbit is the most sensitive species, with monkeys and man showing similar responses to topical detergents and surfactants (27,28). Similar observations of increased ocular sensitivity in rabbits compared to monkeys have been described using surfactants or sodium hydroxide topically (16). One study utilizing surfactants in a number of laboratory species found that the rabbit, hamster, and mouse showed the most sensitivity, followed by the guinea pig and rat, with the dog, cat, rhesus monkey, and chicken showing the least sensitivity (29). Interestingly, one of these studies found that if the irritatant was confined to the rabbit cornea and did not contact the conjunctiva, the degree of ocular irritation was less than when the conjunctiva was also irritated and the degree of response more closely resembled that seen in the monkey. This would suggest that irritation of the conjunctiva plays a significant role in determining the frequently observed sensitivity of the rabbit to ocular toxins (16).

There is also evidence that the rabbit cornea may be more easily traumatized by irritants than other species. Benzalkonium chloride (BAK) 0.01%, when applied to the cornea of the rabbit in a hydroxyethylcellulose vehicle, causes corneal epithelial damage that is not seen in dogs. In part this may relate to the contact time achieved using a viscous vehicle, since neither BAK nor the vehicle alone causes corneal injury in either species (17).

Despite the studies mentioned above, other studies have found that rabbits have a low sensitivity to certain soaps (30), and that the human eye is considerably more sensitive to the riot-control substances dibenzoxazepine (CR) and o-chlorobenzylidine malononitrile (CS) than rabbits, guinea pigs, or rats (31–33). It therefore appears that although species differences exist in responses of the cornea and conjunctiva to topically applied toxins, this may be influenced by the type and formulation of toxin used. In general, however, the response of the monkey eye to surface-applied toxins is most similar to that in man.

Little is known of the neural reflexes and inflammatory mediators involved in producing the signs of ocular inflammation observed in the conjunctiva or cornea when toxins are applied to the ocular surface. Even less is known about species differences. As Bito (34) has pointed out, there are differences in the appearance of perilimbal hyperemia in response to corneal irritation in different species. Some differences may be less real than easy to observe, as in monkeys where the perilimbal conjunctiva may be more difficult to see than in rabbits or rodents because of the narrow primate palpebral fissure and ocular pigmentation in the primate eyelids and uvea. The time course of development of perilimbal hyperemia (involving the conjunctival or episcleral vasculature) in humans after corneal irritation may parallel the time course of development of uveal hyperemia in rabbits associated with blood-aqueous barrier breakdown. Similar axon reflexes with release of neuropeptides and other inflammatory mediators might be involved in causing conjunctival and episcleral hyperemia as are involved in the anterior uvea (see below) (35).

Inflammatory mediators involved in conjunctival vasodilatation that might therefore act as inflammatory mediators released in response to ocular irritation include histamine in man, rabbit, and guinea pig (36–39), some arachidonic acid metabolites including certain prostaglandins in the guinea pig (40,41), and sulfido-leukotrienes in the guinea pig and hamster (41–44). Most studies of conjunctival inflammatory mediators have centered on allergic responses and there is no certainty that the same mediators are involved or are involved to the same extent in toxic reactions of the conjunctiva.

In the cornea there is evidence that cyclooxygenase and lipoxygenase, products of arachidonic acid metabolism (prostaglandins, hydroperoxy acids, and leukotrienes), are produced in the cornea after cryogenic injury or herpes infections. Although there are suggestions that some of these products may be involved in stimulating polymorphonuclear (PMN) chemotaxis and angiogenesis in the cornea, the exact role of these mediators is largely unresolved (45–49). Platelet activating factor (PAF) is produced in the alkali-burned rabbit cornea (50), and a PAF antagonist will reduce corneal edema, chemotaxis, and activation on PMNs in the alkali-burned cornea (51,52).

Infiltrates or metabolic by-products have been reported as opacities in the cornea in response to many drugs in various species (14,15). Interpretation of these findings may be complicated in various species by the occurrence of inherited dystrophies and age-related degenerations (12,53–57). In rodents, spontaneously occurring mineralization and degeneration has been reported. These changes may be inherited or related to environmental factors other than toxins (58–60).

In dogs and cats various types of corneal dystrophies are known to occur. In most, inheritance is the suspected etiology and this has been proven in several instances. Epithelial dystrophies may present with epithelial erosions or nonhealing ulcers. These may be initiated by slight trauma to the epithelial surface, which subsequently fails to heal normally. Stromal deposits of lipids are commonly seen as an inherited disease in several canine breeds including the beagle. The deposits often are arranged in a particular geographic pattern and may develop at particular ages in specific breeds, which may help in differentiating them from toxic reactions in the cornea. Progressively worsening corneal edema and bullous keratopathy occurs in several canine breeds due to endothelial dystrophy. Both stromal and endothelial dystrophies causing corneal edema have been described in cats (54,56). Other deposits occasionally seen include mucopolysaccharides and minerals.

Degenerations of the cornea occur in rodents, cats, and dogs. These present as corneal opacification due to mineral or lipid deposits with or without loss of thickness in the corneal stroma (12,55).

ANTERIOR UVEAL VASCULAR CHANGES AND THE BLOOD-AQUEOUS BARRIER

The area of the eye that has received the most study in relation to species differences is the anterior uvea, comprising the iris and ciliary body. The eye responds to many physical and noxious chemical stimuli with an acute irritative response that may persist as anterior uveitis if the stimulus persists. It has become apparent that considerable variation exists between different species in these responses determined by anatomical and pharmacological differences of the anterior segment of the eye (34,35).

The ocular irritative response of the eye consists of anterior uveal hyperemia, constriction of the iris sphincter muscle causing a reduction in pupil size (miosis), breakdown of the blood-aqueous barrier (BAB), and a change (usually a rise) in intraocular pressure (35). Later components of ocular inflammation may represent a continuation of these effects as well as cellular infiltration into the anterior segment of the eye.

The irritative response can be induced by many physical (traumatic), thermal, and chemical stimuli. These include trauma to the eye and paracentesis, chemical irritants such as nitrogen mustard (61) and formaldehyde (62) applied to the cornea, alkali and acid burns of the cornea, and topically applied potential chemical inflammatory mediators such as prostaglandins and arachidonic acid. The same responses can be achieved by laser and x-ray irradiation of the iris or lens (63–65). Clinically important is the effect of bacterial endotoxins (66). Considerable variation exists between different species in the pharmacology of the components of the ocular irritative response. Aspects of these differences have been reviewed elsewhere (35,67,68).

The rabbit is the species most sensitive to ocular irritation among laboratory and domestic species. The initial irritative response is mediated by a neural reflex arc in the rabbit. Stimulation of the fifth (trigeminal) cranial nerve results in an acute ocular irritative response (69), which is largely due to the release of substance P (SP), calcitonin gene-related peptide (CGRP), and possibly other neuropeptides from trigeminal nerve endings in the anterior uvea (70,71). The effects are reduced but not abolished by an SP-inhibitor, suggesting that other chemical mediators may be involved (64). Since the cornea and conjunctiva are densely innervated by the fifth cranial nerve, any irritation of these tissues by chemicals is likely to result in an irritative response in this species. The anatomical components of the neural reflex arc are presumed to be similar in most laboratory and domestic animal species, whereas the magnitude of the response varies widely both experimentally and clinically and is probably determined by differences in the morphology of the blood-aqueous barrier, receptor types in the anterior uvea, and mediators released into the anterior uvea in response to trigeminal stimulation.

The blood-aqueous barrier comprises tight junctions between ciliary and iridal epithelial cells and an endothelial barrier in the iridal capillaries. Together these structures prevent macromolecules from access to the anterior or posterior chambers. Although the basic pattern is similar in most mammals some anatomical differences exist that might affect the relative sensitivity of the BAB to breakdown. The rabbit, which has the most sensitive BAB, has well-developed iridial portions of the ciliary processes, which appear to be the site of BAB breakdown in this species. By contrast, this region of the ciliary processes is poorly developed in primates with a more stable BAB (72–76). Additionally the types of intercellular junctions in the iris vary between species. In the rat, cat, and pig most are of the gap-junction type, whereas in man, monkey, and mouse they are tight junctions (77). Protein accumulation in the aqueous, which is a feature of BAB breakdown, occurs because of disruption of the

BAB structures in the rabbit (78), whereas in primates it rarely occurs in response to acute ocular irritation. Protein entry into the anterior chamber can be achieved in primates after paracentesis of the anterior chamber, but in this situation, which does not closely mimic irritation of the eye by toxins, the flare primarily results from reflux from the iridocorneal angle and Schlemm's canal (34,76,79). The extent of protein production in the anterior chamber resulting in flare differs considerably between species. Marked flare develops rapidly in rabbits and guinea pigs, more slowly and of lesser magnitude in cats, and not to any measurable extent in owl monkeys and ducks after the topical application of nitrogen mustard to the eye (80).

The difference in the stability of the BAB in rabbits compared with other species and especially primates has been demonstrated with both noxious chemical and physical stimuli applied to the eye and with aqueous loss from the eye (paracentesis). This is therefore not a response that is specific for particular toxic stimuli but does vary considerably between species. The sensitivity of the blood-aqueous barrier to breakdown has been hypothesized to correlate with the extent of lateral positioning and exposure of the eyes in the head and thus exposure of the eye to trauma. This varies in the following manner: rabbit > sheep > pig > dog > cat > primates (81). The rabbit, which has a protruding eye, would be quite likely to sustain damage to the cornea. This species needs an ocular defense mechanism that results in rapid breakdown of the BAB, allowing protein (including fibrin) to enter the anterior chamber to help seal any breach in the cornea until healing can occur. Primates at the other end of the spectrum of BAB reaction have eyes that receive some protection from the bony orbit and are thus less likely to sustain severe injury. Should injury occur in primates, production of large amounts of protein in the anterior chamber would severely limit visual acuity in species that rely heavily upon vision for survival (34).

Calcitonin gene-related peptide is a potent vasodilator in the rabbit and cat, and will break down the BAB when injected into the anterior chamber of the rabbit, but not of the cat (82–84).

Prostaglandins may contribute to anterior uveal vasodilation and BAB disruption in some species. In the rabbit, disruption of the BAB has been detected with intracameral injection of PGE_2 (85,86). The production of prostaglandins (PGs) in the aqueous humor may parallel BAB disruption in endotoxin-induced inflammation in the rabbit (87,88), although in at least some studies disruption of the barrier in rabbits and rats precedes production of detectable PG concentrations in aqueous (89,90). PGs probably play a significant although not exclusive role in disruption of the BAB in dogs as shown by studies using cyclooxygenase-inhibiting drugs to control BAB breakdown (68,91–94). PGs are probably less important in disruption of the primate BAB (35,95).

Other mediators including platelet activating factor, interleukin-1α, and tumor necrosis factor (TNF) cause ocular changes that vary with the chemical and include anterior uveal vasodilatation, disruption of the BAB, or protein extravasation into the aqueous in rabbits. Whether these substances are involved in toxic disruption of the BAB in this species or others and how these substances interact with other inflammatory mediators is largely unknown (96–101).

CELLULAR INFILTRATION INTO THE ANTERIOR CHAMBER

Cellular infiltration into the anterior uvea and subsequently the aqueous is a common feature of spontaneous and experimental inflammatory disease. Cellular infiltration into the anterior uvea and aqueous may differ in magnitude in different species in much the same manner as BAB breakdown. The pharmacology of chemotaxis of polymorphonuclear leukocytes into the aqueous appears similar in several species studied. In at least rabbits, guinea pigs, and cats, leukotriene B_4 (LTB_4) injected into the anterior chamber causes marked PMN chemotaxis (86,102–104). In rabbits and rats, the appearance of PMNs in endotoxin uveitis appears to parallel the rise of LTB_4 concentrations in the aqueous (89,90). In rabbits, interleukin-1, interleukin-1_{α}, and TNF may cause cellular infiltration (99–101,105,106). The role of these mediators in other species is as yet undetermined.

MIOSIS

Constriction of the pupil (miosis) is a characteristic feature of acute ocular irritation and prolonged uveitis in many species. Miosis may be considered an undesirable toxic side effect of various ocular medications in man. For instance, cholinergic drugs (pilocarpine, demecarium bromide) used in glaucoma therapy result in miosis and painful ciliary spasm (107). In evaluating new prostaglandin analogues for glaucoma therapy, an important consideration has been to develop drugs that reduce intraocular pressure without causing toxic side effects including miosis, disruption of the blood-aqueous barrier, and reduced uveoscleral outflow due to ciliary muscle contraction (108).

Miosis results from contraction of the iris sphincter muscle located around the free margin of the iris. The two major iris muscles are the circular sphincter muscle and the radial dilator muscle. In mammals, the sphincter muscle is a smooth muscle type with muscarinic cholinergic receptors (unlike lower vertebrates such as birds and reptiles where the sphincter has nicotinic cholinergic receptors). There are very considerable differences between vertebrate species in the pharmacology of miosis in response to ocular irritation.

Nitrogen mustard applied to the eyes causes miosis in the rabbit, cat, and owl monkey, but not the guinea pig or duck (80,109,110). Additionally miosis in the cat and to a lesser extent the rabbit is reduced by pretreatment with indomethacin, although this has no effect on miosis in the owl monkey. These observations underlie the very complex differences between various species in the response of the iris sphincter muscle to particular toxic substances that irritate the eye. It seems clear, however, that as with disruption of the BAB, miosis is a nonspecific response of the eye caused by neurotransmitters, neuromodulators, or inflammatory agents released or synthesized in ocular tissues in response to trauma or chemical or physical irritation. Although we are far from a complete understanding of the various interactions between inflammatory mediators that result in irritation-induced miosis, evidence from both *in vitro* and *in vivo* experiments is accumulating that suggests interspecies differences in the sensitivity of the iris sphincter to various mediators, in part reflecting species differences in either the presence or density of chemical receptors (111).

The early literature of miosis studied the effects of noxious substances applied to or injected into the eye. Extracts of rabbit, cat, or dog iris with prostaglandin-like activity contracted smooth muscle (112–114). PG-like activity was occasionally measured in the aqueous humor at the time miosis was observed and prostaglandins injected into the eyes of rabbits and cats apparently caused miosis (115–117). Prostaglandins thus became early candidates as mediators of the miotic response. It is now known that miosis is a result of complex interactions that probably involve at least acetylcholine, neuropeptides (particularly the neurotransmitter substance P), norepinephrine, and products of arachidonic acid metabolism (prostaglandins and leukotrienes).

Prostaglandin $F_{2\alpha}$ contracts the iris sphincter muscle in the cow, dog, and cat but not man, pig, or rabbit, whereas PGA2 causes iris sphincter contraction in the cow and pig, but not man, cat, dog, or rabbit. Among these species leukotriene D_4 contracts the iris sphincter only in the cow and cat (118, 119). Similarly, *in vivo* it appears that PGF_{2a} causes miosis when applied topically or injected intracamerally into the canine or feline eye. The bovine iris sphincter muscle is also contracted by PGA_2, PGE_2, and PGE_1. The feline eye is less sensitive to miotic effects of PGE_2 (120–122). The rabbit pupil is not significantly constricted by prostaglandins (85,123) and in early studies that suggested otherwise miosis may have resulted from ocular cannulation or PG-induced release of other mediators, notably neuropeptides from nerve endings of the trigeminal nerve in the uvea (122,124). *In vitro* studies in the rat also suggest that although there is no direct miotic effect of PGs, they may cause the release of other sphincter-contracting mediators (125). In nonhuman primates $PGF_{2\alpha}$ has either no miotic effect or one that is very slight (126–128). Although miosis has been reported in human eyes in response to topical PGs there is also evidence that suggests that PGs have little miotic effect in man (122,129).

Substance P (SP) is present in the uveal tract of several mammalian species. It contracts the iris sphincter muscle in the rabbit, cow, and pig (130,131) but not in the cat, dog, or baboon (131,132). In man SP has variable effects, and although alone it does not appear to contract the iris sphincter (131), contraction may occur in the presence of an enkephalinase inhibitor, suggesting that the peptide enkephalinase may regulate SP-induced iris sphincter contraction in man (133).

The differences in response of the iris sphincter muscle may reflect the action of these various mediators via specific receptors on second messenger systems in the smooth muscle, which appears to be species dependent. Two second messenger systems are present in the iris sphincter—one involved production of inositol triphosphate (IP3) in the muscle cell, the other production of adenosine 3′,5′-cyclic monophosphate (cAMP). IP3 production mobilizes calcium and causes muscle contraction by myosin light chain (MLC) phosphorylation; cAMP inhibits MLC phosphorylation and thus tends to relax the muscle. Acetylcholine stimulates muscarinic receptors and causes IP_3 production in all mammalian iridal sphincter muscles so far tested, thus causing contraction. The differential effects of other agonist or inflammatory mediators on either receptor/second messenger system will determine whether the muscle contracts or relaxes (118). Thus, in considering effects of drugs on the pupil only muscarinic cholinergic drugs, inhibitors of their production, or specific receptor antagonists can be expected to universally affect most mammalian species in a similar fashion. The other mediators listed above that cause iris sphincter contraction are also associated with production of IP_3 in the muscle cell (111,118,119,132) and the variability in receptor and second messenger types among different species will affect the pupil response to particular toxins.

CHANGES IN INTRAOCULAR PRESSURE

Nitrogen mustard applied to the eyes of rabbits, guinea pigs, and cats causes an acute rise of intraocular pressure (IOP), which is biphasic during the first 24 hr in the first two species. A small increase in IOP is also seen in ducks, but not in owl monkeys. These changes in IOP are variably affected by indomethacin, suggesting that prostanoids play at least some role in regulating the changes in IOP in these species, although the exact nature of their involvement differs between species (80,109,110). The rise of IOP is probably not specific for topically applied ocular toxins since similar changes occur in rabbits and dogs following laser damage of the iris or lens (64,93).

The variation in IOP change in different species probably reflects differences in the mechanisms of aqueous production, anatomy of the anterior uveal vasculature, and aqueous outflow anatomy and pharmacology. The increase in IOP after Nd:YAG lasing of the eye is probably due to increased ocular blood flow causing an increase in the fluid volume of the ciliary processes, increased ultrafiltration of aqueous, and an influx of extravasate into the eye associated with disruption of the blood-aqueous barrier (BAB) (35). Additionally, later in ocular inflammation the trabecular meshwork of the iridocorneal angle becomes swollen and protein entering the eye due to disruption of the BAB and inflammatory cells entering the aqueous from the uvea may block outflow through the trabecular meshwork. Subsequent changes in the IOP may reflect the morphological and pharmacological differences in aqueous outflow. In toxicology studies the effects of drugs on the outflow of aqueous may vary between species.

The outflow of aqueous from the eye is via one of two routes: (a) the conventional or iridocorneal outflow, namely the trabecular meshwork, and some form of scleral venous plexus and aqueous veins into the general venous circulation (24); and (b) the uveoscleral route across the iris root and anterior face of the ciliary muscle, between the ciliary muscle bundles, into the suprachoroidal space and out through the sclera (134,135). Differences in the anatomy of the iridocorneal angle exist between the various mammalian species used in experimental studies (136).

The relative contribution of these two outflow pathways vary between species, with the uveoscleral accounting for 30% to 65% in nonhuman primates, 13% in rabbits, 3% in cats, 15% in dogs, and 4% to 14% in man (24).

It has been speculated that increases in IOP associated with obstruction of iridocorneal outflow in ocular inflammation may be minimized by increasing uveoscleral outflow (137). The effects of drugs on the IOP must thus be weighed both against the relative contributions of the outflow pathways in different species and the normal pharmacological control of IOP via the two main outflow routes. For instance, $PGF_{2\alpha}$ and its analogues are known to lower IOP in several mammalian species including the dog, cat, subhuman primates, man, and rabbit, acting primarily by increasing uveoscleral outflow. This effect can be markedly reduced in the dog by cyclooxygenase inhibitors, which reduce PG production in the irritated eye (93,138). PGE2 injected intracamerally will markedly elevate IOP in the rabbit (presumably by increasing uveal vasodilation and disrupting the BAB), but only slightly in monkeys and cats, and in the latter species only with much higher doses than used in the rabbit (139,140). It is possible that in other species drugs that affect PG production may have quantitatively different effects on IOP depending on the uveoscleral contribution to outflow.

Other species differences in IOP regulation in the irritated eye will be determined by other inflammatory mediators released. CGRP is released from trigeminal nerve endings in rabbits in response to ocular irritation (141). CGRP injected into the rabbit eye causes vasodilatation, breakdown of the BAB, and a rise in IOP. Conversely, CGRP injected into the feline eye causes a fall in IOP possibly by increasing outflow facility from the eye (142). Platelet activating factor applied topically to rabbit eyes also increases IOP, an effect that can be abolished with a PAF receptor antagonist, although no studies have been reported using PAF in other species.

Changes in IOP in response to drugs applied to the eye or given systemically might be affected by the existence or predisposition of existing glaucoma or an anatomical predisposition to develop elevated IOP. Species in which spontaneous, inherited glaucoma occurs include man, dogs, and rabbits. Glaucoma as a primary disease is by contrast very rare in rodents, subhuman primates, and cats, although it may occur secondary to intraocular inflammation (12). In man the commonest form of glaucoma is the chronic, open-angle type. Although this type occurs in some breeds of dog, including beagle, narrow-angle glaucoma is also commonly encountered in this species (143). In New Zealand white rabbits a recessively inherited glaucoma has been described similar to congenital glaucoma in man due to an abnormally developed anterior chamber angle (144). Dogs and rabbits should be screened for normal IOP and undergo gonioscopic examination of the iridocorneal angle in any studies where drugs might affect IOP.

AQUEOUS HUMOR

The aqueous humor is secreted and drained at equal rates. These are similar for most animals studied, but highest in cats. Intraocular pressures show slight variations in the different species (145). The biochemical composition of the aqueous humor is generally similar to plasma but with low concentrations of protein. The aqueous is made up of electrolytes, glucose, oxygen, amino acids protein, immunoglobulin, ascorbate, urea, and lactate. Concentrations are similar in most mammals and have been reviewed by Wilkie and Wyman (11). Amino acid transport systems present in rabbits may be missing in primates, cats, and dogs. Little is known of changes in aqueous humor composition except increased protein concentration in response to toxins.

LENS

The most frequent toxic reaction of the lens is the development of cataracts. Cataracts have been seen in most of the laboratory species, although often the etiology is undetermined. Numerous examples of toxic cataracts are known in many species of animal; however, there is little evidence that any particular species is more prone to develop toxic cataracts than any other (14). Some species may be less likely overall to develop cataracts than others, however, and presumably differences in lens biochemistry may account for this. For instance, cataracts of any form are seen less frequently in cats than dogs, and cats are very rarely affected with diabetic cataracts. The time period required for the lens to develop cataractous change may vary between species with any particular toxin, making direct comparisons difficult (146). Differences between species in the development of cataracts may reflect postnatal lens growth. For instance the lens in dogs and humans continues to growth throughout adult life whereas the bovine, rabbit, and rat lens changes little in size. Variations in specific sensitivity to cataract development may also reflect differences in lens metabolism and differences in the chemical composition of the lens in different species (11,147).

Normal variations in the appearance of the lens may be confused with toxic changes, at least in rodents and dogs. The suture lines in dogs, cats, and man have a Y-shaped appearance. In dogs during the first few months of life the suture lines may be very prominent and although this may be less so at a year of age, the posterior sutures may again appear during the second year of life (12). This may be confused with either inherited or toxic cataracts involving the lens sutures.

Inherited cataracts are seen most commonly in dogs and rodents. In rats cataracts at various locations have been associated with aging (148,149). The incidence of unilateral posterior lens opacities in normal laboratory rats is surprisingly high (5% to 10%) and may increase with age (12). Many opacities in the rat lens appear in the posterior cortex, which may also be the site of development of toxic cataract. Animals must be screened before the study to rule out the presence of any preexisting lesions. Rodents under anesthesia may develop lens opacities of the anterior lens cortex. This may be due to aqueous dehydration or cooling and is reversible when blinking is resumed (150). Various inherited cataracts have been described in certain strains of mice, which may become apparent in early postnatal life or in adult animals depending upon the strain of mouse (151-153).

In dogs the commonest cause of cataracts is inheritance, and a considerable number of different types of cataracts have been reported in particular breeds (154). In some the appearance of the cataract and age of onset is characteristic enough to imply an inherited etiology, for instance the posterior polar subcapsular cataracts seen in the Labrador or golden retriever at 6 to 8 months of age (155). In other breeds the appearance and age of onset are not characteristic for inherited cataract, although the frequency with which cataracts occur in the breed would be sufficient to suggest an inherited etiology, for instance cortical cataracts in the American cocker spaniel (156). An average incidence of 3.7% of beagles in a research colony were found to have some unilateral or bilateral lens opacities (157).

RETINA AND CHOROID

Various differences in the anatomy of the retina and choroid in domestic and laboratory species are likely to affect the response of the retina and choroid to toxic injury.

The choroid in several species is modified anteriorly to form a tapetum lucidum. In the dog, cat, and ferret this is formed by a layer of cells containing electron-dense rods. In horses and other ungulates the layer is fibrous, comprising layers of collagen. Biochemically the tapetum varies between species, also. In the cat the tapetal rods have a high concentration of riboflavin, whereas in the dog and ferret tapetum has a high concentration of zinc and cysteine (24). The tapetum may vary in color as seen ophthalmoscopically between and within any species and with the age of the animal (158). This may be significant in toxicity studies since there are drugs such as ethambutol that can also cause color changes in the tapetum (158). An inherited tapetal degeneration has been reported in the beagle (159).

The vasculature of the choroid and retina differ between species. In primates the arterial supply to the retina is via a central retinal artery. In other species with retinal vasculature the retinal arterial supply is via the short posterior ciliary arteries forming cilioretinal arteries. Various retinal patterns are present in mammals: holangiotic vasculature in primates, cats, dogs, rodents and cattle arises from the central retinal arteries or cilioretinal vessels and extends into the inner retinal layers throughout the retina; merangiotic vasculature arises from cilioretinal vessels and radiates into the horizontal quadrants of the retina; paurangiotic vessels are small and numerous and radiate only a small distance from the optic nerve into the retina; the anangiotic pattern is a retina that lacks blood vessels. The relative contribution of the underlying choroid to retinal nutrition depends upon the extent of retinal vascularization. Animals with minimal retinal vascularization have thinner retinas to facilitate diffusion of nutrients and waste products from the choroid (11).

Primates possess an area of especially high cone density in the retina—the fovea centralis, which lacks rod photoreceptors and blood vessels. Carnivores have a comparable area of increased cone density temporal to the optic disc.

Retinal degeneration occurs commonly in several laboratory species and man, although very rarely in any other primates. Retinal degeneration may be inherited, age or environment related, or due to nutritional deficiencies. These various etiologies should be recognized as potential causes of retinal atrophy in animals that will be used for any long-term toxicological studies. Inherited retinal degenerations occur in many breeds of dog, cats, rats, and mice. Inherited degenerations can primarily involve the retinal pigment epithelium (RPE) or the neural retina and may develop as disease in early postnatal life and progress rapidly or later in adult animals with slower progression. Most inherited retinal degenerations affect the rod photoreceptors initially and then progress to involve the cones and ultimately the remaining retinal neurons.

In man several different types of retinal dystrophy/degeneration have been reported. Some of these have an inherited basis, others are associated with other systemic and metabolic diseases (160,161).

In the dog and mouse various primary retinal degenerations involve the photoreceptors. Early-onset retinal degenerations (photoreceptor dysplasia) may vary between breeds or strains in the inheritance locus and biochemical defects involved. Where biochemical abnormalities are known in dogs and rodents they have been shown to involve the guanosine 3′,5′-cyclic monophosphate (cGMP) phosphodiesterase involved in visual transduction (162–164). Late-onset retinal degenerations in dogs, which are similar to some forms of inherited retinitis pigmentosa in man, involve the same gene locus in several different breeds (165). Abnormalities of photoreceptor membrane lipids have been detected in some poodles with late-onset retinal degeneration (166). Similar inherited retinal degenerations are also seen in the cat (167,168).

Retinal degeneration associated with a retinal pigment epithelial dystrophy is also seen in the dog. The diseased RPE accumulates lipopigment and the neural retina subsequently undergoes slow degeneration (169).

Photoreceptor dysplasia also occurs in mice. As in the dog, these are diseases seen in young animals with rapid progression. The best characterized are the rd and rds strains (170,171).

Retinal degenerations have also been reported in the rat. The best documented degeneration is seen in the RCS rat. The disease is a primary retinal pigment epitheliopathy. Failure of the RPE to phagocytose shed photoreceptor outer segments results in accumulation of membranous debris between retina and RPE and subsequent retinal atrophy in the early postnatal period (172). Retinal degenerations have occasionally been reported in other strains of rat that may not be inherited. Defining the etiology of retinal degeneration in this species can be problematic since degenerations associated with old age and exposure to high light levels have also been reported (12).

Phototoxic retinal degeneration may influence the interpretation of toxicologic studies in rodents. Rats and mice are particularly sensitive to light-induced retinal degeneration. In part this may be due to the prevalence of studies performed in albino strains of these species. Various other factors influencing the rate and severity of light-induced degeneration include the use of mydriatics, age (older animals are more susceptible), sex (females are more susceptible), environmental temperature (retinal degeneration proceeds more rapidly at higher temperatures), and maintenance of the animals on a continuous rather than cyclic lighting regime (4,12,173,174).

Other retinal degenerations that may be confused with toxic reactions in the retina of laboratory species include nutritional retinal degeneration due to taurine deficiency in cats (175) and vitamin E deficiency in dogs (176).

OCULAR ALBINISM

The presence or lack of pigment in the eye may have various effects on the response of the eye to toxins. This becomes significant in that albinism is an inherited trait in several mammalian species, and particularly in some that are routinely used in laboratory studies.

Albinism is inherited in man and among species used for toxicity experiments—rats, mice, and rabbits. Although true complete albinism does not occur in the dog, cat, or other domestic species, reduced ocular pigmentation does occur in certain breeds and lines. Since albino rabbits and rats are commonly used for testing potentially toxic drugs, it is important to ask whether the lack of pigment will affect the type of reaction that might be expected in man, a species that usually has a well-pigmented eye.

Rubin (177) has recently thoroughly reviewed the significance of ocular pigmentation in ocular toxicity testing. A lack of melanin pigment has been associated with reduced visual performance in man (178), and physiological differences have been observed in experimental animals (177). For instance, in albino rabbits, mice, and rats dark adaptation thresholds are higher than in their pigmented counterparts (179), and albino rats and rabbits lack an electroretinographic c-wave (180–183).

Toxicological studies on the retina and orbital glands in albino rodents can be affected by the increased sensitivity of the retina in albinos to light-induced degeneration (184,185). Additionally the effects of aging-related retinal degeneration is more pronounced in albino rats than pigmented strains (186).

It is known that certain chemicals can be absorbed by pigment and therefore accumulate in pigmented ocular tissues (187,188). This accumulation of chemical in the eye may predispose the pigmented ocular tissue to more injurious effects from the chemical than in nonpigmented albino strains. Various possible effects of the presence or lack of pigment on ocular reactions to chemicals as outlined below are suggested by Rubin (177).

The albino animal may be more susceptible to chemical toxicity than pigmented animals. For instance, retinal degeneration occurs in albino but not pigmented rats given vinyl δ-aminobutyric acid (GABA) (189). Conversely, pigmented animals may be more susceptible to toxic injury than albinos. Pigmented rats are more susceptible to naphthalene cataracts since they possess enzymes required for cataract development that are lacking in albino rats. Uveal degeneration and ocular phthisis has been seen in pigmented rats but not in albinos administered a herbicide (177).

Although some chemicals may be accumulated in pigmented ocular tissues, toxicity may occur regardless of whether pigment is present or not and also may affect nonpigmented parts of the eye. This is the case with amopyroquin, which causes retinal degeneration in pigmented dogs and albino rats (190) and in chloroquine- and chlorpromazine-induced keratopathies (191,192).

Finally, there are examples where, despite accumulation of chemicals in pigmented tissue, no ocular toxic reactions are detected in either pigmented or albino animals. This is true for certain antimalarials (193), beta blockers (194), and certain other drugs in clinical use (195).

To avoid the effects of pigmentation or its absence on toxicological studies, it is essential to use both pigmented and albino strains of the test species wherever possible.

There are many unresolved issues in comparative toxicology of the eye. It is obvious that, ideally, studies of ocular drug reactions should be performed in the species to which the information will be most relevantly applied in the clinical setting. Since the primate appears to react like man in most respects, it would seem to be a logical choice as an experimental model for toxicological and drug side effects studies. However, there are considerable ethical and cost considerations in using primates in toxicological research, at least in part due to the often precarious status of many primate species in the wild.

The use of rodents and rabbits should continue to be the mainstay of toxicological research whenever possible. Use of dogs and cats, however, may be considered when the results are applicable to the clinical veterinary situation.

REFERENCES

1. Slatter DH. *Fundamentals of veterinary ophthalmology*, 2nd ed. Philadelphia: W.B. Saunders, 1990.
2. Gelatt KN. *Veterinary ophthalmology*, 2nd ed. Philadelphia: Lea & Febiger, 1991.
3. Tabbara KF, Cello RM. *Animal models of ocular diseases*. Springfield, IL: Charles C. Thomas, 1984.
4. Naash MI, LaVail MM, Anderson RE. Factors affecting the susceptibility of the retina to light damage. *Prog Clin Biol Res* 1989;314:513-522.
5. Walls GL. *The vertebrate eye and its adaptive radiation*. Bloomfield Hills, MI: Cranbrook Institute of Science, 1942.
6. Duke-Elder S. The eye in evolution. In: *System of ophthalmology, vol 1*. St. Louis: C.V. Mosby, 1958.
7. Prince JH, Diesem CD, Eglitis I, Ruskell GL. *Anatomy and histology of the eye and orbit in domestic animals*. Springfield, IL: Charles C. Thomas, 1960.
8. Berman ER. *Biochemistry of the eye*. New York: Plenum Press, 1991.
9. Davson H. *Physiology of the eye*, 5th ed. New York: Pergamon Press, 1990.
10. Havener WH. *Pharmacology of the eye*. Berlin: Springer-Verlag, 1984.
11. Wilkie DA, Wyman M. Comparative anatomy and physiology of the mammalian eye. In: Hobson DW, ed. *Dermal and ocular toxicology: fundamentals and methods*. 1991;433-491.
12. Bellhorn RW. Laboratory animal ophthalmology. In: Gelatt KN, ed. *Veterinary ophthalmology*, 2nd ed. Philadelphia: Lea & Febiger, 1991;656-679.
13. Peiffer RL, Armstrong JR, Johnson PT. Animals in ophthalmic research: concepts and methodologies. In: Gay WI, ed. *Methods of animal experimentation*. New York: Academic Press, 1981;140-235.
14. Grant WM. *Toxicology of the eye*, 3rd ed. Springfield, IL: Charles C. Thomas, 1986.
15. Fraunfelder FT, Meyer SM. *Drug-induced ocular side effects and drug interactions*, 2nd ed. Philadelphia: Lea & Febiger, 1982.
16. Buehler EV, Newmann EA. A comparison of eye irritation in monkeys and rabbits. *Toxicol Appl Pharmacol* 1964;6:701-710.
17. Durand-Cavagna G, Delort P, Duprat P, Bailly Y, Plazonnet B, Gordon LR. Corneal toxicity studies in rabbits and dogs with hydroxyethylcellulose and benzalkonium chloride. *Fundam Appl Toxicol* 1989;13:500-508.
18. Prince JH. *The rabbit in eye research*. Springfield, IL: Charles C. Thomas, 1964.
19. Hackett RB, Stern ME. Preclinical toxicology/safety considerations in the development of ophthalmic drugs and devices. In: Hobson DW, ed. *Dermal and ocular toxicology: fundamentals and methods*. 1991;607-626.

20. Kaswan RL, Salisbury MA. A new perspective on canine keratoconjunctivitis sicca: treatment with ophthalmic cyclosporine. *Vet Clin North Am [Small Anim Pract]* 1990;20:583-613.
21. Lai YL, Jacoby R, Bhatt P, Jonas A. Keratoconjunctivitis associated with sialodacryoadenitis in rats. *Invest Ophthalmol Vis Sci* 1976;15:538-541.
22. Hunt RD. Dacryoadenitis in the Sprague-Dawley rat. *Am J Vet Res* 1963;24:638—641.
23. Weissbroth SH, Peress N. Ophthalmic lesions and dacryoadenitis: a naturally occurring aspect of sialodacryoadenitis virus infection of the laboratory rat. *Lab Anim Sci* 1977;27:466-473.
24. Samuelson DA. Ophthalmic anatomy and embryology. In: Gelatt KN, ed. *Veterinary ophthalmology*, 2nd ed. Philadelphia: Lea & Febiger, 1991;3-123.
25. Daston GP, Freeberg FE. Ocular irritation testing. In: Hobson DW, ed. *Dermal and ocular toxicology: fundamentals and methods.* 1991;509-539.
26. Hellauer HF. Sensibilitat und acetylcholingehalt der hornhaut verschiedenier tiere und des menschen. *Z vergleichende Physiol* 1950;32:303-310.
27. Beckley JH. Comparative eye testing: man vs. animal. *Toxicol Appl Pharmacol* 1965;7:93-101.
28. Beckley JH, Russell TJ, Rubin LF. Use of the rhesus monkey for predicting human response to eye irritants. *Toxicol Appl Pharmacol* 1969;15:1-9.
29. Gersbein LL, McDonald JE. Evaluation of the corneal irritancy of test shampoos and detergents in various animal species. *Food Cosmet Toxicol* 1992;15:131-134.
30. Gaunt F, Harper KH. The potential irritancy to the rabbit eye of certain commercially available shampoos. *J Soc Cosmet Chem* 1964;15:209-230.
31. Ballantyne B, Swanston DW. The irritant potential of dilute solutions of ortho-chlorobenzylidene malononitrile (CS) on the eye and tongue. *Acta Pharm Toxicol* 1973;32:266-277.
32. Ballantyne B, Gazzard MF, et al. Ophthalmic toxicology of o-chlorobenzylidene malononitrile (CS). *Arch Toxicol* 1974;32:149-168.
33. Ballantyne B, Swanston DW. The irritant effects of dilute solutions dibenzoxazepine (CR) on the eye and tongue. *Acta Pharm Toxicol* 1974;35:412-423.
34. Bito LZ. Species differences in the responses of the eye to irritation and trauma: a hypothesis of divergence in ocular defense mechanisms, and the choice of experimental animals for eye research. *Exp Eye Res* 1984;39:807-829.
35. Unger WG. Mediation of the ocular response to injury and irritation: peptides versus prostaglandins. *Prog Clin Biol Res* 1989;312:293-328.
36. Eakins KE, Bhattacherjee P. Histamine, prostaglandins and ocular inflammation. *Exp Eye Res* 1977;24:299-305.
37. Abelson MB, Allansmith MR, Friedlander MH. Effects of topically applied decongestant and antihistamine. *Am J Ophthalmol* 1980;90:254-257.
38. Abelson MB, Soter NA, Simon MA, Dohlman J, Allansmith MR. Histamine in human tears. *Am J Ophthalmol* 1977;83:417-418.
39. Stock EL, Roth SI, Kim ED, Walsh MK, Thamman R. The effect of platelet-activating factor (PAF), histamine, and ethanol on vascular permeability of the guinea pig conjunctiva. *Invest Ophthalmol Vis Sci* 1990;31:987-992.
40. Woodward DF, Ledgard SE. Effect of LTD_4 on conjunctival vasopermeability and blood-aqueous barrier integrity. *Invest Ophthalmol Vis Sci* 1985;26:481-485.
41. Woodward DF, Hawley SB, Williams LS, et al. Studies on the ocular pharmacology of prostaglandin D_2. *Invest Ophthalmol Vis Sci* 1990;31:138-146.
42. Woodward DF, Ledgard SE. Comparison of leukotrienes as conjunctival microvascular permeability factors. *Ophthalmic Res* 1985;17:318-320.
43. Garceau D, Ford-Hutchinson AW. The role of leukotriene D_4 as a mediator of allergic conjunctivitis in the guinea-pig. *Eur J Pharmacol* 1987;134:285-292.
44. Gary RK, Woodward DF, Nieves AL, Williams LS, Gleason JG, Wasserman MA. Characterization of the conjunctival vasopermeability response to leukotrienes and their involvement in immediate hypersensitivity. *Invest Ophthalmol Vis Sci* 1988;29:119-126.
45. Bazan HEP. Corneal injury alters eicosanoid formation in the rabbit anterior segment in vivo. *Invest Ophthalmol Vis Sci* 1987;28:314-319.
46. Bazan HEP, Birkle DL, Beuerman RW, Bazan NG. Inflammation-induced stimulation of the synthesis of prostaglandins and lipoxygenase-reaction products in rabbit cornea. *Curr Eye Res* 1985;4:175-179.
47. Birkle DL, Sanitiato JJ, Kaufman HE, Bazan NG. Arachidonic acid metabolism to eicosanoids in herpes virus-infected rabbit cornea. *Invest Ophthalmol Vis Sci* 1986;27:1443-1446.

48. Srinivasa BD, Kulkarni PS. The role of arachidonic acid metabolites in the mediation of the polymorphonuclear leukocyte response following corneal injury. *Invest Ophthalmol Vis Sci* 1980;19:1087-1093.
49. Benezra D. Neovasculogenic ability of prostaglandins, growth factors and synthetic chemoattractants. *Am J Ophthalmol* 1978;86:455-461.
50. Bazan HEP, Reddy STK. Production of platelet-activating factor (PAF) in the cornea after stimulation. *Invest Ophthalmol Vis Sci* 1989;30(suppl):404.
51. Bazan HEP, Sridevi TK, Woodland JM, Bazan NG. The accumulation of platelet activating factor in the injured cornea may be interrelated with the synthesis of lipoxygenase products. *Biochem Biophys Res Commun* 1987;149:915-920.
52. Bazan HEP, Braquet P, Reddy STK, Bazan NG. Inhibition of the alkali burn-induced lipoxygenation of arachidonic acid in the rabbit cornea in vivo by a platelet activating factor antagonist. *J Ocul Pharmacol* 1987;3:357-365.
53. Kenyon KR, Fogle JA, Grayson M. Dysgeneses, dystrophies and degenerations of the cornea. In: Duane TD, ed. *Clinical Ophthalmology*. Philadelphia: Harper & Row, 1986;1-56.
54. Cooley PL, Dice PF. Corneal dystrophy in the dog and cat. *Vet Clin North Am [Small Anim Pract]* 1990;20:681-692.
55. Whitley RD. Canine cornea. In: Gelatt KN, ed. *Veterinary ophthalmology*, 2nd ed. Philadelphia: Lea & Febiger, 1991;307-356.
56. Nasisse MP. Feline ophthalmology. In: Gelatt KN, ed. *Veterinary ophthalmology*, 2nd ed. Philadelphia: Lea & Febiger, 1991;529-575.
57. Crispin SM. Corneal dystrophies in small animals. *Vet Ann* 1982;22:298-310.
58. Bellhorn RW, Korte GE, Abrutyn D. Spontaneous corneal degeneration in the rat. *Lab Anim Sci* 1988;38:46-50.
59. Losco PE, Troup CM. Corneal dystrophy in Fischer 344 rats. *Lab Anim Sci* 1988;38:702-710.
60. Van Winkle TJ, Balk MW. Spontaneous corneal opacities in laboratory mice. *Lab Animal Sci* 1986;36:248-255.
61. Jampol LM, Axelrod A, Tessler H. Pathways of the eye's response to topical nitrogen mustard. *Invest Ophthalmol Vis Sci* 1976;15:486-489.
62. Butler JM, Unger WG, Hammond BR. Sensory mediation of the ocular response to neutral formaldehyde. *Exp Eye Res* 1979;28:577-589.
63. Unger WG, Perkins ES, Bass MS. The response of the rabbit eye to laser irradiation of the iris. *Exp Eye Res* 1974;19:367-377.
64. Stjernschantz J, von Dickhoff K, Oksala O, Seppa H. A study of the mechanism of ocular irritation following YAG laser capsulotomy in rabbits. *Exp Eye Res* 1986;43:641-651.
65. Bito LZ, Klein EM. The unique sensitivity of the rabbit eye to x-ray-induced ocular inflammation. *Exp Eye Res* 1981;33:403-412.
66. Eakins KE. Prostaglandin and non-prostaglandin mediated breakdown of the blood aqueous barrier. *Exp Eye Res* 1977;suppl.483-498.
67. Bhattacherjee P, Paterson CA. Inflammatory mediators in models of immunogenic and non-immunogenic inflammation of the anterior segment of the eye. In: Bazan NG, ed. *Lipid mediators in eye inflammation*. Basel: Karger, 1990;65-82.
68. Millichamp NJ, Dziezyc J. Mediators of ocular inflammation. *Prog Vet Comp Ophthalmol* 1991;1:41-58.
69. Stjernschantz J, Geijer C, Bill A. Electrical stimulation of the fifth cranial nerve in rabbits: effects on ocular blood flow, extravascular albumin content and intraocular pressure. *Exp Eye Res* 1979;28:229-238.
70. Bill A, Stjernschantz J, Mandahl A, Brodin E, Nilsson G. Substance P: release on trigeminal nerve stimulation effects in the eye. *Acta Physiol Scand* 1979;106:371-373.
71. Stjernschantz J, Sears M, Mishima H. Role of substance P in the antidromic vasodilation, neurogenic plasma extravasation and disruption of the blood-aqueous barrier in the rabbit eye. *Arch Pharm* 1982;321:329-335.
72. Raviola G. The structural basis of the blood-ocular barriers. *Exp Eye Res* 1977;suppl:27-63.
73. Kozart DM. Light and electron microscopic study of regional morphologic differences in the processes of the ciliary body in the rabbit. *Invest Ophthalmol Vis Sci* 1968;7:15-33.
74. Smelser GK, Pei YK. Cytological basis of protein leakage into the eye following paracentesis. An electron microscopic study. *Invest Ophthalmol Vis Sci* 1965;4:249-263.

75. Ohnishi Y, Tanaka M. Effects of pilocarpine and paracentesis on occluding junctions between the nonpigmented ciliary epithelial cells. *Exp Eye Res* 1981;32:635–647.
76. Bartels SP, Pederson JE, Gaasterland DE, Armaly MF. Sites of breakdown of the blood aqueous barrier after paracentesis of the rhesus monkey eye. *Invest Ophthalmol Vis Sci* 1979;18:1050–1060.
77. Szalay J, Nunziata B, Henkind P. Permeability of the iridal blood vessels. *Exp Eye Res* 1991;21:531–543.
78. Unger WG, Cole DF, Hammond B. Disruption of the blood-aqueous barrier following paracentesis in the rabbit. *Exp Eye Res* 1975;20:255–270.
79. Raviola G. Effects of paracentesis on the blood-aqueous barrier: an electron microscope study on *Macaca mulatta* using horseradish peroxidase as a tracer. *Invest Ophthalmol Vis Sci* 1974;13:828–858.
80. Klein EM, Bito LZ. Species variations in the pathophysiologic responses of vertebrate eyes to a chemical irritant, nitrogen mustard. *Invest Ophthalmol Vis Sci* 1983;24:184–191.
81. Bito LZ. A physiological approach to glaucoma management: the use of local hormones and the pharmacokinetics of prostaglandin esters. *Prog Clin Biol Res* 1989;312:329–347.
82. Unger WG, Terenghi G, Ghatei MA, Butler JM, Polak JM, Bloom SR. Calcitonin gene-related polypeptide as a mediator of the neurogenic ocular injury response. *J Ocul Pharmacol* 1985;1:185–195.
83. Oksala O, Stjernschantz J. Effects of calcitonin gene-related peptide in the eye. *Invest Ophthalmol Vis Sci* 1988;29:1006–1011.
84. Oksala O. Effects of calcitonin gene-related peptide and substance P on regional blood flow in the cat eye. *Exp Eye Res* 1988;47:283–289.
85. Bito LZ, Nichols PR, Baroody RA. A comparison of the miotic and inflammatory effects of biologically active polypeptides and prostaglandin E_2 on the rabbit eye. *Exp Eye Res* 1982;34:325–337.
86. Bhattacherjee P, Paterson CA. Further investigation into the ocular effects of prostaglandin E_2, leukotriene B_4 and formyl-methionyl-leucyl phenylalanine. *Exp Eye Res* 1990;51:93–96.
87. Bhattacherjee P. Release of prostaglandin-like substances by *Shigella* endotoxin and its inhibition by nonsteroidal anti-inflammatory compounds. *Br J Pharmacol* 1975;54:489–494.
88. Fleisher LN, McGahan MC. Time course for prostaglandin synthesis by rabbit lens during endotoxin-induced ocular inflammation. *Curr Eye Res* 1986;5:629–634.
89. Csukas S, Paterson CA, Brown K, Bhattacherjee P. Time course of rabbit ocular inflammatory response and mediator release after intravitreal endotoxin. *Invest Ophthalmol Vis Sci* 1990;31:382–387.
90. Herbort CP, Okumura A, Mochizuki M. Endotoxin-induced uveitis in the rat. *Graefes Arch Clin Exp Ophthalmol* 1988;226:553–558.
91. Regnier A, Whitley RD, Benard P, Bonnefoi M. Effect of flunixin meglumine on the breakdown of the blood-aqueous barrier following paracentesis in the canine eye. *J Ocul Pharmacol* 1986;2:165–170.
92. Krohne SDG, Vestre WA. Effects of flunixin meglumine and dexamethasone on aqueous protein values after intraocular surgery in the dog. *Am J Vet Res* 1987;48:420–422.
93. Millichamp NJ, Dziezyc JD, Rohde BH, Chiou GCY, Smith WB. Acute effects of anti-inflammatory drugs in Nd:YAG laser induced uveitis in the dog. *Am J Vet Res* 1991;52:1279–1284.
94. Dziezyc J, Millichamp NJ, Keller CK, Smith WB. The effect of $PGF_{2\alpha}$ and LTD4 on pupil size, intraocular pressure and blood-aqueous barrier in the dog. *Am J Vet Res* 1991;in press.
95. Bito LZ, Camras CB, Gum GG, Resul B. The ocular hypotensive effects and side effects of prostaglandins on the eyes of experimental animals. *Prog Clin Biol Res* 1989;312:349–365.
96. Verbey NL, Van Delft JL, Van Haeringen NJ, Braquet P. Platelet-activating factor and laser trauma to the iris. *Invest Ophthalmol Vis Sci* 1989;30:1101–1103.
97. Bussolino F, Carenini AB, Carenini BB, Arese P. Platelet-activating factor and cytokines mediate and amplify the inflammatory response at site of microvascular injury. In: Bazan NG, ed. *Lipid mediators in eye inflammation*. Basel: Karger, 1990;130–148.
98. Rubin RM, Rosenbaum JT. The role of platelet activating factor in ocular inflammation. In: Handley DA, Saunders RN, Houlihan WJ, et al., eds. *Platelet-activating factor in endotoxin and immune diseases*. New York: Marcel Dekker, 1990;189–205.
99. Rubin RM, Rosenbaum T. Platelet-activating factor antagonist inhibits interleukin 1-induced inflammation. *Biochem Biophys Res Commun* 1988;154:429–436.

100. Rosenbaum JT, Howes E Jr, Rubin RM, Samples JR. Ocular inflammatory effects of intravitreally injected tumor necrosis factor. *Am J Pathol* 1988;133:47-53.
101. Fleisher LN, Ferrell JB, McGahan MC. Ocular inflammatory effects of intravitreally injected tumor necrosis factor-alpha and endotoxin. *Inflammation* 1990;14:325-335.
102. Bhattacherjee P, Eakins KE, Hammond B. Chemotactic activity of arachidonic acid lipoxygenase products in the rabbit eye. *Br J Pharmacol* 1980;73:254P-255P.
103. Bhattacherjee P, Hammond B, Salmon JA, Stepney R, Eakins KE. Chemotactic response to some arachidonic acid lipoxygenase products in the rabbit eye. *Eur J Pharmacol* 1981;73:21-28.
104. Stjernschantz J, Sherk T, Borgeat P, Sears M. Intraocular effects of lipoxygenase pathway products in arachidonic acid metabolism. *Acta Ophthalmol* 1984;62:104-111.
105. Bhattacherjee P, Henderson B. Ocular responses to interleukin-1 injected into the anterior chamber of the rabbit. *Invest Ophthalmol Vis Sci* 1987;28(suppl):200.
106. Kulkarni PS, Srinivasan BD. Cachectin: a novel polypeptide induces uveitis in the rabbit eye. *Exp Eye Res* 1988;46:631-633.
107. Havener HA. *Ocular pharmacology*. St. Louis: Mosby, 1966.
108. Bito LZ. A physiologic approach to the development of new drugs for glaucoma. *Ophthalmol Clin North Am* 1989;2:65-76.
109. Camras CB, Bito LZ. The pathophysiological effects of nitrogen mustard on the rabbit eye. I. The biphasic intraocular pressure response and the role of prostaglandins. *Exp Eye Res* 1980;30:41-52.
110. Camras CB, Bito LZ, The pathophysiological effects of nitrogen mustard on the rabbit eye. II. The inhibition of the initial hypertensive phase by capsaicin and the apparent role of substance P. *Invest Ophthalmol Vis Sci* 1980;19:423-428.
111. Tachado SD, Akhtar RA, Yousufzai SYK, Abdel-Latif AA. Species differences in the effects of substance P on inositol triphosphate accumulation and cyclic AMP formation, and on contraction in isolated iris sphincter of the mammalian eye: differences in receptor density. *Exp Eye Res* 1991;53:729-739.
112. Ambache N. Properties of irin, a physiological constituent of the rabbit's eye. *J Physiol* 1957;135:114-132.
113. Ambache N, Kavanagh L, Whiting J. Effect of mechanical stimulation on rabbits' eyes: release of active substance in anterior chamber perfusates. *J Physiol* 1965;176:378-408.
114. Ambache N, Kavanagh L, Whiting J. Some differences in uveal reactions between cats and rabbits. *J Physiol* 1990;182:110-130.
115. Eakins KE, Whitelocke RAF, Perkins ES. Release of prostaglandins in ocular inflammation in the rabbit. *Nature* 1972;239:248-249.
116. Waitzman MB, King CD. Prostaglandin influences on intraocular pressure and pupil size. *Am J Physiol* 1967;212:329-334.
117. Beitch BR, Eakins KE. The effects of prostaglandins on the intraocular pressure of the rabbit. *Br J Pharmacol* 1969;37:158-167.
118. Yousufzai SYK, Chen A-L, Abdel-Latif AA. Species differences in the effects of prostaglandins on inositol triphosphate accumulation, phosphatidic acid formation, myosin light chain phosphorylation and contraction of iris sphincter of the mammalian eye: interaction with the cyclic AMP system. *J Pharmacol Exp Ther* 1988:247:1064-1072.
119. Yousufzai SYK, Tachado SD, Abdel-Latif AA. Species differences in the effects of leukotriene D4 on inositol trisphosphate accumulation, cyclic AMP formation and contraction in iris sphincter of the mammalian eye. *Prostaglandins* 1990;39:227-240.
120. Bito LZ, Draga A, Blanco J, Camras CB. Long-term maintenance of reduced intraocular pressure by daily or twice daily topical application of prostaglandins to cat or rhesus monkey eyes. *Invest Ophthalmol Vis Sci* 1983;24:312-319.
121. Bito LZ, Baroody RA, Miranda OC. Eicosanoids as a new class of ocular hypotensive agents. 1. The apparent therapeutic advantages of derived prostaglandins of the A and B type as compared with primary prostaglandins on the E, F, and D type. *Exp Eye Res* 1987;44:825-837.
122. Miranda OC, Bito LZ. The putative and demonstrated miotic effects of prostaglandins in mammals. *Prog Clin Biol Res* 1989;312:171-195.
123. Kulkarni PS, Srinivasan BD. The effect of intravitreal and topical prostaglandins on intraocular inflammation. *Invest Ophthalmol Vis Sci* 1982;23:383-392.
124. Unger WG, Butler JM. Neuropeptides in the uveal tract. *Eye* 1988;2:S202-S212.
125. Hayashi MT, Miranda OC, Bito LZ, Baroody RA. Specific, non-specific, direct, and indirect miotic effects of prostaglandins (PGs). *Invest Ophthalmol Vis Sci* 1986;27(suppl):248.(abstract)

126. Camras CB, Podos SM, Rosenthal JS, Lee P-Y, Severin CH. Multiple dosing of prostaglandin $F_{2\alpha}$ or epinephrine on cynomolgus monkey eyes. 1. Aqueous humor dynamics. *Invest Ophthalmol Vis Sci* 1987;28:463-469.
127. Crawford K, Kaufman PL, Gabelt BT. Effects on topical PGF2a on aqueous humor dynamics in cynomolgus monkeys. *Curr Eye Res* 1987;6:1035-1044.
128. Lee P, Podos SM, Severin C. Effect of prostaglandin $F_{2\alpha}$ on aqueous humor dynamics of rabbit, cat, and monkey. *Invest Ophthalmol Vis Sci* 1984;25:1087-1093.
129. Camras CB, Miranda OC. The putative role of prostaglandins in surgical miosis. *Prog Clin Biol Res* 1989;312:197-210.
130. Soloway MR, Stjernschantz J, Sears M. The miotic effect of substance P on the isolated rabbit iris. *Invest Ophthalmol Vis Sci* 1981;20:47-52.
131. Unger WG, Tighe J. The response of the isolated iris sphincter pupillary muscle to substance P. *Exp Eye Res* 1984;39:677-684.
132. Abdel-Latif AA, Yousufzai SYK, Tachado SD. Differential effects of PGF2α, PGA2, LTD_4, and substance P on formation of cAMP and IP_3 and on contraction in iris sphincters of different mammalian species. *Invest Ophthalmol Vis Sci* 1990;31(suppl):247.
133. Anderson JA, Malfroy B, Richard NR, Hernandez EV, Lucas C, Binder PS. Substance P contracts the human iris sphincter, a response regulated by endogenous enkephalinase. *Invest Ophthalmol Vis Sci* 1989;30(suppl):269.
134. Bill A. Blood circulation and fluid dynamics in the eye. *Pharmacol Rev* 1975;55:383-417.
135. Barrie KP, Gum GG, Gelatt KN. Morphological studies of uveoscleral outflow in normotensive and glaucomatous beagles with fluorescein labelled dextran. *Am J Vet Res* 1985;46:89-97.
136. Tripathi RC. Comparative physiology and anatomy of the aqueous outflow pathway. In: Favson H, Graham LT, eds. *The eye*, vol 5. New York: Academic Press, 1974;163.
137. Kaufman PL, Crawford K, Gabelt BT. The effects of prostaglandins on aqueous humor dynamics. *Ophthalmol Clin North Am* 1989;2:141-150.
138. Millichamp NJ, Dziezyc JD. Control of the ocular irritative response in the dog: a comparison of flunixin meglumine and flurbiprofen. *Am J Vet Res* 1991;52:1452-1455.
139. Eakins KE. Increased intraocular pressure produced by prostaglandins PGE_1 and E_2 in the cat eye. *Exp Eye Res* 1970;10:87-92.
140. Kelly RGM, Starr MS. Effects of prostaglandins and a prostaglandin antagonist on intraocular pressure and protein in the monkey eye. *Can J Ophthalmol* 1971;6:205-211.
141. Wahlestedt C, Hakanson R, Beding B, Brodin E, Ekman R, Sundler F. Intraocular effects of CGRP, a neuropeptide in sensory nerves. In: Hakanson R, Sundler F, eds. *Tachykinin antagonists*. New York: Elsevier Science, 1985;137-146.
142. Oksala O, Stjernschantz J. Increase in outflow facility of aqueous humor in cats induced by calcitonin gene-related peptide. *Exp Eye Res* 1988;47:787-790.
143. Gelatt KN. The canine glaucomas. In: Gelatt KN, ed. *Veterinary ophthalmology*, 2nd ed. Philadelphia: Lea & Febiger, 1991;396-428.
144. Hanna BL, Swain PB, Sheppard B. Recessive buphthalmos in the rabbit. *Genetics* 1963;47:519-529.
145. Gum GG. Physiology of the eye. In: Gelatt KN, ed. *Veterinary ophthalmology*, 2nd ed. Philadelphia: Lea & Febiger, 1991;124-161.
146. Barnett KC, Noel PRB. The eye in general toxicity studies. In: Piggot PV, ed. *Evaluation of drug effects on the eye*. London: F.J. Parsons, 1968.
147. van Heyningen R. Experimental studies on cataract. *Invest Ophthalmol Vis Sci* 1976;15:685-697.
148. Taradach C, Regnier B, Perraud J. Eye lesions in Sprague-Dawley rats: types and incidence in relation to age. *Lab Anim* 1981;15:285-287.
149. Balazs T, Ohtake S, Noble JF. Spontaneous lenticular changes in the rat. *Lab Anim Sci* 1970;20:215.
150. Fraunfelder FT, Burns RP. Effect of lid closure in drug-induced experimental cataracts. *Arch Ophthalmol* 1966;76:599-601.
151. Kador PF, Fukui HN, Fukushi S, Jernigan HM, Kinoshita JH. Philly mouse: a new model of hereditary cataract. *Exp Eye Res* 1980;30:59-68.
152. Kuck JFR, Kuwabara T, Kuck KD. The Emory mouse cataract: an animal model for human senile cataract. *Curr Eye Res* 1981;1:643-649.
153. Russell P, Tsunematsu Y, Huang FL, Kinoshita JH. Tissue culture of lens epithelial cells from normal and Nakano mice. *Invest Ophthalmol Vis Sci* 1977;16:243-246.
154. Gelatt KN. The canine lens. In: Gelatt KN, ed. *Veterinary Ophthalmology*, 2nd ed. Philadelphia: Lea & Febiger, 1991;429-460.

155. Curtis R, Barnett KC. A survey of cataracts in golden and Labrador retrievers. *J Small Animal Pract* 1989;30:277-286.
156. Yakely WL. A study of hereditary cataracts in the American cocker spaniel. *J Am Vet Med Assoc* 1978;172:814.
157. Rubin LF. *Inherited eye diseases in purebred dogs.* Baltimore: Williams & Wilkins, 1989.
158. Rubin LF. *Atlas of veterinary ophthalmoscopy.* Philadelphia: Lea & Febiger, 1974.
159. Bellhorn RW, Bellhorn MB, Swarm RL, Impellizzeri CW. Hereditary tapetal abnormality in the beagle. *Ophthalmic Res* 1975;7:250-260.
160. Weleber RG. Retinitis pigmentosa and allied disorders. In: Ryan SJ, Ogden TE, eds. *Retina*, vol 1. St. Louis: C.V. Mosby, 1989;299-420.
161. Bateman JB, Lang GE, Maumenee IH. Genetic metabolic disorders associated with retinal degenerations/dystrophies. In: Ryan SJ, Ogden TE, eds. *Retina*, vol. 1. St. Louis: C.V. Mosby, 1989;421-445.
162. Millichamp NJ. Retinal degeneration in the dog and cat. *Vet Clin North Am [Small Anim Prac]* 1990;20:799-835.
163. Lee RH, Lieberman BS, Hurwitz RL, Lolley RN. Phosphodiesterase-probes show distinct defects in rd mice and Irish Setter dog disorders. *Invest Ophthalmol Vis Sci* 1985;26:1569-1579.
164. Woodford BJ, Liu Y, Fletcher RT, et al. Cyclic nucleotide metabolism in inherited retinopathy in collies: a biochemical and histochemical study. *Exp Eye Res* 1982;34:703-714.
165. Aguirre GD, Acland GM. Variation in retinal degeneration phenotype inherited at the prcd locus. *Exp Eye Res* 1988;46:663-687.
166. Wetzel MG, Fahlman C, Maude MB, et al. Fatty acid metabolism in normal miniature poodles and those affected with progressive rod-cone degeneration (PRCD). *Prog Clin Biol Res* 1989;314:427-440.
167. Barnett KC, Curtis R. Autosomal dominant progressive retinal atrophy in Abyssinian cats. *J Hered* 1985;76:168-170.
168. Narfstrom K. Progressive retinal atrophy in the Abyssinian cat: clinical characteristics. *Invest Ophthalmol Vis Sci* 1985;26:193-200.
169. Aguirre GD, Laties A. Pigment epithelial dystrophy in the dog. *Exp Eye Res* 1976;23:247-256.
170. Sanyal S, De Ruiter A, Hawkins RK. Development and degeneration of retina in rds mutant mice: light microscopy. *J Comp Neurol* 1980;194:193-207.
171. Sidman R, Green M. Retinal degeneration in the mouse. Localization of the rd locus in linkage group XVII. *J Hered* 1965;56:23.
172. Dowling JE, Sidman RL. Inherited retinal dystrophy in the rat. *J Cell Biol* 1962;14:73-109.
173. Noell WK, Walker VS, Kang BS, Berman S. Retinal damage by light in rats. *Invest Ophthalmol Vis Sci* 1966;5:450-473.
174. O'Steen WK, Anderson KV, Shear CR. Photoreceptor degeneration in albino rats: dependency on age. *Invest Ophthalmol Vis Sci* 1974;13:334-339.
175. Hayes KC, Carey RE. Retinal degeneration associated with taurine deficiency in the cat. *Science* 1975;188:949-950.
176. Riis RC, Sheffy BE, Loew E, Kern TJ, Smith JS. Vitamin E deficiency retinopathy in dogs. *Am J Vet Res* 1981;42:74-86.
177. Rubin LF. Albino versus pigmented animals for ocular toxicity testing. *Lens Eye Toxic Res* 1990;7:221-230.
178. Creel D, O'Donnell FE Jr, Witkop CJ Jr. Visual system anomalies in human ocular albinos. *Science* 1978;201:931-933.
179. Balkema GW. Elevated dark-adapted thresholds in albino rodents. *Invest Ophthalmol Vis Sci* 1988;29:544-549.
180. Weidner C. The c-wave in the erg of albino rat. *Vision Res* 1976;16:753-763.
181. Graves A, Green DG, Fisher LJ. Light exposure can reduce selectively or abolish the c-wave of the albino rat electroretinogram. *Invest Ophthalmol Vis Sci* 1985;26:388-393.
182. Dodt E, Echte K. Dark and light adaptation in pigmented and white rat as measured by erg threshold. *J Neurophysiol* 1961;24:427-445.
183. Reuter JH. The electroretinogram of albino and pigmented rabbits. *Doc Ophthalmol* 1974;11:483.
184. Williams RH, Howard AG, Williams TP. Retinal damage in pigmented and albino rats exposed to low levels of cyclic light following a single mydriatic treatment. *Curr Eye Res* 1985;4:97-102.
185. Reiter RJ. Comparative effects of continual lighting and pinealectomy on the eyes, the harderian glands and reproduction in pigmented and albino rats. *Comp Biochem Physiol* 1973;44A:503.

186. Weisse I, Loosen H, Peil H. Age-related retinal changes—a comparison between albino and pigmented rats. *Lens Eye Toxic Res* 1990;7:717-739.
187. Potts AM. The reaction of uveal pigment *in vitro* with polycyclic compounds. *Invest Ophthalmol* 1964;3:405-416.
188. Havener WH. *Ocular pharmacology*, 5th ed. St. Louis: C.V. Mosby, 1983.
189. Butler WH, Ford GP, Newberne JW. A study of the effects of vigabrabin on the central nervous system and retina of Sprague Dawley and Lister-hooded rats. *Toxicol Pathol* 1987;15:143-148.
190. Kurtz SM, Kaump DH, Schardein JL, Roll DE, Reutner TF, Fisken RA. The effect of long-term administration of amopyroquin, a 4-aminoquinoline compound, on the retina of pigmented and nonpigmented laboratory animals. *Invest Ophthalmol* 1967;6:420.
191. Francois J, Maudgal MC. Experimental chloroquine keratopathy. *Am J Ophthalmol* 1965;60:459-464.
192. Rubin LF, Murchison TE, Barron CN. Chlorpromazine and the eye of the dog. A chronic study. *Exp Mol Pathol* 1970;13:111-117.
193. Kuhn H, Keller P, Kovacs E, Steiger A. Lack of correlation between melanin affinity and retinopathy in mice and cats treated with chloroquine or flunitrazepam. *Graefes Arch Clin Exp Ophthalmol* 1981;216:177-190.
194. Poynter D, Martin LE, Harrison C, Cook J. Affinity of labetalol for ocular melanin. *Br J Clin Pharmacol* 1976;3:711-720.
195. Howard RD, McDonald CJ, Dunn B, Creasey WA. Experimental chlorpromazine cataracts. *Invest Ophthalmol* 1969;8:413-421.

Ophthalmic Toxicology, edited by
George C. Y. Chiou. Raven Press, Ltd.,
New York © 1992.

4

In Vivo Eye Irritation Test Methods

Brooks H. Rohde

*Department of Medical Pharmacology and Toxicology,
and Institute of Ocular Pharmacology,
Texas A & M University College of Medicine,
College Station, Texas 77843*

DRAIZE TEST

Introduction

Although *in vitro* methods have been developed to replace the older *in vivo* methods, the Draize test and other *in vivo* methods are still the most widely used eye irritation tests for determining the safety of cosmetics, consumer products, pharmaceuticals, and industrial chemicals.

The need to test these products for eye irritation was made plain in the early 1930s, when an eyelash dye containing *p*-phenylene-diamine was brought into the United States market. It was soon discovered that this product developed supersensitivity in external structures of the eye, which could lead to corneal ulceration and vision loss (1). Reaction to and outrage at these occurrences led to the development of occular irritation test methods to predict eye irritation in humans. In 1944, Friedenwald and his associates (2) published a method using albino rabbits as test animals. This method was modified by Draize et al. (3) to provide an overall scoring system (Table 1). The Draize test has become the most widely used method for studying eye irritation since 1944; however, numerous other *in vivo* eye irritation tests have been developed to better test the eye irritation potential of different groups and types of chemicals (4–6).

The Draize test has several major problems: (a) Different people read the same response differently (7,8). It is difficult to standardize subjective readings even though two sets of standards have been published by the Food and Drug Administration (9) and Consumer Product Safety Commission (10) to provide guidance for comparison. (b) Different people use different methods to instill test materials into the eyes. Some researchers instill test materials into cul-de-sacs and then allow animals to blink and spread the material across the corneal surface, whereas others instill the test material directly onto the surface of the cornea. (c) Different people use

TABLE 1. *Scale of weighted scores for grading the severity of ocular lesions*

I. Cornea	
A. Opacity—degree of density (area that is most dense is taken for reading)	
Scattered or diffuse area—details of iris clearly visible	1
Easily discernible translucent areas, details of iris slightly obscured	2
Opalescent areas, no details of iris visible, size of pupil barely discernible	3
Opaque, iris invisible	4
B. Area of cornea involved	
One-quarter (or less) but not zero	1
Greater than one-quarter—less than one-half	2
Greater than one-half—less than three-quarters	3
Greater than three-quarters up to whole area	4
Score equals A × B × 5 Total maximum = 80	
II. Iris	
A. Values	
Folds above normal, congestion, swelling, circumcorneal injection (any one or all of these or combination of any thereof), iris still reacting to light (sluggish reaction is positive)	1
No reaction to light, hemorrhage; gross destruction (any one or all of these)	2
Score equals A × 5 Total maximum = 10	
III. Conjunctive	
A. Redness (refers to palpebral conjunctivae only)	
Vessels definitely injected above normal	1
More diffuse, deeper crimson red, individual vessels not easily discernible	2
Diffuse beefy red	3
B. Chemosis	
Any swelling above normal (includes nictitating membrane)	1
Obvious swelling with partial eversion of the lids	2
Swelling with lids about half closed	3
Swelling with lids about half closed to completely closed	4
C. Discharge	
Any amount different from normal (does not include small amount observed in inner canthus of normal animals)	1
Discharge with moistening of the lids and hairs just adjacent to the lids	2
Discharge with moistening of the lids and considerable area around the eye	3
Score (A × B × C) × 2 Total maximum = 20	

The maximum total score is the sum of all scores obtained for the cornea, iris, and conjunctivae. (Reproduced with permission from Draize et al., ref. 3.)

different experimental designs. As a result, it is difficult to compare results of one set of readings with another and comparisons can be very misleading.

The Draize test also poses logistic difficulties: large numbers of rabbits are necessary, making the tests very expensive; the tests are time-consuming; and there is today much popular pressure against putting rabbits through so much discomfort as the Draize test is believed to produce. Today, many rabbits are used to prove that potential nonirritants really are nonirritants *in vivo*. Skin tests are usually performed before eye irritation studies. If skin tests show irritation, then no eye tests will be carried out; the substance under study has already been proven an irritant. If skin tests show no effect or only a mild effect, then eye irritation tests will be done. Although substances that irritate the skin are almost certain to irritate the eyes, there is always the possibility that substances having little or no effect on the skin will be anomalously irritating to the eyes. As an example, soaps and shampoos may irritate the eyes but not the skin; they must be tested to assure that they are not so dangerous and inflammatory that they cannot be marketed. Unfortunately, the popular image (almost never accurate today) is of a rabbit having its eyes burned out with a strong corrosive, held immobile while racked with pain. The populists play up the tragedy of a blinded rabbit, though most rabbits are terminated right after their test is completed.

Typical Draize tests are done with rabbits, because rabbit eyes are probably most sensitive to irritations and because rabbits are the cheapest lab animal with large eyes. However, this introduces still another problem: interspecies differences between rabbits and humans (11,12). The two cannot always be directly compared. To bridge the information gap between rabbits and humans, monkeys are occasionally used to obtain the data for comparison with rabbit data and human data (4). Monkeys are much more expensive and difficult to obtain, maintain, and handle than rabbits.

In this chapter various *in vivo* protocols are presented with emphasis placed on different parts of eye tissues, including the whole eye, conjunctiva, cornea, tearing, muscle movement, ocular blood circulation, lens, retina, and skin. Readers are encouraged to read excellent reviews by Gad and Ghengelis (13), Ballantyne and Swanston (14), McDonald and coworkers (15,16), and Chan and Hayes (17).

Rabbit Experiments

Albino rabbits are typically used for Draize eye-mucosa toxicity studies (3-6). The test substance is instilled in one eye; the other eye is treated with vehicle and serves as a control. Normally a series of nine rabbits is used to test one substance. In the first three subjects, the treated eyes remain unwashed. In the second three subjects, the eyes are instilled with the test substance and 2 sec later are washed with 20 ml of lukewarm water. In the last three subjects, the treated eyes are washed with lukewarm water 4 sec after instillation of the test substance.

Ocular reactions are read either with the unaided eye or with the aid of a slit lamp. Readings are typically made 1 hr after the test substance is applied, then after 1, 2, 3, 4, and 7 days, and as long as the lesion persists. A preparation that has elicited corneal and iris lesions that have not cleared by the 7th day is considered a severe eye irritant. The cornea is scored on the basis of the sensitivity of the opacity and the total area involved. The iris is scored on the intensity or degree of inflammation exhibited, and the palpebral and bulbar mucosae are scored on the extent of the chemosis, redness, and discharge. This method has been used widely to study the eye irritation of common household products such as shampoos (18).

Attempts have also been made to evaluate eye irritation with an objective method by using fluorescein (19). The eyes of healthy rabbits are examined with fluorescein before testing and only those eyes showing no preexisting lesions are used. The test contains two phases separated by 6 months. The rabbits are tested and scored clinically in the first phase. In the second phase, in addition to the clinical examination of the cornea, swelling is measured with the transducer of an ultrasonic pachometer. The undiluted test substance is instilled into one eye of each animal while the other eye serves as a blank. The eyes are not washed after administration of the test solution. The eyes are examined and the grade of ocular irritation is recorded at 4 hr and at 1, 2, 3, 4, and 7 days.

Erythema, chemosis, iritis, and corneal opacity are scored according to the Draize scores (5). Corneal swelling (expressed as the percent of corneal swelling; %CS) is calculated according to the formula:

$$\%CS = \left(\frac{\text{corneal thickness at time t}}{\text{corneal thickness at time 0}} - 1 \right) \times 100\%$$

Ocular lesions were considered to be corrosive if the mean scores for corneal opacity (limit score of 4), erythema (limit score of 3), or chemosis (limit score of 4) were equal to or greater than the limit scores.

Monkey Experiments

Based on the idea that the eyes of animals more closely related to humans could more accurately predict human ocular responses to irritant, the ocular responses of rhesus monkeys have been studied (4,20). These results were compared to observations made in rabbits and humans. The compounds instilled into the eyes of rabbits, rhesus monkeys, and human volunteers were a soap suspension (5%) and an experimental all-purpose liquid household cleaner.

To minimize self-trauma in the rabbits, a polyethylene cap was fitted over the head and eyes. The monkeys were placed in restraining boxes so that only the head protruded. They were fed and watered by hand and were not removed during the observation period. Male adult volunteers (ages 23 to 40) were used to gather human data.

In all three species, 0.1 ml of each test material was instilled directly onto the cornea without washing afterward (humans were allowed to wash their eyes 1 to 2 min after instillation). One eye of each subject served as a control. A Zeiss slit-lamp biomicroscope was used for pretest examination of all subjects. The animal subjects were graded according to the Draize system (3). Examinations were also performed at 1 hr and 6 hr postinstillation and daily thereafter. For humans, examination was made at 15 min, 1 hr, 4 or 6 hr, and 24 hr postinstillation. The eyes were stained with fluorescein-impregnated papers for the examinations. Scores were given according to a system more accurate than the Draize test (21). The results were encouraging. Similarities between the reactions in monkeys and humans, which were much closer to each other than either human or monkey reactions were to rabbit reactions, suggest the usefulness of utilizing nonhuman primates in irritation studies.

Similar experiments were also run by Swanston (21). Rabbit, monkey, and human ocular reaction to the instillation of a 5% soap solution and a liquid household cleaner were graded and compared according to a scoring system based on the use of slit-lamp biomicroscopy and fluorescein, and also according to the commonly used Draize visual observation method (3).

Reactions in monkeys were more comparable to human reactions than were those seen in rabbits, based on biomicroscopic observations. Instillation of a 5% soap solution into rabbits' eyes produced almost no corneal epithelium effect. The same material caused corneal epithelial damage to both monkeys and humans. These lesions were not, however, visible without the use of slit-lamp biomicroscopy and/or fluorescein. The detergent composition used for these studies did produce irritation in all three species. However, in this study of the degree of human response predicted by the rabbit studied was much greater than that predicted by the monkey data, which again was more accurate in predicting the nature of the human hazard.

LACRIMATION AND PAIN

Tear gas causes excessive tearing and irritation of the eye tissues mainly because it contains o-chlorobenzylidine malononitrile (CBM), which causes burning, blepharospasm, and excessive lacrimation in the eye. In this study, animals were used to assess the likelihood of damage caused by CBM as a solid, in solution, and as a smoke (22,23). Tear gas is an unusual toxic chemical because it is one that may be deployed intentionally against humans by agents who wish them to recover alive and uninjured when the gas has cleared; it is considered nonlethal force. Its use is very different from that of toxic nerve gas, pesticides, herbicides, and other such nasty concoctions.

Ocular Irritation Tests

Ocular irritation tests were conducted with solutions, solid powders, and smokes of CBM (22). Solutions containing 0.5%, 1%, 2%, and 10% (wt/vol) CBM were used, each one on ten rabbits. Each solution (0.1 ml) was instilled into the conjunctival sac of the right eye and the lids gently held together for a few seconds. Eyes were examined at 10 min, 1 hr, and up to 45 days later. This study highlights another limitation of these experiments: keeping large numbers of rabbits alive and keeping their numbers and data straight for relatively long periods of time.

Four groups of ten rabbits had solid CBM applied to one eye. The groups were treated with 0.5, 1, 2, and 5 mg solid CBM. Finely powdered material was blown into the conjunctival sacs using Pasteur pipettes. Rabbits were examined at 10 min, 1 hr, and daily for 7 days.

Ten rabbits were exposed for 15 min to the pyrotechnic effluent from CBM grenades contained in a 10-m^3 chamber. The grenades contained 25% CBM, 30% potassium chlorate, 30% lactose, and 15% kaolin. The chamber atmosphere was measured at 1-min intervals for its CBM content. The CBM was trapped on a glass fiber pad and was subsequently eluted from the pad with hydrochloric acid in ethanol.

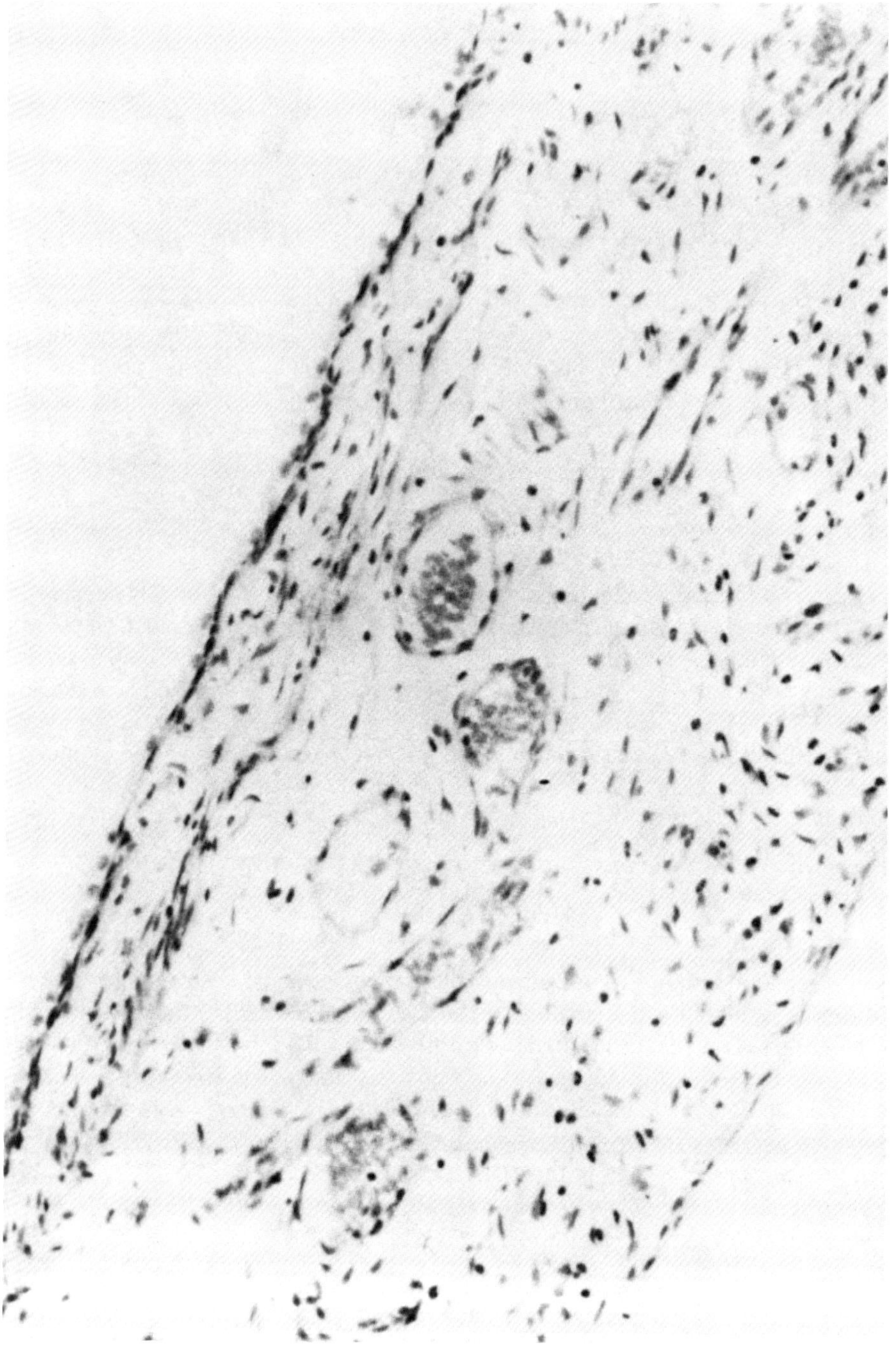

FIG. 1. Photomicrograph of the iris of an eye removed from a rabbit 3 days after 0.1 ml of 10% o-chlorobenzylidine malononitrile (CBM) in polyethylene glycol 300 had been applied to the surface of the eye. There is congestion with a neutrophil infiltration of the stroma. Hematoxylin and eosin ×294. (Reproduced with permission from Ballantyne et al., ref. 22.)

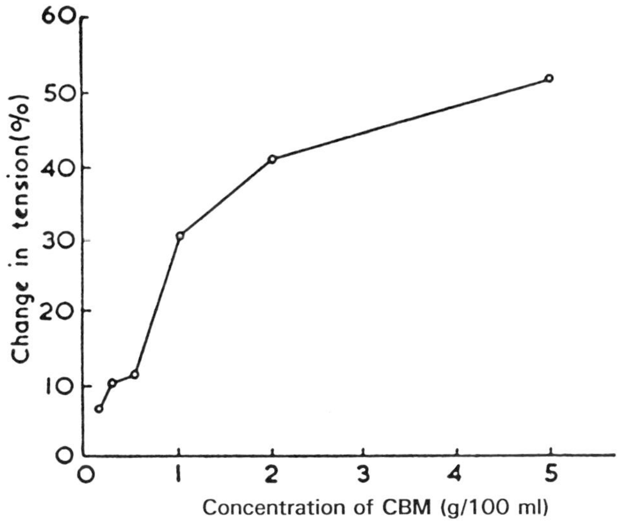

FIG. 2. Effects of different concentrations of o-chlorobenzylidine malononitrile (CBM) applied to the eye in polyethylene glycol 300, on intraocular tension and irritation. (Reproduced with permission from Ballantyne et al., ref. 22.)

The concentration was estimated spectroscopically. Rabbits were examined periodically for 1 week. This is the closest model to human exposure.

A few animals were sacrificed with sodium pentobarbitone while macroscopic lesions were present, but most were sacrificed at the ends of the periods of observation. The eyes were removed, fixed in phosphate-buffered neutral nitrocellulose, and 10-μm sections stained with hematoxylin and eosin.

In the scoring of the effects of CBM on the eye, particular attention was paid to the effects listed in Table 2. A six-point scale was used: 0, no effect; 1, just detectable effect; 2, mild effect; 3, moderate effect; 4, marked effect; and 5, severe effect with complications. Figure 1 shows iritis after CMB exposure. The relationship between the concentration of CBM in polyethylene glycol applied to the eye and the rise in intraocular tension is shown in Fig. 2 (22).

Tear Flow

For the study of tear flow, two dosage schemes were used: (a) in the "worst-case condition" a large eyedrop of full-strength material was used; and (b) in the graded stimuli, the volume or concentration of the eyedrop was controlled and the contact time of the CBM was varied. Since the small drop with a high concentration of the chemical would be diluted more by the tear fluid, it would be better to use a larger drop of known concentration to obtain more consistent data. It should be noted that it

TABLE 2. *Details of the system for scoring various effects on the rabbit eye*

Effect	Grade	Observation
Lachrymation	0	Normal
	1	Slight excess at lower tarsal margin
	2	Slight wetting of periorbital hair
	3	Obvious wetting of lid margins and periorbital hair
	4	Gross wetting of periorbital hair
	5	Gross wetting of hair with fluid running down the face
Blepharitis	0	Eyelids normal
	1	Slight reddening of lid margins
	2	Diffuse redness and slight swelling of lid margins
	3	Diffuse bright redness with moderate thickening of lids
	4	Diffuse bright redness with marked thickening and deformity of lids
	5	Diffuse bright redness with marked thickening and irregular deformity of lid margins and decreased palpebral fissure
Chemosis	0	No swelling of conjunctivae or nictitating membrane
	1	Minimal swelling without eversion of lids
	2	Moderate swelling with slight eversion of lids
	3	Moderate swelling with moderate eversion of lids and swollen tissues encroaching over periphery of cornea
	4	Marked swelling and eversion with tissues almost completely obliterating the cornea
	5	Gross swelling and eversion of lids and complete obliteration of cornea
Congestion of conjunctivae and nictitating membrane	0	Vessels normal
	1	A few injected vessels
	2	Diffuse and moderate dilation of blood vessels
	3	Diffuse and marked dilation, but individual vessels still discernible
	4	Diffuse and gross dilation with individual vessels barely discernible
	5	Diffuse intense redness with no discernible vessels
Sloughing	0	Absent
	1	Patchy detachment of film
	2	Diffuse detachment of fine membrane
	3	Diffuse detachment of film with slight contamination of lachrymal fluid
	4	Obvious stripping of membrane with moderate contamination of lachrymal fluid
	5	Gross detachment of membrane and gross contamination of lachrymal fluid
Iritis	0	Normal iris
	1	Slight injection of blood vessels of iris
	2	Slight thickening of folds with moderate injection but still reacting to light
	3	Moderate thickening of folds with diffuse moderate congestion and slight reduction in response to light
	4	Diffuse and gross erythema with obvious thickening and a sluggish reaction to light
	5	No reaction to light, distorted pupil, gross inflammatory change with hemorrhages
Keratitis	0	Normal cornea
	1	Just detectable haziness of cornea
	2	Obvious opacity of cornea (local or general) but iris clearly visible

TABLE 2. Continued

Effect	Grade	Observation
Keratitis (cont.)	3	Local of general opacity of cornea almost obscuring vision of the iris
	4	Local or general opacity of cornea totally obscuring the iris
	5	Gross opacification of cornea with deformity and/or ulceration
Vascularization of cornea	0	Avascular
	1	Localized ingrowth of vessels for 1 to 2 mm
	2	Generalized ingrowth of vessels for 1 to 2 mm
	3	Generalized ingrowth of vessels for 3 to 4 mm
	4	Ingrowth of vessels to within 1 to 2 mm of center of cornea, but without confluence
	5	Complete vascularization of cornea with confluence of vessels at center of cornea.

(Reproduced with permission from Ballantyne et al., ref. 22.)

is generally the concentration of the drug, but not the total quantity of the drug, that is instilled into the eyes that determines the responses of the eye tissues.

In addition to chemical concentration and eyedrop volume, the dose should also be considered in terms of the kinetics of the chemical in the tear film expressed as contact time. The contact time was measured by instilling a microdrop of fluorescein into the cul-de-sacs of the eyes, and measuring the change of fluorescein concentration by tear fluid with a fluorophotometer.

There were two situations involving tearing: (a) the eyedrop was not irritating and tears did not disturb the normal tear flow; and (b) the eyedrop was irritating to the eyes and resulted in a rapid rate of tear flow. In the first case, in the stimulated eye the fluorescein concentration in the eyedrops decreased exponentially with time, approximately ten fold in 10 min. In the second case, in the stimulated eye the fluorescein in the cul-de-sac was washed out instantaneously. Therefore, when a lower dose of irritating substance was given, it paradoxically caused much greater exposure than high doses since the higher dose toxin was washed out instantaneously, whereas the low dose toxin remained in the eye for several minutes.

Blinking also caused faster loss of the substance instilled into the eyes. To avoid blinking, eyes of a completely anesthetized rabbit could be used. In this case a known amount of eyedrops could be instilled into the cul-de-sac for a known period of time before washing it out. Use of an anesthetized rabbit is more humane when using something that is very irritating.

Pain Alleviation

The substances tested in animal eyes can be divided into three groups; desirable responses to these may or may not include pain. The groups are (a) household or industrial chemicals—pain and lacrimation are desirable for flushing these out; (b) therapeutic drugs—pain is not desirable because of reduced effect and reduced patient compliance; and (c) cosmetics, including shampoos—pain is unwanted.

The threshold of pain in humans is considerably lower than that in rabbits. Therefore, in comparing uncontrolled drops of toxin (as in the Draize test), there may be a hundredfold or a thousandfold less exposure in the human eye than in the rabbit eye. There are two stages of pain response: (a) acute stinging and pain, and (b) chronic soreness. Rabbits should not be allowed to progress to advanced stages of ulceration, even though these stages presumably produce no pain.

Local anesthesia should be made routine. The problem of this interfering with responses to toxicity can be avoided. Although anesthesia could interfere with tearing, relying on comparisons of human and rabbit tearing is not wise in any case. Controlled exposure to the toxin is better. Although anesthetics produce greater permeability of the epithelium, this seems to be the case primarily when dealing with extremely (and unnecessarily) high concentrations.

It has been suggested that antihistamines rather than anesthetics should be used to alleviate pain. However, this would interfere in the inflammatory processes being studied. There is also no evidence that antihistamines actually reduce pain in the cornea.

Pain Testing

Two types of experiments can be performed to test the painfulness of potential toxins. In the first type, the substance is instilled full strength into the eye and painfulness is measured from the animal's reaction. In the second type, dilutions of the agent are gradually increased until a definite mild response is evoked (for example, a full blink). The second way is probably more precise as well as more humane. However, the first method is closer to the way humans accidentally get chemicals and agents in their eyes. Oven cleaners and shampoos are packaged in full strength. Testing the pain threshold by electrophysiological techniques is another possibility. In the future, excitable nerve axons may be grown *in vitro* and their responses measured. Another possibility would be to measure the membrane potential of cultured neuroblasts or neuroblastoma cells, both resting and stimulated, and then adding chemicals to the medium to see how these affect membrane potential and membrane responses to stimulation. This is *in vitro* toxicology, and not strictly ocular toxicology, though eye irritants could be easily tested with this system.

EYE MOVEMENTS

Saccadic Eye Movement

Ocular toxicology can be manifest not only as pain, irritation, and loss of vision, but as dysfunction of the muscles of eye movement or of accommodation, which also leads to impairment of vision. Eye movements can be used to determine the toxic effects of certain chemicals on the eye, particularly those that paralyze muscle movements. Because fine muscle movement, such as eye and face muscles, is more sensitive to muscle paralyzing agents than is coarse muscle movement (such as the limbs and trunk), this is a good *in vivo* model for studying toxic effects of chemicals on the eye.

This research has been carried out on human subjects (24). Following a 3- to 5-hr fast, subjects were fitted with a special pair of eyeglass frames on which were mounted two phototransistors and one infrared source, by which eye movements were monitored. The frame permitted the phototransistors to be closely positioned near the limbus on either side of the eye. The phototransistor outputs were differentially amplified to give a voltage output proportional to reflected infrared light, which gave an accurate indication of eye position. The subject's head rested in a modified ophthalmic examination device viewing an oscilloscope. The dot displayed on the oscilloscope served as the target and only took one of two positions on the screen during the course of the experiments. After calibrating the eye movement detector, data were taken. The target position and the eye position were continuously recorded on a two-channel strip chart recorder and also entered an averaging computer with histogram feature. Histograms of saccadic eye movement latency were computed, typically for between 25 and 100 responses in each histogram position.

Example

For a given subject, two to five histograms were collected under normal conditions (no drug). A prescribed quantity of alcohol was then given in a juice mixer, and consumed as rapidly as possible. Latency histograms were then repeatedly computed at 15-min intervals for periods of 3 to 5 hr following the administration of alcohol. Subjects were instructed to rest with eyes closed during intervals in the experiments.

In normal subjects, data showed the most common range for saccadic eye movement latency to be approximately 200 to 250 msec. The fastest times observed were on the order of 50 msec and the longest times were unbounded. There was therefore considerable variation in normal subjects. In all subjects tested, saccadic eye movement latency increased following administration of alcohol. In one typical subject, the control mean saccadic eye movement latency was 248 msec and the latency increased to 314 msec at maximum blood alcohol levels; this was a 34% increase. This procedure could be used to study the toxicity of other substances that affect eye movement and muscle coordination, and that may have undesirable effects on alertness and reaction time. Besides alcohol, many kinds of medication and drugs, both prescription and over-the-counter, are reported to have the side effect of drowsiness. Subjects taking these agents are cautioned against operating machinery or driving. This procedure could be a quick, noninvasive means of quantitating these side effects, which are of real relevance to leading a normal life in our society. Another potential test would be typing acuity and speed; a great many people now earn a living at a keyboard of some sort. Making and sometimes correcting errors greatly reduces efficiency. The procedure may be useful in screening new formulations and derivatives of drugs that are hoped to have fewer side effects.

Smooth Pursuit Eye Movements

This procedure tests the effects of toxins on a voluntary neurological function. A monocular eye movement monitor was used in this study (25). The experiment and data acquisition were under the control of a real-time computer. The computer presented a target stimulus on a horizontal axis. Each trial consisted of the subject tracking the target for approximately 1 min. Rest periods of 3 to 5 min were given between trials.

Subjects previously screened for normal oculomotor function were asked to come to the laboratory after a 12-hr fast. They were given a standard light lunch, and a control blood alcohol determination was made on a breath analyzer. The control data, which consisted of approximately ten tracking periods, was recorded in the next hour. This was followed by the oral administration of alcohol (2 ml/kg) as a commercially available liquor mixed with a soft drink or fruit juice. Subjects were given 20 min to drink. Fifteen minutes after drinking, the treatment data was collected over the next hour.

The model chosen for this study is shown in Fig. 3A. The model assumed that system output (eye position) was attempting to follow system input (target position) and that the error signal of position was being minimized by a negative feedback loop. A large portion of the output could be accounted for by the presence of a linear element Y (jw) in the forward path. The remaining portion of the output, ϕrr (jw) was

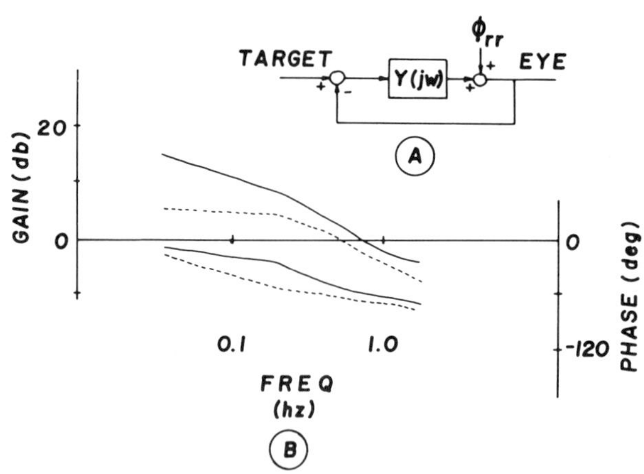

FIG. 3. A: Model of smooth pursuit eye movements, studied in human volunteers. **B:** Bode plot of smooth pursuit eye movements before (*solid*) and after (*dashed*) alcohol. The shift in the Bode plot is consistent with visual impairment produced by alcohol. (Reproduced with permission from Levitt and Jaeger, ref. 24.)

modeled as a noise signal added to the loop (Fig. 3A). This noise was referred to as a remnant. Both Y (jw) and ϕrr (jw) were determined by spectral analysis. Express Y (jw) as a Bode plot (Fig. 3B) shows the amplitude characteristics of the system as a function of frequency (the gain portion of the plot) and the temporal characteristics of the system as a function of frequency (the phase portion of the plot).

Example

The results of this study suggest a general pattern of response. This response indicates that between normal smooth pursuit movements and the saccadic pursuit movements of the severely intoxicated state, there exists a continuum of degraded smooth pursuit movements. A representative plot of Y (jw) in Fig. 3B illustrates one point in this continuum.

OCULAR MICROCIRCULATION

Eye irritants frequently cause vasodilation and increase in ocular circulation, which are not measured in the Draize test. Several techniques are available for the measurement of eye circulation including (a) the microsphere technique (26), (b) laser Doppler velocimetry (27,28), and (c) pulsatile blood flow measurement (29,30).

Microsphere Technique

The microsphere technique can be used to measure blood flow in all parts of the eye tissue (26). However, this technique can be used only for animal research as the animal must be sacrificed at the end of the experiment. Rabbits are anesthetized with pentobarbital. The left femoral artery is cannulated, and PE 90 surgical tubing is inserted into the left ventricle through the right carotid artery. Heparin is administered intravenously to prevent clotting. A bolus of strontium 85 (^{85}Sr)-labeled microspheres or colored microspheres (15.6 ± 0.8 μm sphere diameter) is injected in 0.2 ml saline plus 1% Tween 80 into the left ventricle. Approximately 1 million microspheres are administered. Blood is collected from the femoral artery for 60 sec immediately after injection of the microspheres. The rabbit is then sacrificed with an overdose of pentobarbital. The eyes are removed and dissected into iris, ciliary body, retina, and choroid. The tissues are weighed and, when using ^{85}Sr microspheres, their radioactivities are determined. When using colored microspheres, the number of microspheres in the digested tissues is counted under a microscope using a hemocytometer. The blood flow in the tissues is calculated using the rate of blood flow in the femoral artery and its radioactivity, or the number of colored microspheres, and expressed as μl/min/mg tissue.

Laser-Doppler Velocimetry

Laser-Doppler velocimetry is a relatively new technique for the measurement of retinal blood flow in conscious animals and patients. It is widely used in animal experiments (28) and in some clinics (27).

Although the procedure can be used on conscious animals, rabbits are usually anesthetized to eliminate eye movements. The femoral artery and vein are cannulated to monitor blood pressure through a pressure transducer and physiograph, and for injection of anesthetic and drugs. Drugs were injected in 1.5 ml saline; controls were injected with only saline. The beam of laser light from the laser-Doppler depends on the average velocity and cell density in the measured volume.

Pulsatile Blood Flow Method

The pulsatile blood flow measured with oculosphygmography is noninvasive and easily workable (29). Rabbits are placed in restraining boxes and a drop of tetracaine is applied to the cornea. Then a Langham pneumatic probe, a modified tonometer, with a special tip for rabbit corneal curvature is applied to the eye. It measures the quick pulsations in intraocular pressure produced by the flow of blood in the ocular vessels when pressure is applied to the eye. The probe is connected to a pressure transducer and a computer system that deduces ocular blood flow from the intraocular pressure fluctuations.

CORNEA

Measurement of Corneal Thickness with Pachometer

As foreign materials that enter the eye contact the cornea directly, the injury of the cornea can be used as a good indicator of the eye toxicity/irritancy of the foreign materials. One manifestation of corneal injury is thickening of the cornea. The swelling of the cornea by eye irritants can be measured with instruments, particularly with a Nikon model CS-2 slit-lamp microscope equipped with a Nikon pachometer (31,32). Healthy rabbits were used in this study. The corneal thickness of the untreated animals was measured; several hours later, the test substance (0.1 ml) was instilled in the lower conjunctival sac of the left eye of each rabbit. The right eye was the control. During observations, rabbits were restrained in canvas restraining bags with their heads exposed. The changes in the cornea, iris, conjunctiva and in corneal thickness were recorded on days 1, 2, 3, 4, 7, 10, 14, and 21 after dosing. The pachometer horizontally split the image into two halves. The convex edge of the lower image was aligned with the concave edge of the upper image. The amount of rotation required to align the images was proportional to the corneal thickness. Measurements were made as close to the apex as possible with the lamp perpendicular to the surface. Rabbits were anesthetized by injecting ketamine intramuscularly to sedate them just prior to measurement. Corneal swelling was expressed as:

$$\% \text{ swelling} = \left(\frac{\text{average corneal thickness (mm) on observation day}}{\text{average corneal thickness (mm) prior to intillation}} - 1 \right) \times 100\%$$

Example

Linear concentration-response relationships were obtained from seven alcohols using Draize scoring and percentage corneal swelling. The relationship between the ratio of corneal thickness (treated eye/untreated eye) and the duration of corneal cloudiness were also established by calculating correlation coefficients and slopes for each observation day. From these it was determined that maximum correlation and slope occurred on day 3 after treatment. Therefore, day 3 is the ideal day to use pachometry.

Measurement of Corneal Injury with Fluorescein Staining

Fluorescein Staining Time

Fluorescein is commonly used in ocular irritation studies to stain corneal epithelial defects. This study was undertaken to investigate fluorescein staining times that would eliminate or minimize staining of normal corneas (33). Male and female New Zealand albino rabbits were used. Biomicroscope examination revealed no corneal abnormalities in the rabbits chosen before treatment was started. Rabbits were divided into four groups and their corneas were exposed to fluorescein for 15 sec, 30 sec, 1 min, and 4 min; in this procedure 2% fluorescein sodium was instilled into the lower conjunctival sac of each eye. After exposure the eyes were flushed with sterile isotonic saline and examined with a slit lamp equipped with a cobalt filter. Drawings were made and the amount of staining was graded (0 = none, 1 = slight, 2 = moderate, and 3 = high). The eyes were examined daily for 2 weeks, and then the rabbits were anesthetized with ketamine. The right corneas of the rabbits were lightly scratched with a 20-gauge needle, exposed to fluorescein, and examined immediately and after another 48 hr. It was found that normal corneas exposed to fluorescein for 15 sec had the lowest average staining intensity scores. That means exposing eyes to fluorescein for 15 sec only will produce the lowest number of false-positive identifications of eye lesions.

Chemical Burns on the Cornea

Chemical burns on the cornea due to industrial chemicals are frequent occurrences in industrial plants. Understanding the cornea and eye irritancy of these chemicals is essential for treatment (34,35).

Eyes of normal rabbits were screened for lack of anomalies by exposing them to

5% aqueous fluorescein sodium for 20 sec and flushing with distilled water. After a 2-hr interval to allow eyes to return to normal, 0.005 ml of an undiluted test chemical was applied to the center of one cornea while the lids were retracted. After 1 min, the lids were released. The other eye served as a control. Eighteen to 24 hr later, the eyes were examined with a slit lamp for signs of irritation, then stained with fluorescein, and corneal injuries were scored. Some of the treated eyes were not washed following instillation of the test substance. Others were irrigated with tap water 20 sec after instillation (this mimics the industrial eyewash fountain). The eyes were examined for any immediate signs of discomfort after instillation of the test substance. Grading and scoring of ocular irritation was done according to the standard Draize grades (3). The eyes were examined and grades of ocular reaction were recorded at 1 hr, and 1, 2, 3, 4, and 7 days after exposure. If necessary, readings were taken on days 10 and 14. After all observations were recorded and photographed 1 day after exposure, all corneas were further examined with the aid of fluorescein sodium. The diagrams of the staining patterns of the corneal area were recorded. The Federal Hazardous Substances Act (FHSA) regulations were used to designate a test substance as an eye irritant. A classification scale of ocular responses based on severity and persistence described in National Academy of Sciences publication 1138 (36), which derived from that reported by Green (37), was used to further define and classify the extent of irritation (35).

Rat Cornea

Rats could be used instead of rabbits for a large number of corneal lesion experiments (38). In one study, rats were administered with drug solutions (treated) or saline (control) once a day for a week. The animals were housed singly at 22°C, 55% relative humidity, and light intensity of 60 lux. The anterior eyes were examined daily using a photo-slit lamp. Fluorescein paper strips were used to carry out intravital staining of the corneal surface. On day 7, rats were sacrificed and the bulbi were fixed in Susa-fixative and embedded in paraplast to preserve them for further examination.

Lacrimal secretion was studied in 18 male and 18 female rats. A strip of litmus paper was inserted in the region of the temporal lid angle and after 1 min the length of the dampened portion of the paper strip was estimated. After a 1-week control period, clonidine was given orally over a 4-day period to two groups of rats. The lacrimal secretion was measured 0.5 and 4 hr after dosing in group I, and 2 and 6 hr after dosing in group II. Drug-induced exophthalmus was quantified using rats placed in the lateral position in front of a fixed-position reflex camera. Exposures were made prior and at 20 and 60 min subsequent to drug administration. The distance between the plane of the lids and the corneal vertex was measured. The effect of the drug on the frequency of blinking and wiping was examined both prior and subsequent to treatment with the drug over a 1-hr period.

Clonidine, at doses from 0.3 mg/kg orally on up, resulted in corneal lesions.

Amitriptyline did not cause any alterations in the cornea. Clonidine produced corneal opacities and intracellular edema of epithelial basal cells in the opaque areas.

Intrastromal Application of Chemicals

Test materials can be given directly to the stroma by intrastromal injection or by applying them topically to an epithelium-lacking cornea (39). In the study described here, three series of experiments were performed:

1. Normal rabbits were kept in rabbit holders, which allowed the use of an ether cone during the experiment. The rabbit corneas were kept bathed in a test solution for 10 min by allowing 1 drop of solution to fall from a buret directly onto the upper portion of the cornea approximately every 2 sec.
2. The rabbit corneal epithelium was removed by the application of ox bile or a 1% solution of sodium glycocholate, or mechanically by means of a cotton pledget mounted on a toothpick and previously dipped in collodion. Then the corneas were irrigated as above.
3. One-tenth cubic centimeter of the test solution was injected directly into the corneal stroma with a 25-gauge needle and a tuberculin syringe. General anesthesia was used in all experiments.

A numerical method of quantitative evaluation of the response was used to record reactions. In this method, 0 designates no symptoms, 1 indicates slight, 2 moderately severe, 3 severe, and 4 extremely severe symptoms.

LENS

Accommodation

Accommodation is a combined response of the lens, ciliary muscle, and iris to foreign materials added to the eye. Measurement of accommodation affected by foreign materials is a sensitive method for detecting chemical stimuli on the eyeball (24).

The accommodation portion of the Triple Function Ocular Monitor was used in this study. This device was capable of simultaneously monitoring accommodation, eye vergence, and pupil movement. The human subject was seated in a modified ophthalmic examination device, and the head was secured with elastic Velcro straps. The subject was presented with either a near target or a far target. The response of the lens, along with information about which target was illuminated, was recorded on a strip chart recorder. From the strip chart record, measurements of the latency of the response and the duration of the dynamic portion of the response were made manually. Positive accommodation involved changing focus from far to near; the reverse was negative accommodation. The experiments were conducted in a light-tight room.

Example

Subjects were instructed not to eat or drink 3 hr prior to coming to the laboratory. After a warm-up period on the focusing task, control data were taken. Subjects were then given alcohol in juice. One hour after the alcohol was consumed, treatment data were collected. Blood alcohol levels were periodically estimated with an intoxilyzer during the experiment. Sets of approximately 25 positive and 25 negative accommodative responses were collected during the course of a falling blood alcohol level.

The findings showed significant differences in the accommodative response only when the blood alcohol levels exceeded approximately 0.05%. These differences persist up to the maximum blood alcohol levels used in these experiments. Increases in latency and duration of response were approximately 10% to 40% above normal control values after administration of alcohol.

The effects of alcohol on the frequency response of the pupil were also determined. They determined the transfer characteristics of the pupillary system by introducing sinusoidally modulated light from a glow modulator tube into the eye of the subject using a maxwellian view. The response of the pupil was measured by infrared reflection techniques. By taking data at a number of frequencies, a Bode plot was constructed for the system. The stimulus and response were recorded on a strip chart recorder.

The subjects came to the laboratory after a 12-hr fast and were given a light lunch. Normal data was collected, and subjects were then given an appropriate dose of alcohol. Twenty minutes after the ingestion was completed, the treatment data were collected. Periodic blood alcohol levels were determined by a breath analyzer. The results showed that both gain and phase of the pupillary responses were degraded by alcohol.

Cataract Formation

Cataracts can be induced by ultraviolet (UV) light (40), by chemicals (41,42), and by diseases such as diabetes (43).

Cataractogenesis by UV Irradiation

This study (40) was undertaken to establish a new cataract model for animal studies in which the cataractogenic agent is short-wave UV radiation (280 to 315 nm; UV-B). This model has few side effects and does not interfere with the absorption of drugs in the lens.

Rats weighing 60 to 80 g were divided into three groups. Group I was exposed daily to 1.08 J/cm^2 from an SUP lamp for 18-min sessions. After one dosage of 0.36 J/cm^2 given in one 6-min session, group II underwent the same procedure as group I, but the daily UV-B dose was smaller by a factor of 3. Group III served as a control.

Animals in small cages, no more than two to a cage, were placed underneath UV-B lamps. Rat food and water were removed during irradiation. Pupils were dilated by application of 1% atropine prior to exposure to UV-B.

Eyes were examined with a Zeiss photo-slit lamp at 2-week intervals. Drawings were made, and both eyes of each pair were subjected to Scheimpflug photography. Animals were sacrificed after 3 and 6 weeks. Lenses were fixed in 2.5% glutaraldehyde and processed in glycol methylacrylate. Lenses were sectioned on a Reichert-Supercut microtome and slices of 1.5 μm were taken.

Keratitis and vascularization were observed in all group I animals. "Tumors" of irregular epithelial cells were evolved in group I animals. UV-B could produce cataracts in a short time (6 to 8 weeks) and produced no significant differences in body weight.

Cataractogenesis by Chemicals

Many drugs and environmental chemicals are bioactivated by enzyme systems such as cytochrome P-450 and prostaglandin synthetase to potentially toxic reactive intermediates. Naphthalene is one of many polycyclic aromatic hydrocarbons that may be bioactivated by the cytochrome P-450 monoxygenase enzymes to a potentially toxic, reactive arene oxide intermediate. If not immediately detoxified, the arene oxide intermediate, or possibly a quinone derivative, may bind covalently to lenticular macromolecules resulting in cellular toxicity, which may be expressed as a cataract (42).

New Zealand white or chinchilla pigmented rabbits were tested in this experiment. Either a single injection of naphthalene (2,000 mg/kg in corn oil, i.p.) or multiple smaller injections (1,000 mg/kg/day, i.p., for 2 days) were used. Whereas the cataract generated by the single higher dose injection was progressive, leading to permanent, 100% opacification, the opacity generated by the lower multiple dosing regime was reversible and was not detectable 2 weeks after initial observation. Cataract formation could be measured with ^{13}C-, ^{31}P-, or ^{1}H-nuclear magnetic resonance (NMR) spectroscopy or imaging as presented in the chapter by Rohde, "*In Vitro* Methods in Ophthalmic Toxicology." It was also detected with a photo-slit lamp and results were documented by drawings and by photography. Although there were no opacities or lens abnormalities seen in the control groups treated with solvent alone, there were considerable opacities developed in naphthalene-treated groups (42).

Cataractogenesis Due to Diabetes

Brown-Norway rats were used in three groups: group C, control; group D, diabetes; and group DS, diabetes and sorbinil treatment (44). Streptozotocin (70 mg/kg) in a single injection was used to provoke diabetes in groups D and DS. Sorbinil (25 mg/kg) was given orally every 2 days to group DS. During the entire 6-week experiment, controls of blood glucose level showed values of at least 280 mg/100 ml blood. Slit-lamp examinations and Scheimpflug photos were made before, during, and at the end of the experiments in case of possible changes in opacity. After the experiments were completed, the lenses were dissected from the eyes and lens weights were measured. The lenses were sectioned by a frozen-sectioning technique (45). Lenses were quick-frozen with dry ice on a microtome sample holder, with the posterior side of the lens facing downward. The lenses were cut into sections in a cryostat at −20°C. Thirty to forty sections were united to one fraction. The fractions were homogenized by hand and centrifuged at 11,000 × g. Supernatants and sediments of each fraction were lyophilized, and the amounts of water-soluble and water-insoluble crystallins and their ratios determined. The fraction dry weight was calculated by addition of water-soluble and water-insoluble crystallins.

The water-soluble crystallins of each fraction or layer of the three groups were separated by polyacrylamide thin-layer isoelectric focusing. The samples were stained for proteins with Coomassie Brilliant Blue W, quantity 300 μg protein, and for glycoproteins with periodic acid-Schiff reagant, quantity 800 μg protein. The proteins of each crystallin class were determined by densitometry with transducing light and calculated in percent from the fraction dry weight.

The lens wet weights of the diabetes (D) group and of the diabetes-sorbinil (DS) group were significantly diminished by 5 mg ($2p < 0.003\%$) partly due to hydration in group D and dehydration in group DS.

The dry weight content (in milligrams) was lower in groups D and DS than in group C. The percent dry weight in group D was lower than in groups C and DS. The water content in groups D and DS was lower than in group C, but the percent lens water was higher in group D but lower in group DS than in the control. The ratio of wet weight over dry weight was higher for group D and for group DS, compared to group C.

RETINA

The retina is extremely sensitive to physicochemical stimuli as it contains ample neurons and photocells. Drug-induced oculotoxicity is thus detectable by measuring the retinal changes with electroretinography (ERG) (46) and visual evoked responses (47).

Electroretinography

The most important ion in the ERG studies in potassium (K^+), and the potassium channel. The b-wave component of the electroretinogram and the subsequent oscillatory b-wave component are both mediated by potassium shifts in the retina, and are sensitive to alcohol. It has been found that the b-wave is a Müller glial cell response, that Müller cells in the cerebral cortex act as K^+ electrodes, and that there are a variety of changes in extracellular potassium in the frog retina in response to various stimuli.

The frog retina is a common model for ERG studies. In a common procedure (46) the frog is paralyzed by injecting tubocurare perisacrally. The eye is gently proptosed using blunt probes so that the nictitating membrane is forced down. A subminiature

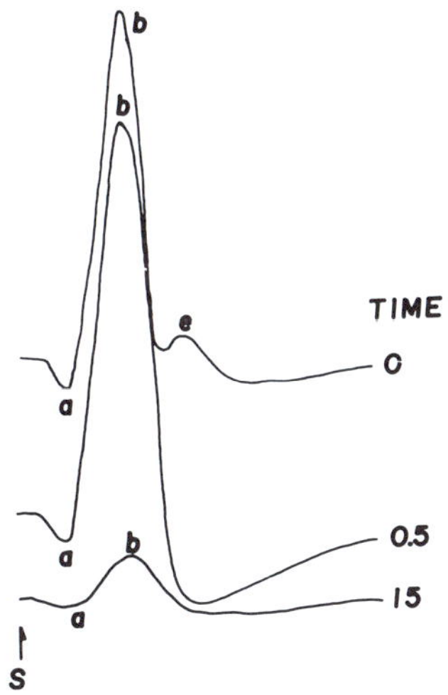

FIG. 4. Alcohol was applied topically to the skin of the frog. The b-wave (b) increases, then decreases, whereas the b′-wave (e) disappears. Time is in days of alcohol treatment. (Reproduced with permission from Levitt and Jaeger, ref. 24.)

needle electrode is inserted subcutaneously on the dorsal midline approximately 5 mm posterior to the eyes as a reference electrode. A slightly modified human ear-clip electrode is attached to a rear leg for a ground electrode. The frog is then placed in a Ganzfeld full-field stimulating apparatus. Cotton wick electrodes coupled to silver-silver chloride electrodes are moistened with normal saline and placed on the corneas, using micromanipulators. An adaptive light is set at 10 foot-lamberts. Flash stimuli are delivered at various intensities, using a xenon flash tube. The electroretinograms are amplified and displayed on a storage oscilloscope and analyzed with an averaging computer. Use of this procedure allows the ERG to be taken without actually puncturing the eye or retina. Besides the obvious advantage of the frog's superficial eye placement, the use of tubocurare for paralysis instead of a general anesthetic eliminates some effects of anesthetics on neuronal activity in the retina.

This procedure was used to test the effects of acute and chronic alcohol. For acute alcohol studies, frogs were injected with a "cocktail" of normal saline and 95 ethanol (5% to 40% ethanol) intraperitoneally prior to monitoring the ERG over time. For chronic alcohol studies, frogs were given daily soakings in 1% to 3% alcohol solutions for periods of 30 to 45 min. (Frogs do not drink fluids but absorb liquids through their skin.) ERGs were periodically taken and monitored over several weeks to several months. It was found that chronic exposure to alcohol gradually reduces the b-wave and abolishes the b′-wave (Fig. 4). On removal from the chronic treatment, the b′-wave returned after 1 to several days.

Human Studies

A study of the effects of acute ethanol ingestion on the human ERG was conducted in a hospital clinical electroretinography laboratory (46). Subjects came to the laboratory after an overnight fast and were given a light lunch. They were then fitted with Burian-Allen corneal electrodes. Stimulation was accomplished with a Ganzfeld full-field stimulator with adapting light and xenon flash tube. Control responses were taken on the first visit to the laboratory; responses following ingestion of alcohol were recorded on a second visit. A follow-up ERG was sometimes taken within several days.

Visual Evoked Responses

A need has developed for techniques that will evaluate the effects of toxins on the central nervous system and will be sensitive, easily applied, and quantitative. The visual evoked response (VER) of the brain shows promise. Exposure of the eyes of an anesthetized animal to bright light produces a reproducible perturbation in the electroencephalogram (the VER). An example of the use of the VER in toxicology is a study of the effects of heavy metals (lead and cadmium) on the development of the VER of rat pups (47).

Rats were exposed to low levels of lead via the dam's milk during their suckling period. Experimental dams consumed 0.2% lead acetate solution during lactation, whereas control dams received tap water.

Visual evoked response testing was performed on 84 rat pups (9 to 20 days old) and on 12 adult rats (90 to 100 days old). Animals were anesthetized by intraperitoneal injections of pentobarbital sodium. VERs were evoked by brief light flashes produced by a Grass photostimulator placed in front of the rat's head and adjusted to maximum intensity, and were recorded from the exposed occipital cortex. Responses were electronically averaged for analysis. In adult animals the recovery function of the P1N1 wave was determined on acute experiments using equal intensity-paired flashes.

VERs of lead-treated rats appeared to follow the same maturational sequence as the control animals but were delayed in appearance. Alterations in the waveform were evident from approximately 30% of the rats. No differences in amplitude were noted in the standard VER testing, but significantly greater latencies were obtained for most of the potentials measured (P1, N1, P2, N2) at all ages.

SKIN TESTS

Good correlation of dermal irritation and ocular irritation would allow a reasonable prediction of eye irritation from skin irritation tests. As a result, eye irritation tests could be avoided for chemicals that potentially cause severe eye damage. Draize testing would be carried out only if the eye irritation of a chemical is predicted to be mild or nonirritating. It should be used mainly for safety assurance rather than for toxicity determination (3,48). Unfortunately, people are likely to come in contact with irritants and even corrosives (like oven cleaners) in their daily life and work, so a knowledge of the kind of ocular damage these chemicals produce is needed to predict the best form of emergency treatment.

Acute Toxicity

In a typical experiment (48), a rubber sleeve is made from rubber dam and constructed so that the ends, reinforced with an additional strip of dam, fit snugly around the trunk of an animal. The ends are tucked, permitting the central portion to "balloon" and furnish a reservoir for the dose. The animals are prepared by clipping the skin of the trunk free of hair and may be further prepared by making epidermal abrasions longitudinally over the area of exposure 2 cm apart. Twenty-four hours later the sleeve is slipped onto the animal, which is then placed in a comfortable but immobilized position in a multiple animal holder. The doses of liquids or solutions are calculated on the basis of body weight and are introduced under the sleeve. Exposures to the agent are for 24 hours.

In the testing of materials with unctuous characteristics that adhere readily to the skin, a 20-mesh wire screen is usually employed instead of the rubber sleeve. The screen is padded and raised approximately 2 cm from the exposed skin. In the case of finely divided amorphous or crystalline solids the material is first evenly distributed on a strip of gauze that is then secured over the area of exposure. The sleeve is fitted over the gauze.

At the end of the 24-hr period of exposure the sleeves or screens are removed, the volume of unabsorbed liquids and solutions, if any, is measured, and the skin reactions are noted immediately. The animals are checked for gross symptoms and are then transferred to individual metabolism cages where they are observed for a minimal period of 2 weeks. Body weight, food consumption, and gross symptoms of systemic effects are checked daily. Observations for changes in blood morphology are made. The tissues of animals that die several days after exposure and of those sacrificed (sometimes because of severe poisoning) are examined for histopathology.

Subacute Toxicity (20-Day or 90-Day Experiments)

In these experiments relatively large doses are applied daily by inunction to an uncovered area of the clipped skin. The area inuncted is approximately 10% of the total surface of the animal. The material is gently rubbed into the skin with a glass rod; this involves manipulation of the hair shafts and mild pressure. The animals are observed for 2 weeks following the final exposure. The same observations for gross symptoms, urine, tissues, and so on are made as in the acute experiments.

Compounds differing widely in chemical structure and behavior may be readily absorbed through the skin. It should be noted also that certain compounds that are judged to be only slightly toxic by acute exposure to the skin may be severely damaging upon repeated exposure (20- or 90-day).

ACKNOWLEDGMENT

This chapter was written with the assistance of Feng Zhao, who performed the literature searches and made copies of the papers.

REFERENCES

1. McCally AW, Farmer AG, Loomis EC. Corneal ulceration following use of lash lure. *JAMA* 1933;101:1560-1561.
2. Friedenwald JS, Hughes WF, Herrmann H. Acid-base tolerance of cornea. *Arch Ophthalmol* 1944;31:279.
3. Draize JH, Woodward G, Calvery HO. Methods for the study of irritation and toxicity of substances applied topically to the skin and mucus membranes. *J Pharmacol Exp Ther* 1944;82:377-390.
4. Green WR, Sullivan JB, Hehir RM, Scharpf LG, Dickenson AW. *A systematic comparison of chemically induced eye injury in the albino rabbit and rhesus monkey.* New York: Soap and Detergent Association, 1978.
5. Draize JH, Kelley EA. Toxicity to eye mucosa of certain cosmetic preparations containing surface-active agents. *Proc Sci Sect Toilet Goods Assoc* 1952;17:1-4.
6. Draize JH. Dermal toxicity. In: *Appraisal of the safety of chemicals in foods, drugs and cosmetics.* Austin, TX: Assoc. Food and Drug Officials of the United States, 1959;44-59.
7. Weltman AS, Sparber SB, Jurtshuk T. Comparative evaluation and the influence of various factors on eye-irritation scores. *Toxicol Appl Pharmacol* 1965;7:308-319.
8. Baldwin HA, McDonald TO, Beasley CH. Slit-lamp examination of experimental animal eyes. II. Grading scales and photographic evaluation of induced pathological conditions. *J Soc Cosmet Chem* 1973;24:181-195.
9. Food and Drug Administration. *Illustrated guide for grading eye irritation by hazardous substances.* Washington, DC: FDA, 1965.
10. Consumer Product Safety Commission. *Illustrated guide for grading eye irritation caused by hazardous substances.* 16CFR 1500. 1976.
11. Griffith JF, Nixon GA, Bruce RD, Reer PJ, Bannan EA. Dose-response studies with chemical irritants in the albino rabbit eye as a basis for selecting optimum testing conditions for predicting hazard to the human eye. *Toxicol Appl Pharmacol* 1982;55:501-513.
12. Freeberg FE, Nixon GA, Reer PJ, et al. Human and rabbit eye responses to chemical insult. *Fundam Appl Toxicol* 1986;7:626-634.
13. Gad SC, Ghengelis CP. Ocular irritation testing. In: *Acute toxicology testing.* Caldwell NJ: Telfand Press, 1988;51-80.
14. Ballantyne B, Swanston DW. The scope and limitations of acute eye irritation tests. In: Ballantyne B, ed. *Current approaches to toxicology.* Bristol: John Wright and Sons, 1977;139-157.
15. McDonald TO, Seabaugh V, Shadduck JA, Edelhauser HF. Eye irritation. In: Marzulli FN, Maibach HI, eds. *Dermatoxicology*, 3rd ed. Washington DC: Hemisphere, 1987;641-696.
16. McDonald TO, Hiddeman JW, Howe WE, Robertson SM. Ocular safety evaluation: alternatives and the future. In: Marzulli FN, Maibach HI, eds. *Dermatoxicology*, 3rd ed. Washington DC: Hemisphere, 1987;697-710.
17. Chan PK, Hayes AW. Assessment of chemically induced ocular toxicity: a survey of methods. In: Hayes AW, ed. *Toxicology of the eye, ear and other special senses.* New York: Raven Press, 1985;103-143.
18. Bell M, Holmes PM, Nisbet TM, Uttley M, Van Abbe NJ. Evaluating the potential eye irritancy of shampoos. *Int J Cosmet Sci* 1979;1:123-131.
19. Jacobs GA, Martens MA. An objective method for the evaluation of eye irritation *in vivo*. *Food Chem Toxicol* 1989;27:255-258.

20. Beckley JH, Russell TJ, Rubin LF. Use of the rhesus monkey for predicting human responses to eye irritants. *Toxicol Appl Pharmacol* 1969;15:1-9.
21. Swanston DW. Eye irritancy testing. In: Balls M, Riddell RJ, Worden AN, eds. *Animals and alternatives in toxicity testing*. New York: Academic Press, 1983;337-366.
22. Ballantyne B, Gazzard MF, Swanston DW, Williams P. The ophthalmic toxicology of d-chlorobenzylidine malononitrile (CS). *Arch Toxicol* 1974;32:149-168.
23. Maurice D. Chairman's introduction: pain and acute toxicity testing in the eye. In: Goldberg AM, ed. *Alternative methods in toxicology vol 3: In vitro toxicology*. New York: Mary Ann Liebert, 1985;341-354.
24. Levitt J, Jaeger R. Effects of alcohol on eye movements. In: Merigan WH, Weiss B, eds. *Neurotoxicity of the visual system*. New York: Raven Press, 1980;90-95.
25. Jaeger RJ, Yao JHK. Analysis of drug-induced changes in smooth pursuit eye movements. *Proceedings of the 28th Annual Conference on Engineering in Medicine and Biology*. Chevy Chase, MD: Alliance for Engineering in Medicine and Biology, 1975;321.
26. Chiou GCY, Yan HY. Effects of antiglaucoma drugs on the blood flow in rabbit eyes. *Ophthalmol Res* 1986;18:265-269.
27. Robinson F, Riva CE, Grunwald JE, Petrig BL, Sinclair SH. Retinal blood flow autoregulation in response to an acute increase in blood pressure. *Invest Ophthalmol Vis Sci* 1986;27:722-726.
28. Yan HY, Chiou, GCY. Effects of L-timolol, D-timolol, haloperidol and domperidone on rabbit retinal blood flow measured with laser doppler method. *Ophthalmol Res* 1987;19:45-48.
29. Raitta C, Tolonen M. Microcirculation of the eye in workers exposed to carbon disulfide. In: Merigan WH, Weiss B, eds. *Neurotoxicity of the visual system*. New York: Raven Press, 1980;73-86.
30. Chiou GCY, Zhao F, Shen ZF, Li BHP. Effects of D-timolol and L-timolol on ocular blood flow and intraocular pressure. *J Ocular Pharmacol* 1990;6:23-30.
31. Kennah HE, Hignet S, Laux PE, Dorko JD, Barrow CS. An objective procedure for quantitating eye irritation based upon changes of corneal thickness. *Fundam Appl Toxicol* 1989;12:258-268.
32. Morgan RL, Sorenson SS, Castle S. Prediction of ocular irritation by corneal pachymetry. *Food Chem Toxicol* 1986;25:609-613.
33. Hickey TE, Beck GL, Botta JA. Optimum fluorescein staining time in ocular irritation studies. *Toxicol Appl Pharmacol* 1973;26:571-574.
34. Carpenter CP, Smyth HF. Chemical burns of the rabbit cornea. *Am J Ophthalmol* 1946;29:1363-1372.
35. Gad SC, Walsh RD, Dunn BJ. Correlation of ocular and dermal irritancy of industrial chemicals. *J Toxicol Cutan Ocular Toxicol* 1986;5:195-213.
36. NAS Committee for Revisions of NAS Publication 1138. Dermal and eye toxicity tests. In: *Principles and procedures for evaluating the toxicity of household substances*. Washington, DC: National Academy of Sciences, 1978;41.
37. Green WR. *A systemic comparison of chemically induced eye injury in the albino rabbit and rhesus monkey*. New York: Soap and Detergent Association, 1978.
38. Weisse I, Hoefke W, Grenberg S, Galda W, Stotzer H, Kreuzer H. Ophthalmological and pharmacological studies after administration of clonidine in rats. *Arch Toxicol* 1978;41:89-98.
39. Friedenwald JS, Hughes WF, Herrmann H. Acid-base tolerance of the cornea. *Arch Ophthalmol* 1944;31:279-283.
40. Tuffs A, Weneger A, Hockwin D. Pilot studies on cataractogenesis by UV irradiation. *Concepts Toxicol* 1987;4:276-284.
41. Koch HR, Doldi K, Hockwin D. Naphthalene cataracts in rats. Association of eye pigmentation and cataract development. *Doc Ophthalmol Proc Ser* 1976;8:293-303.
42. Lubek BM, Kubow S, Basu PK, Wells PG. Cataractogenicity and bioactivation of naphthalene derivatives in lens culture and in vivo. In: Lerman S, Tripathi RC, eds. *Ocular toxicology*. New York: Marcel Dekker, 1990;203-209.
43. Piatigorsky J. Intracellular ions, protein metabolism and cataract formation. *Curr Top Eye Res* 1980;3:1-39.
44. Bours J. Ahrend MHJ, Weneger A, Hockwin D. Glycosylated crystallins in microsection of diabetic rat lenses. *Concepts Toxicol* 1987;4:350-359.
45. Hockwin D, Ahrend MJH, Bours J. Correlation of Scheimpflug photoscopy of the anterior eye segment with biochemical analysis of the lens. Application of a frozen-sectioning technique to investigate differences in protein distribution of single lens layers. *Graefes Arch Clin Exp Ophthalmol* 1986;224:265-270.

46. Levett J, Jaeger R. Effects of alcohol on retinal potentials. In: Merigan WH, Weiss B, eds. *Neurotoxicity of the visual system.* New York: Raven Press, 1987;87–89.
47. Cooper GP, Fox DA, Howell WE, Laurie RD, Tsang W, Lewkowski JP. Visual evoked responses in rats exposed to heavy metals. In: Merigan WH, Weiss B, eds. *Neurotoxicity of the visual system.* New York: Raven Press, 1987;203–218.
48. Williams SJ. Prediction of ocular irritancy potential from dermal irritation test results. *Food Chem Toxic* 1984;22:157–161.

Ophthalmic Toxicology, edited by
George C. Y. Chiou. Raven Press, Ltd.,
New York © 1992.

5

In Vitro Methods in Ophthalmic Toxicology

Brooks H. Rohde

*Department of Medical Pharmacology and Toxicology,
and Institute of Ocular Pharmacology,
Texas A & M University College of Medicine,
College Station, Texas 77843*

A modified Draize eye irritation test has been routinely mandated for use by manufacturers to study the safety of their products for marketing (1). The testing guidelines of the Organization for Economic and Cooperative Development (OECD) specify the rabbit eye irritation test to be used for these studies (2). Since the United States is a member of OECD, the rabbit eye irritation test is considered the official model for eye irritation studies (3).

The rabbit eye irritation test has several problems: (a) it lacks objective and accurate quantitation for the grading system; (b) it is opposed by animal welfare groups and many other individuals, primarily but not exclusively because of the pain involved; and (c) it is a slow, expensive, and time-consuming process. Therefore, alternative *in vitro* methods as substitutes for *in vivo* tests are now actively being sought. These methods have focused on the use of enucleated eyes, isolated eye tissues or non-eye tissues, and cultured eye or non-eye cells.

It should be noted that no single *in vitro* method can be used as a complete alternative to the rabbit eye irritation test; the eye *in vivo* is a complex system capable of producing a wide variety of actions due to injurious stimuli and insults. Reactions may vary because of chemical irritation, direct physical irritation, damage to corneal or conjunctival cells, release of histamine or prostaglandins, and even because of prior medication of the animal. *In vitro* methods are, in general, capable of evoking and measuring a single aspect of eye irritation rather than replicating the multiple aspects of eye irritation produced *in vivo*. Therefore, the safety of certain groups of chemicals must be evaluated with several *in vitro* methods to obtain a complete and accurate picture of their irritation potential in living animal eyes.

A wide variety of *in vitro* methods are now available as alternatives to the *in vivo* Draize test (3). Some particularly promising methods include (a) release of plasminogen activator from rabbit corneal cells (4); (b) cytotoxicity of chemicals to rabbit corneal cells or effects of chemicals on cell cloning (5–7); (c) necrosis of embryonic chick chorioallantoic membrane (8,9); (d) inhibition of uridine uptake measured with mouse fibroblast cells (6,10); (e) ^{51}Cr-release measured from murine mastocytoma cells (11); and (f) Madin-Darby canine kidney cells in culture (12).

There are both advantages and disadvantages to *in vitro* methods. The advantages include the following: (a) they allow a large number of observations to be measured in a quantitative way; (b) they are easily controllable and reproducible, and are particularly suitable for studies on dose-response relationships and pharmacokinetics; (c) they can be carried out in a relatively short period of time as compared to *in vivo* methods; (d) they are painless and devoid of the variability among animals; (e) they are in general less expensive than *in vivo* methods; and (f) some methods involve the use of no living animals. Disadvantages include the following: (a) they are unable to produce the complete irritation reaction produced by *in vivo* methods; (b) they are unable to mimic the tearing and pain that are common phenomena in human eye irritation; (c) they are still in the development stage and are not widely accepted by regulatory agencies; (d) they lack a large data base for comparison; and (e) they are devoid of the recovery or healing stages found in *in vivo* eye irritation experiments. In addition, in many instances it is difficult to extrapolate the *in vitro* data to *in vivo* eye irritation, even if the tissues and cells used are obtained from the same species, because *in vitro* systems represent only a small aspect of the complicated *in vivo* eye system and function. It is even more difficult to extrapolate *in vitro* data obtained from animal tissues or cells to the living human eye system. Furthermore, effective concentrations obtained from *in vitro* experiments are hard to relate to the effective irritation doses in *in vivo* systems, as the slope of the dose-response relationship in these two systems can be quite different. Most *in vitro* assays measure acute toxicity and are not suitable models for evaluating the long-term toxicity and carcinogenicity effects of potential eye irritants.

Despite these difficulties, development of *in vitro* alternative methods to *in vivo* eye irritation test methods is urgently needed. Increasing numbers of chemicals that are developed for ocular and cosmetic uses require eye irritation tests. *In vitro* methods will provide a workable way to meet the large demand in a humane way.

It is most important that a valid relationship between an *in vitro* method and the *in vivo* Draize test should be established. In some instances the relationship might be valid only for testing certain classes of chemicals; in these cases, the limitation of the *in vitro* method ought to be clearly indicated. Although a false-positive result obtained with an *in vitro* method is unacceptable, a false negative obtained with an *in vitro* method is even worse, indicating an unsafe product is safe. To minimize these problems, the dose-response relationship must be promptly established for all *in vitro* method experiments.

To establish fully the relationship between *in vitro* and *in vivo* tests, large numbers of chemicals of various classes must be tested *in vitro* and the results compared with the known data from Draize rabbit ocular irritation tests. The ranking of these chemicals established by *in vitro* testing should match as closely as possible the Draize's ocular irritancy test in rabbit eyes.

ISOLATED RABBIT EYE

In order to mimic the *in vivo* Draize test, rabbit eyes are enucleated immediately after death and placed in a temperature-controlled chamber where they are superfused with normal saline solution (13,14). Test substances are applied topically to the eyes and the effects are observed with a slit-lamp biomicroscope.

This method has a number of advantages over other possible *in vitro* systems: (a) The system will identify materials that have the potential to be extremely irritant to the *in vivo* eye. Such materials cause direct, clearly visible damage to the *in vitro* cornea following a very short period of contact. (b) The system investigates the effect of the products or chemicals in the form in which they might enter the human eye. The system does not need to rely on dilution or solubilization of the material to ascertain whether the product is particularly toxic to cells. (c) As materials are applied directly onto the cornea, the system can be used for a very wide range of irritants, from corrosive materials to totally nonirritating materials. The test's versatility across this wide range of irritants is of considerable advantage; it is doubtful whether other *in vitro* systems would be able to cope adequately with products that differ so widely in their irritation potentials. An example to illustrate this advantage is sodium hydroxide. It must be present at a misleadingly high concentration in cell culture to cause a toxic effect, and therefore it appears to be less of a hazard than it actually is *in vivo* (14).

Method

This method was developed mainly by Burton and coworkers (13). The eyes of rabbits were examined using a slit-lamp biomicroscope and the initial corneal thickness was measured with depth measurement attachment #1 for the slit lamp. Then the rabbits were killed by an overdose of pentobarbital sodium. Immediately after death each animal was laid on its side and one drop of isotonic NaCl was applied to the surface of the eye to prevent drying during dissection. The eyeball was enucleated carefully to avoid touching the surface of the cornea or cutting the optic nerve too close to the eyeball.

Any eye that had abnormalities or had been damaged during dissection was discarded. Eye viability was determined by application of 2% fluorescein sodium dye to the corneal surface for a few seconds followed by rinsing with isotonic NaCl solution. Eyes that were significantly swollen after dissection, that stained with fluorescein dye, or showed any other signs of damage were rejected.

Enucleated eyes were mounted in a perspex clamp with the cornea positioned vertically and placed in a temperature-controlled (32°C ± 1°C) superfusion chamber (13,14). Normal saline solution was pumped into the chamber through a stainless steel tube at a rate of 0.10 to 0.15 ml/min. It dripped onto the cornea at the limbus and flowed down over the corneal surface. The chamber was enclosed in a water jacket through which water was pumped at approximately 4 l/min from a temperature-controlled water bath. The saline was passed through tubing within the water jacket so that it was warmed to the correct temperature before entering the chamber. The chamber wall was made of black perspex, providing a suitable background for slit-lamp observation. Readers are referred to the original reports (13,14) for more details and illustrations of the superfusion chamber.

Enucleated eyes were reexamined using the slit lamp to ensure that they had not been damaged during dissection. The corneal thickness was also measured. Enucleated eyes were left in the chambers for 45 to 75 min to equilibrate. Then the saline superfusion was stopped. Test substances (2 drops or 50 μl) were applied to the eye with a 1-ml syringe so that the cornea was continuously bathed with the test substances for 10 sec. The corneal solution was then rinsed thoroughly with warm isotonic saline solution (20 ml) and the saline superfusion immediately restarted. Solids were tested by applying 50 mg for 10 sec and then rinsing as before.

The eyes were reexamined at intervals for up to 4 hr after the application of the test substances and any changes in the normal appearance of the cornea were carefully noted. The corneal thickness was also measured, either in terms of instrument units (1 unit = 0.8 mm) or as corneal swelling, which was expressed as

$$\left(\frac{\text{corneal thickness at time t}}{\text{corneal thickness before treatment}} - 1\right) \times 100\%$$

Examples

Sodium Hydroxide

The examples chosen were compounds known to cause dose-dependent ocular irritation and corneal damage as determined by the Draize test and by most other tests. Sodium hydroxide caused rapidly developing and intense opacity of the anterior stroma of the cornea. The areas of opacity had well-defined margins. The epithelium remained relatively clear, but was permeable to fluorescein. The corneal thickness was increased by 50% in 4 hr.

Ethanol

Ethanol caused opacity in the epithelium and increased permeability to fluorescein. Areas of the epithelium became detached from the cornea. Stromal opacity and edema developed gradually. The increase in corneal thickness after 4 hr was 65%.

Acetone

Acetone caused slight opacity of the epithelium, probably representing the loss of some of the surface layers of cells, and increased permeability to fluorescein. There was little stromal opacity. Corneal thickness after 4 hr increased by 20%.

ISOLATED CORNEAL PREPARATIONS

The cornea is the part of the eyeball that is in direct contact with chemicals that enter the eye topically and is directly exposed to toxic radiation. Therefore, *in vitro* methods to determine toxic responses induced by chemicals, pollutants, and radiation on the cornea ought to be developed in order to reduce or eliminate the need for the *in vivo* Draize test. There are at least four methods of *in vitro* corneal preparations that have been developed, including the Eytex method, corneal opacity method, corneal cup method, and cornea fluorescent probe method.

Eytex Method

The Eytex method (15,16) was developed by the National Testing Corporation and can reduce or eliminate the need for the Draize test. This method is a corneal opacification assay to predict ocular irritation of chemicals and formulations based on alterations in a protein matrix reagent. There is a high degree of correlation between results from the *in vitro* Eytex method and the *in vivo* Draize method. The Eytex method is quantitative and reproducible, and may allow more uniform testing results. This method, however, measures only chemical irritancy; facts of *in vivo* irritation such as abrasion, allergy, and sensitization, or the ability to heal after irritation must be measured by other means.

The Eytex method can rapidly identify irritants, which can be eliminated from further testing by *in vivo* methods. This method can identify increased ocular irritancy and can follow product stability by monitoring breakdown products. It can also identify and quantitate anti-irritants in personal care products.

Methods

The protein matrix is extracted from jack bean powder, and does not require the sacrifice of any animal or sampling of any animal tissue. Fine ground jack bean meal is soaked in saline solution with acetate buffer and ethylenediaminetetraacetic acid (EDTA) added. The mixture is filtered and pH adjusted to 8.0 with sodium borate. The mixture is again filtered and the filtrate, or protein matrix, is analyzed for composition and then lyophilized. A prototype method has been used to establish a relationship between ocular irritants and their ability to produce opacity *in vitro*. Additional studies have been conducted to establish a direct relationship between ocular irritation of known irritants and their ability to cause aggregation or denaturation of certain proteins *in vitro*.

An Eytex kit consists of the protein matrix reagent, six calibrators, a dilution buffer, distilled water, and special 1-ml cuvettes. Equipment needed includes a colorimeter, cuvette rack, and dispensing pipettes; this represents a much smaller investment than most methods and certainly much smaller than is needed for the Draize test. Samples of soluble test solutions (30, 50, or 100 µl) or soluble solids (30,

50, or 100 mg) are added directly to the Eytex reagent. The membrane partition assay (MPA) protocol is used for insoluble chemicals; samples are placed in a membrane cut that is permeable to molecules of 16,000 daltons or less and that separates the sample from the reaction chamber with the Eytex reagant. The standard and MPA vessels are incubated at 25°C for 1 hr or 24 hr. A set of calibrators defines the relationship of the optical density produced in the Eytex reagent with the Draize score and three known controls are assayed for internal assay control. Optical density after incubation is converted to Eytex/Draize equivalents (Eytex score) and the substance is classified as an irritant or nonirritant.

Examples

The scientific validation of the Eytex method has been pursued by the National Testing Corporation in many ways. A study presented at the 1987 Center for Alternatives to Animal Testing (CAAT) symposium showed Eytex results to have a 96% correlation with *in vivo* Draize test results.

In 1987, studies of the Eytex method were conducted in 12 industrial, military, university, and independent laboratories. Each lab chose between 5 and 60 materials for testing. The *in vitro* results exhibited an overall substantial equivalence of 89% to the *in vivo* test results. It was determined that the ability of the assay to discriminate between irritants and nonirritants was 99% (17).

A two-lab, double-masked study of 70 products (including furniture polish, laundry detergent, air freshener, insect repellent, shampoos, and first-aid creams) was conducted by S.C. Johnson and Son. A 93% predictive value of the Eytex method was demonstrated (18).

In a study by Avon, different products, including cosmetics, bubble baths, and moisturizers, were tested. There was a 100% concordance of the Eytex method with the Avon study (19).

In 12% of the samples in these studies the Eytex method overpredicted irritancy. A new rapid membrane assay (RMA) used together with the Eytex method estimates the irritancy of compounds such as highly ethoxylated surfactants correctly (20); the earlier MPA underestimated their irritancy. In these studies, advantages observed of the Eytex method included lower costs, reduction in animal use, and an increased capability to test undiluted products.

Opacity of Isolated Cornea

The opacitometer (20) was designed and constructed to monitor corneal opacity development. Readers are directed to the original reference (20) for an illustration and detailed description of the opacitometer. The perspex corneal holders allow the cornea to be firmly clamped with 5 ml of solution in contact with the front (epithelial) and 5 ml with the rear (endothelial) part. The opacitometer allows a beam of white light to be directed through the cornea in its holder to a photocell. The instrument is first calibrated by shining the light beam through an empty holder. The voltage recorded is set at 25 V before each reading by adjusting the variable register. To eliminate reflections and scatter, all surfaces of the opacitometer are mat black. Dark current is small with this system; a voltage of below 0.005 V is recorded with the lamp off. With a cornea in place, development of opacity is indicated by a drop in the voltage measured. All incubations are carried out at 32°C, the cornea being bathed in Tyrode solution with or without surfactant on both sides.

Methods

The corneas were removed from fresh whole bovine eyes and were washed with Tyrode solution (21). For some preparations the epithelium was scraped off gently before the cornea was removed from the eyeball; in other preparations the endothelium and Descemet's membrane were scraped off after first removing the rear of the eyeball, removing the lens, and everting the cornea over a second eyeball. Some corneas were used with both epithelium and Descemet's membrane removed. Holders, designed to allow contact of either or both surfaces with Tyrode solution or sodium lauryl sulfate (NaLS) solutions of various concentrations, were filled with Tyrode solution and placed in a Muir opacitometer. The voltage was adjusted to 2.5 V. The Tyrode solution was discarded and a cornea fixed in the chamber. Then Tyrode solution or NaLS solution was placed on one or both sides of the cornea. The holder, with cornea and solutions, was placed again in the opacitometer and the voltage recorded (V1). Corneas were then incubated for 4.5 hr. The solutions on both sides of the cornea were then replaced with fresh Tyrode's solution and the voltage recorded again (V2). Since a drop in voltage indicates the development of opacity in the cornea, the results were expressed as percent opacity:

$$\left(\frac{V1 - V2}{V1}\right) \times 100\%$$

where V1 − V2 = 0 represents zero opacity and V1 − V2 = 2.5 represents 100% opacity.

Examples

In one study (20) control corneas showed no opacity for 8 hr and then became more opaque over 24 hr. Care had to be taken to use fresh Tyrode solution as solutions became turbid with time. Sodium dodecyl sulfate (NaDS) at 1 mM caused almost complete opacity by 8 to 12 hr, whereas sodium lauryl sulfate (NaLS) at 1 mM caused opacity to fall more slowly, leveling off at 0.5 at 20 hr. Opacity with both surfactants was concentration-dependent, with NaDS much more potent as an irritant; this contrasts to its lower toxicity to cultured cells (22).

Another study of isolated corneas exposed to NaLS (21) showed that opacity developed primarily in the stroma, in a concentration-dependent manner, and was greatest when epithelium and endothelium were removed. Igarashi (21) thought that opacity was due to a reaction of NaLS with stromal proteins.

Corneal Cup Method

Leukocyte Chemotactic Factor Production

Corneas are prepared from fresh bovine eyes as illustrated in Fig. 1 (23,24). The attached lens and most of the iris are removed and the resulting "corneal cup" is then washed twice in saline and maintained in cold minimal essential medium (MEM) until used. The cup is mounted in a paraffin well with the epithelial surface facing upward and covered by tissue culture MEM. Using the corneal cup model, the capability of corneal tissues to produce leukocyte chemotactic factor (LCF) in response to inflammatory chemicals and/or leukocyte mediated injury to corneal epithelium can be evaluated. The production of LCF is a response of cells to irritation and damage, and is proportional to the degree of cell damage. The migration of leukocytes in response to supernatants containing released LCF provides a method of quantitating this damage. It is a valuable model because cells in the epithelium of the corneal cup, like cells *in vivo*, may produce LCF for some time after very brief exposure to an irritating chemical or physical insult.

Leukocyte Production

The epithelial surfaces of isolated bovine corneal cups were treated with 1 N NaOH for 35 sec at room temperature. The NaOH was then removed, and the epithelial surfaces were washed once with MEM and incubated with fresh serum-free MEM for 1, 2, 4, and 6 hr at 37°C in a 5% CO_2 atmosphere. At various time points experimental and control supernatants from the epithelial surfaces were removed and assayed for chemotactic activity using a modified Boyden chamber (24,25). This protocol imitated the effects of an alkali burn followed by eye washing; the formation of LCF is a measure of cell damage and cell repair. A Boyden chamber is a small cylinder divided into two parts by a micropore membrane. In this study the pores were of 5 μm diameter. Substances that will or will not attract leukocytes are placed in the bottom compartment while a leukocyte suspension is placed in the top compartment. If the cells are attracted to the bottom compartment they attempt to cross the membrane and are caught in the pores. After incubating for a fixed time (1 hr for neutrophils, 5 hr for mononuclear cells) the filter is removed, fixed in pure isopropyl alcohol, stained with hematoxylin, and cells are counted on a glass slide using a microscope with an Optomax image analyzer.

Unfractionated leukocytes were isolated from fresh bovine blood by a modified procedure of Boyum (26,27). Sodium citrate-dehydrate was used as an anticoagulant. Methycellulose was mixed with citrated blood and the blood was centrifuged. The white, buffy leukocyte layer on the pellet of erythrocytes was pipetted off and

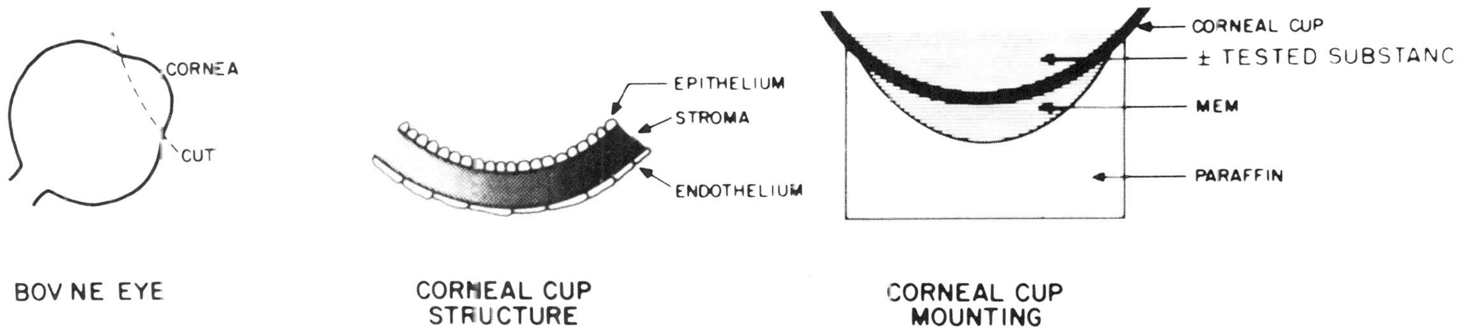

FIG. 1. Diagrammatic representation of the isolation and preparation of the cornea and the corneal cup model. (Reproduced with permission from Elgebaly et al., ref. 24.)

contaminating erythrocytes were lysed. Isolated leukocytes were washed twice by resuspension in isotonic saline followed by recentrifugation. The unfractionated leukocytes were then suspended in sterile saline and layered over 3 ml of Ficoll/Hypaque mixture in a tube and centrifuged at 800 × g at room temperature. Mononuclear cells were found on top of the separation fluid, whereas neutrophils were sedimented at the bottom of the tube. The isolated leukocytes were resuspended in serum-free MEM for leukocyte chemotactic activity assay using modified Boyden chambers (28). Cell migration in response to the putative chemoattractants was expressed as

$$\text{maximum chemotactic response} = \left(\frac{CI_{experimental} - CI_{HBSS}}{CI_{C5\,fragment} - CI_{HBSS}} \right) \times 100\%$$

where CI is the chemotactic index (distance traveled on the filter × cell number), C5 fragment is the positive control for 100% chemotactic response, and HBSS is Hank's balanced salt solution (a blank with no attractant property).

Example

The effects of supernatants obtained from NaOH-treated bovine corneas on the migration of neutrophils or mononuclear cells *in vitro* are shown in Fig. 2. After 2 hr of incubation, significant levels of chemotactic activity for both cell types were detected. Less activity, however, was found in supernatants of corneas incubated for 4 or 6 hr. The observed decline in the chemotactic activity is probably due to the release of LCF deactivators and/or inhibitors (24).

Epithelial/Leukocyte Interactions

Not only will irritated cells release LCF, but leukocytes attracted to the epithelium will adhere, penetrate, and damage the corneal epithelium. The corneal cup can be used to model this kind of irritation and damage (23). The isolated bovine leukocytes and leukocyte lysates, both prepared in MEM, were added separately to the epithelial surfaces of isolated bovine corneal cups. The cups were incubated and at time intervals of 5, 10, 20, 60, 120, and 180 min samples were taken for light and ultrastructural evaluations to assess the status of corneal epithelial cells.

Example

Histological and ultrastructural evaluation had indicated that leukocyte-epithelial cell interactions are characterized by five successive stages (23):

Stage 1: Brief interactions of leukocytes with epithelial cells (0 to 20 min) demon-

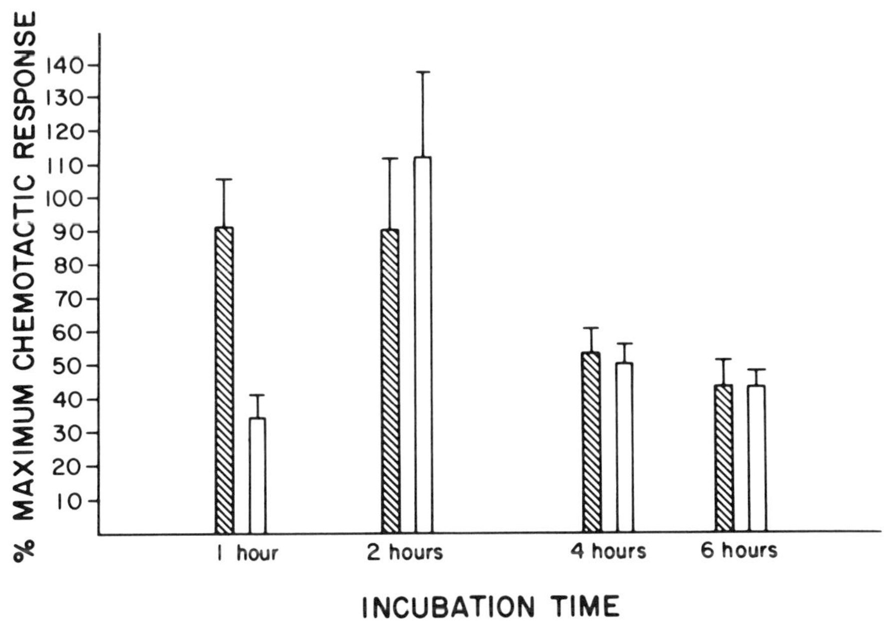

FIG. 2. Mononuclear cell and neutrophil chemotactic activity present in supernatants of bovine corneas exposed to 1 N NaOH for 35 sec, washed once with MEM, and then incubated with MEM for 1, 2, 4, and 6 hr. The figure represents the mean of four experiments ± standard deviation. (Reproduced with permission from Elgebaly et al., ref. 24.) ▨ Mononuclear cell response to supernatants obtained from NaOH-treated corneas; □ PMN response to supernatants obtained from NaOH-treated corneas. (MEM-treated corneas produced low levels of LCF of maximum activity of 10%.)

strated tight adhesion of leukocytes to the epithelial surface, but no significant alteration of the corneal epithelial cell structure was observed.

Stage 2: As the duration of leukocyte contact with epithelial cells increased (20 to 60 min), leukocytes penetrated beneath the superficial layer of epithelium.

Stage 3: In this period, leukocyte penetration beneath the epithelial layer induced mild to severe injury to corneal epithelial cells and caused detachment of several superficial layers.

Stage 4: Phagocytosis of dead epithelial cells by leukocytes was observed following 20 to 60 min exposures.

Stage 5: After 2 to 3 hr of postleukocyte exposure, significant damage to the entire epithelial layer was observed.

The damage to the epithelial cell layer was proportional to the concentration of leukocytes applied. Intact leukocytes are necessary to induce epithelial cell injury; lysates were ineffective. Direct leukocyte-epithelial contact plays a role in stimulating the synthesis and release of effector inflammatory mediators.

Cornea Fluorescent Probe Method

Increases in permeability of the epithelium of living rabbit cornea to ^{24}Na parallel inflammatory response (29). This suggests that permeability might be used as a measure of corneal injury. Permeability can be measured using a fluorescent probe.

Method

Two fluorescent dyes, fluorescein and sulforhodamine B (SRB), were investigated in the first experiments. The dyes were dissolved in saline at neutral pH to make 10% solutions. Adult pigmented mice were killed using T61 euthanasia solution (American Hoechst Corp., Somerville, NJ) (30). Immediately after death the eyes of the mice were proptosed by pulling down the skin below the ears and clamping it beneath the neck. The test substance was placed on one eye so as to cover the cornea. After 1 min it was washed off with saline. Then a drop of fluorescent dye solution was applied to both corneas and then washed off after 1 min. With a slit-lamp fluorophotometer, measurements of the fluorescence of the corneas were made at four points around a circle imagined halfway between the apex and periphery. The measurements were averaged. This averaged out regional differences in fluorescent dye uptake. Six animals were used for each substance tested. Each animal was scored as the ratio of the average fluorescent measurement from the control cornea to that from the test (drug-treated) cornea. To evaluate the method, a variety of substances were tested, including NaOH, benzalkonium chloride, Tween-20, Tween-80, propacaine, and water. Tween-20 increases permeability to fluorescein, whereas Tween-80 does not. This method may be promising as a cheap and rapid screening test for substances with acute ocular toxicity. It does require the sacrifice of mice but does not involve the application of irritants to the eyes of a live animal. A simple fluorometric device was reported to be under development in 1986, which would make it unnecessary to acquire an expensive slit-lamp fluorophotometer (30).

ISOLATED LENS PREPARATION

Numerous chemicals and physical stimuli can cause cataracts. Frequently, biochemical changes in the lens occur long before cloudiness of the lens can be diagnosed with the naked eye. Therefore, new technologies have been developed to detect the biochemical changes that occur in the lens after eye irritation. Methods include nuclear magnetic resonance spectroscopy (MRS), nuclear magnetic resonance imaging (MRI), scanning lens monitor, and fluorescence spectroscopy. *In vitro*, lens metabolism and enzyme activities can also be analyzed for detection of biochemical abnormalities caused by eye irritation.

MRS and MRI

Nuclear magnetic resonance spectroscopy (MRS) and imaging (MRI) have received attention as both *in vivo* and *in vitro* methods for monitoring lens metabolism, hydration, and T_1 and T_2 pulse relaxation (31–33). Nuclear magnetic resonance techniques were developed from the observation that nuclei of certain isotopes (including protium, ^{13}C, and ^{31}P) absorb energy from a magnetic field at discrete wavelengths. The wavelength of energy perturbation is constant under a constant environment and shifts reproducibly with changes in the environment, revealing the environment of the atoms absorbing energy and something of the structure of the molecule they belong to. The time that certain molecules take to release energy after absorbing distinct quanta of energy from a magnetic pulse (T_1 and T_2 pulse relaxation times) are sensitive to changes in the environments of these molecules and provide a reproducible means of assessing changes in environment. MRS and MRI are superior over traditional observation with a slit-lamp microscope in many aspects including (a) objective data generated, (b) speed of getting data, and (c) various aspects of the studies allowed depending on the nuclei used. Nuclear magnetic resonance (NMR) has the advantage of being usable noninvasively; it can measure quantitatively otherwise unobservable parameters pertinent to lens integrity, such as the small subtle alterations in protein structure in the lens with changes in the interaction of proteins with the surrounding water, or lens hydration (32). Low molecular weight phosphorus compounds have very sharp ^{31}P-NMR-spectra, whereas phosphorus bound to high molecular weight compounds have broad diffuse spectra (31), so levels of inorganic phosphate (Pi) and adenosine triphosphate (ATP) can be monitored through NMR.

^{31}*P-MRS Study*

^{31}P-MRS was used to monitor lenticular organophosphate metabolism and the ability to maintain lens viability *in vitro* (31,32). Enucleated bovine globes were rendered aphakic by intracapsular lens extraction. A large (160° to 180°) limbal incision was made superiorly, the zonular fibers cut, and the lens removed using forceps. Following lens extraction, a thin-walled glass phantom, approximately the geometry and size of the lens, filled with 120 mM NaC1, was inserted into the lens cavity. The phantom, filled with only saline or with phosphate solutions, would be used to calibrate the instrument and determine optimum experimental conditions. Corneal tissue was excised from the globe through an incision that extended circumferentially at the limbus. The iris was removed by way of the incision made for the lens extraction. Then the limbal incision was closed with silk sutures.

Method

A Nicolet Magnetics NT-200 spectrometer, equipped with a 4.7-cm wide-bore Oxford superconducting magnet interfaced with a Nicolet 1180 computer system, was used. In a typical experiment, a globe covered with Saran wrap to retard tissue dehydration was mounted in the probe of the instrument with the anterior pole proximal to the surface coil. Position was assessed by the use of thin feeler gauges and the graduated scale of the globe holder. The probe was positioned in the magnet, and air at 5°C was blown over the globe to stabilize ocular tissue metabolite levels. The probe was carefully tuned to 80.96 MHz for each tissue sample. Shimming was accomplished using the water proton resonance in the tissue. Water line widths of 20 to 40 Hz were usually attained. This is a standard procedure for setting up the instrument prior to making a spectrum of an unknown sample. A 20- or 30-Hz exponential line-broadening factor was employed. Chemical shift values are expressed in parts per million (ppm) relative to internal tissue glycerolphosphorylcholine (GPC) (+0.49 ppm). This was accomplished by using the tissue water proton resonance was an intermediate standard. GPC is an internal standard for this procedure; the instrument is able to take the spectrum of the naturally occurring ^{31}P.

Titration curves relating the chemical shift of phosphorus-containing metabolites to pH were obtained using lens homogenates diluted by the addition of a small amount of 120 Mm NaC1 to reduce solution viscosity, followed by adjustment to the desired pH. Titration measurements were made at 80.96 MHz using a conventional saddle-coil probe. Typical spectrometer parameters are the following: pulse width, variable; 2,000 data points per free induction decay; sweep width, ±4000 Hz; and repetition time, 0.378 sec.

Example

A bovine globe phantom containing 10 mM inorganic phosphate (Pi) and 120 mM NaC1 in the lens compartment, and with both the anterior and posterior compartments filled with 120 mM NaC1, was used to obtain an initial kRF pulse duration with maximized signal-to-noise for the lens compartment when used with a 3.8-cm diameter surface coil (Fig. 3). It was possible to "focus" the coil on the lens compartment of the eye (31) and subtract the signal from an aphakic globe, which represents other parts of the eye. Sharply defined signals of lens Pi, and alpha, beta, and gamma phosphate moieties of ATP could be determined. Interestingly, the iris contains almost no detectable phosphates of any kind.

^{13}C-MRS Study

It has been found (33) that there is a direct correlation between the relative concentration of gamma-crystallin fraction in the lens and the degree of acrylamide incorporation and its ability to affect the cold cataract phenomenon. Localized alterations in the density of packing of lens proteins leads to changes in transparency. A classic example of this is the cold cataract phenomenon, which can be reversed by warming. It is known that certain reagents such as acrylamide can prevent the cold cataract phenomenon.

Carbon13 is an isotope that occurs naturally; however, the concentrations are not high enough to be used for MRS analysis. Therefore, exogenous carbon13 such as

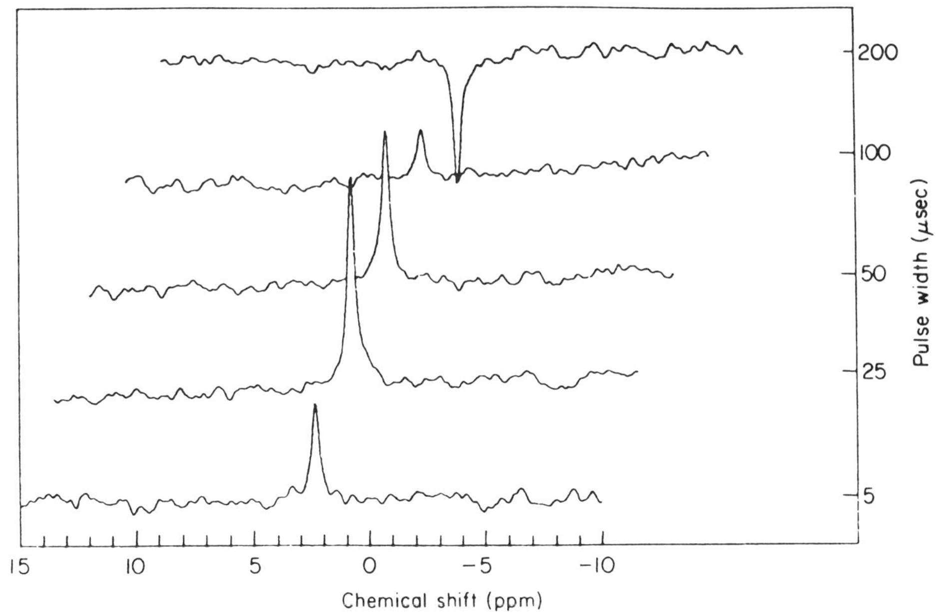

FIG. 3. ^{31}P NMR spectra, acquired using different RF pulse duration times, of a bovine globe phantom containing 10 mM P_i and 120 mM NaCl (plus a trace amount of $MnCl_2$ to reduce the sample T_1 to ca. 1 sec) in the lens compartment; the anterior and posterior compartments contained 120 mM NaCl. The surface coil diameter was 3.8 cm. All other spectral acquisition parameters are described in Materials and Methods. (Reproduced with permission from Schleich et al., ref. 31.)

^{13}C-glucose has to be added. To study lens protein packing by MRS, lenses were placed in sample tubes and ^{13}C and ^{1}H-MRS were obtained at 75 and 46 MHz. Lenses were incubated in a medium of balanced salt solution with a bicarbonate buffer containing 7 mM glucose, 0.75 mM L-glutamine, 2 mg/dl potassium penicillin G, and 2 mg/dl streptomycin sulfate. The medium was gassed with 95% oxygen–5% CO_2 to maintain oxygen tension and regulate pH. The incubations were maintained at controlled temperatures; to prevent the cold cataract, 5% acrylamide was added. For deuterated experiments, the components of the incubation media were added to deuterium oxide (D_2O) solutions. The pH was maintained at preincubation levels. Deuterium has no MRS spectrum so peaks due to solvent water or protons exchangeable with solvent water will disappear. Buffering is important because deuterium oxide is not equivalent to water in its acidity behavior.

Method

Water-proton transverse relaxation rates were measured on lenses to which 1.3 mM dextran-magnetite had been added to the solution outside the lens. The transverse magnetization decay was obtained by signal averaging the output from a Spin-lock CPS-2 pulsed spectrometer, employing the CPMG pulse sequence and sampling echo maxima. Data analysis was performed on a DEC system-10 computer, and temperature was controlled at ±1.0°C by a YSI Model 72 Proportional Temperature Controller employing thermally regulated nitrogen gas. Control of temperature is important because heat can alter protein-solvent interactions and even denature some proteins, and the probes generate heat. The amount of acrylamide in the lenses was estimated with ^{13}C-MRS to measure the loss of acrylamide from the incubating solution by using dioxane as a reference and by measuring area ratios.

Example

For diabetic cataract studies, the lenses were incubated in 35.5 mM glucose for 48 hr. The ^{13}C-sorbitol peaks grow taller and taller over the time period; growth of the peaks can be blocked by certain aldose reductase inhibitors such as flavonoids.

MRI

MRI is an established tool in clinical imaging, but has largely been limited to whole body imaging (34,35). Aguayo and coworkers (36) were able to use the technique for ova of frogs and on a mouse eye, obtaining a clear image of the interior of an intact eye without invading the eye in any way.

Fluorescence Spectroscopy

Tryptophan (TRP) in lens proteins can be made to produce fluorescence that can be detected with fluorescence spectroscopy. This fluorescence allows the study of the lens proteins, their structural integrity, and their relationship with their solvent medium, and is particularly useful in studying phenomena like cold cataract. Acrylamide is a neutral quencher of TRP fluorescence in the interior of proteins, whereas iodide does not significantly quench TRP fluorescence in native proteins due to surface charges. Prevention of cold cataract with acrylamide can be studied with TRP fluorescence in lenses incubated with either acrylamide or iodide. MRS of ^{13}C-labeled acrylamide is used to monitor which crystallins are most affected, using the techniques presented in the previous section.

Method

Fresh human lenses of various ages were used in the study presented here. Five percent acrylamide (20% of which is ^{13}C-labeled) was added to Earle's media containing 5.5 mM glucose. A similar amount of iodide was used in a parallel study. The lenses remained clear during the 2-hr incubation (37°C). The effects of exposing one lens to low-level broadband UV radiation were compared with the contralateral lens incubated in the dark. Both fluorescence and NMR spectra were recorded (37). After incubation the lenses were scanned with a Farand MKII spectrometer. The lenses were dialyzed against Earle's media overnight at 37°C and the fluorescence and NMR spectra were repeated. One percent acrylamide or iodide was used for the fluorescence and NMR spectra were repeated. One percent acrylamide or iodide was used for the fluorescence-quenching studies. Afterward the proteins were extracted and separated.

Example

In lenses incubated with acrylamide in the dark, there was a marked diminution in the TRP fluorescence intensity compared with its preincubation levels. TRP fluorescence returned to at least 75% of its preincubation level after overnight dialysis, indicating the acrylamide was not covalently bound to proteins. In contrast, when the lens was exposed to UV radiation there was marked quenching and the lens never recovered to its preincubation fluorescence, even after overnight dialysis, indicating the acrylamide was covalently bound. UV light alone, without acrylamide, had no effect on fluorescence. It was also observed that the degree of acrylamide photobinding decreased progressively with age as did the extent of acrylamide incorporated in the dark. NMR also showed the most acrylamide binding in young lenses. Iodide had no quenching effect in the intact lens but had a little effect on extracted alpha and beta crystallins, which do have some exposed tryptophan residues.

Scanning Lens Monitor

Lenses can develop opacities due to exposure to various chemicals, including high glucose concentrations. The opacities can be detected with the scanning lens monitor (38). Results correlate well with the development of the sorbitol peak in the lens detected with ^{13}C-MRS as described previously.

Lenses isolated from freshly enucleated rat eyes were quickly rinsed with sterile phosphate buffered saline (PBS) solution and placed in normal medium (M199 containing 10% fetal calf serum and 0.1% glutamine). Lenses were then transferred to sterile clear-plastic culture tubes containing 3 ml of normal glucose medium (5.5 mM glucose) or high glucose medium (55 mM glucose) and incubated at 37°C in a water jacketed incubator with 5% carbon dioxide.

Lenses were examined after 21 hr of culturing using the scanning lens monitor. Kevex hardware/software was also used to analyze the intensity distributions of lens light projections. Wide-beam white light from a tungsten light source was projected through rat lenses onto an opaque white plastic screen. On the opposite side of this screen an RCA video camera was focused on the light image and fed into a Colorado

Video unit. The video signal was modulated and calibrated by the Colorado unit and the same setup conditions were held for imaging of lenses.

After 21 hr of incubation, lenses in normal medium were clear, whereas lenses in high glucose medium had developed opacities. A scanning lens monitor generated plots of focal length as a function of distance from the optical center. Kevex imaging of lens light projections revealed differences in intensity distributions between 5.5 mM and 55 mM glucose lenses. The system allowed the lens opacities produced by culturing in high glucose medium to be detected not only qualitatively but also quantitated.

Lens Metabolism and Enzyme Activities

Lens metabolism and lens enzyme activities can be changed by eye irritation. Therefore, detection of these changes can measure eye irritation and intoxication.

Each lens of one pair (bovine or porcine) was laid into an Erlenmeyer flask containing a culture medium (39). The compound to be tested was added to the medium of one lens of the pair; the other lens was not treated and served as the control. After 20 to 24 hr of incubation (this may be prolonged even to 96 hr) at 37°C, lenses were taken out of the medium and were prepared for analysis.

Numerous parameters might be analyzed in a single lens, provided that the lens extract was divided in a proper way. In a deproteinized extract, energy-rich compounds such as the free adenine nucleotides, carbohydrates, intermediates of glycolysis, glutathione, and the coenzymes nicotinamide-adenine dinucleotide, reduced (NADH) and nicotinamide-adenine dinucleotide phosphate, reduced (NADPH) in both their oxidized and reduced states might be determined. In the aqueous extract, most enzymes catalyzing the breakdown of carbohydrates are found; their catalytic activities, kinetic properties, and heat labilities might be measured. Not all of the above parameters can be determined in a single lens. Frequently only a few of the parameters are altered by an experimental compound and will need to be tested further.

Many enzyme activities can be determined in lens homogenates, allowing a detailed picture of normal lens metabolism and pertubations of metabolism by specific compounds to be obtained (40). In one protocol, lenses were dissected from the eye, weighed, and frozen at −28°C. Samples of the different layers were obtained using a newly constructed slicing instrument. With this technique layers down to 0.25 mm can be obtained. The layers were weighed and worked up into a 10% homogenate. This was centrifuged at 11,630 × g for 30 min and the supernatants were taken for the determination of enzyme activities and protein concentrations. The authors determined the activities of key enzymes of several metabolic pathways: aldose reductase (AR) and sorbitol dehydrogenase (SDH) for the sorbitol pathway, phosphofructokinase (PFK) and aldolase (ALD) for glycolysis, and glutathione reductase (GR) and glutathione peroxidase (GPX) as representatives for the protection of the lens against oxidative stress. The enzyme activities were expressed as specific activities (mU/mg water-soluble protein).

Some results using incubated lenses have been negative (39). Many eyedrops contain potassium iodide (KI) which is said to protect protein -SH groups from oxidation and to reduce disulfides produced by oxidation. However, KI had no effect on the distribution and numbers of any oxidized or reduced -SH groups in bovine lenses after incubation.

Another study using cultured lenses dealt with aldose reductase inhibitors (40). Aldose reductase catalyzes the first step in the conversion of glucose to sorbitol, which in turn is converted to fructose. An excess of glucose (as in diabetes) produces an excess of sorbitol, which disturbs the lens's osmotic balance and leads to sugar cataracts. It was possible to study the levels of glucose and fructose, of ATP and adenosine monophosphate (AMP), and of glutathione in its oxidized and reduced states in lenses and determine that different aldose reductase inhibitors may have very different effects on these ratios.

Calcium Accumulation

Human cataracts do not necessarily have high calcium accumulations; however, high and low calcium levels *in vitro* are cataractogenic to cultured lenses (41). These authors showed that calcium accumulation is often a secondary change in human cataractogenesis. Lens calcium levels are not elevated prior to the first appearance of cataract, but are greatly elevated in severe cataracts. It is hoped that studies of lens calcium accumulation will give a greater understanding of cataractogensis.

Methods

Emory mice are used in many cataract studies because they develop cataracts spontaneously. Lenses were removed from the enucleated eyes of Emory mice and were cleaned and weighed under conditions chosen to minimize contamination with extraneous calcium. A lens pair was treated with 0.8 N KOH in a microcentrifuge tube. The lenses were dissolved with occasional vigorous vortex-mixing at room temperature over several days. More 0.8 N KOH was added and the solution was mixed well. The resulting lens extract was suitable for direct calcium determination.

The total protein was determined by a bicinchoninic acid (BCA) procedure (42). Calcium was determined by a modified calcium fluoremetry procedure (43). An aliquot of the initial lens extract was diluted with KOH to give suitable calcium concentrations for fluorometry. The tubes for the procedure had been carefully cleaned by soaking in a special cleaning solution (nitric acid and sodium bichromate) followed by rinsing with distilled water. This removed most extraneous calcium. The tubes were read in a Turner model 111 fluorometer, and a calibration curve was constructed for each batch of calcium stock solution.

Example

There was no age-dependent increase in calcium in the normal mouse lens (cataract-resistant strain). Since cataractous changes precede the first detectable increases in calcium, calcium accumulation was thought to be a secondary event. It would still be useful to demonstrate that calcium accumulation is secondary to cataract formation with an animal model. Calcium levels went up as cataracts developed in Emory mice, but did not go up significantly in mice with late-forming cataracts until the cataracts actually developed. In addition, mercaptopropionylglycine, a calcium chelating agent, failed to prevent development of cataracts in Emory mice (44) and could not remove the calcium from old cataracts. The data all confirmed that calcium accumulation in cataracts is secondary to the development of the cataract and is due in part to tight binding of calcium to proteins.

Special Ca^{2+},K^{+} Channels

The apical membrane of the chick lens epithelial cell has been shown to contain several varieties of K^{+} selective channels, including a large conductance channel activated by internal Ca^{2+} and depolarization (the Ca^{2+},K^{+} channel). Rae and Cooper (45) have examined the changes in these channels with maturation. Their technique shows the possibility of using not only chicks but chick embryos as model systems for studying the lens.

Two different types of preparations were used. For 5 to 7 day chick embryos, explants were used. Capsule-epithelial preparations were attached to 35-mm petri dishes by making four cuts through the epithelia with a scalpel blade. For embryos older than 7 days and for chicks after hatching, the lens was excised from its ciliary body attachments. The dissections were done in a sodium aspartate Ringer solution because this resulted in many viable cells. The lens was decapsulated and the capsule and epithelium were pinned with stainless steel insect pins to a Sylgard cylinder. This was fitted into an acrylic chamber for visualization under a compound microscope. Single channel currents were recorded and the data was digitized into a pulse code modulated videocassette recorder or into an INDEC computer interface.

Example

From day 5 of the embryo until hatching the apical membrane of the lens epithelium contained primarily large conductance Ca^{2+},K^{+} channels. A new maxi-K^{+} channel appeared about the same time the Ca^{2+},K^{+} channels disappeared. The function of these channels *in vivo* proved something of a mystery to Rae and Cooper (45). They speculated that one channel is somehow converted into another; if so this would suggest that the interconversion of channels is a model for studying lens maturation and a site at which potential ocular teratogens could be tested. Beebe and Feagans (46) suggested that changes in potassium ion permeability might be important for the differentiation of fiber cells from epithelial cells even in adult lenses; therefore, the effect of potential ocular toxins on this receptor could provide a measure of their potency in inhibiting lens repair after injury.

Distribution of Cholesterol, Phospholipid, and Protein

The lens tissue normally has a cholesterol to phospholipid molar ratio of 3.5:1.0. It has been found that if this ratio is reduced or elevated, cataracts result (47). In this study (48), the regional distribution of cholesterol, phospholipid, and protein content were determined in human and bovine lenses.

Human lenses were excised from eyes obtained 4 hr postmortem and were frozen in liquid nitrogen. A 5.5-mm diameter thin-walled trephine was placed in a hand drill and used to remove a core sample from the frozen lens (warmed to −20°C in a freezer prior to taking the sample). This sample was divided into four sections. Core sections and surrounding tissue from lenses of about the same age were pooled. Lipid was extracted at 0°C under a stream of argon. Buffer B contained urea and dithiothreitol buffered with tris/HCl (pH 7.4). Ice cold buffer B was added to each of the pooled lens sections and was homogenized with a teflon douncer jacketed in ice. Lipid was extracted with cold chloroform/methanol, mixed, and centrifuged. The lower phase was removed and evaporated under argon. This dried extract was rectified to remove any denatured lipoprotein with ice cold chloroform and KC1. The bottom phase was then removed and assayed for phospholipid and cholesterol.

Protein was determined by the Peterson (49) modification of the Lowry assay. Two standard curves were made consisting of aliquots of bovine diluted lens homogenate. The protein concentration was determined by dividing the slope of the sample curve by the slope of the standard curve. This was necessary as differences in protein composition may alter the apparent protein concentrations measured by the ordinary Lowry method.

Lipid phosphorus was determined using a modified Bartlett (50) assay. Two standard curves were made with inorganic phosphorus. Aliquots of lipid extract were dried under argon before assaying.

Cholesterol was determined by a modification of the Huang et al. (51) assay. Aliquots of lipid extract were dried under argon before assay. Cholesterol detection reagent was added to the dried samples and sonicated for 5 min.

ISOLATED RETINA PREPARATIONS

Although chemicals that contact the eye topically do not penetrate well enough into the eyeball to reach the retina in the back of the eye, photostimulation from the frontal part of the eye (which can lead to phototoxicity) and retinal toxicity caused by systemic drugs are rather common occurrences. Therefore, the isolated perfused bovine eye can be used as a model for the study of acute retinal toxicity.

Electroretinography (ERG) is a measurement of the total neuronal activity of retinal cells, and is said to measure "the objective and functional response of the retina" to light (52). It follows that any inflammatory mediator that can alter the ERG "may be a messenger between ocular inflammatory impairments and visual function."

Bovine eyes were enucleated immediately following exsanguination (52,53). A branch of the ophthalmociliary artery feeding the retina was identified and cannulated with a 22-gauge needle. The cannula was secured with a small clamp and the residual blood flushed with Hank's balanced salt solution containing heparin. Subsequently, the eyes were attached to a peristaltic pump set at a rate of 1.2 to 1.3 ml/min.

The cannulated eye was placed in a stand equipped with an overhead Grass flash unit before a recording electrode was implanted through its cornea. One reference electrode was placed midway down the globe and a ground electrode was connected to the stump of the severed optic nerve. The eyes were continuously perfused and dark adapted before further experimentation. For the determination of the stability of the preparation, electronic flashes were given at 15-min intervals and ERG responses recorded until expiration of the preparation. The responses to changing oxygen tension were tested by stopping the perfusion. Photic flashes were administered at 1-min intervals until extinction of the ERG; at this time an additional 20 min of ischemia was maintained. The effects of reperfusion were determined by recording ERG responses to photic stimuli at 1-min intervals.

At the conclusion of each experiment the eye was perfusion fixed through the attached cannula for 5 min. Retinas from these eyes were carefully dissected and immersion fixed for 2 hr in 2% paraformaldehyde-glutaraldehyde solution. Small rectangular pieces were carefully dissected, placed in specimen vials, washed overnight in cacodylate buffer, postfixed in osmium tetroxide, and dehydrated in ascending concentrations of ethanol before being embedded in Araldite 502. The polymerized blocks were sectioned at 1-μm or 800-nm thickness and stained for light or electron microscopy, respectively.

Isolated retinas could be kept viable for several hours and reproducible ERGs recorded. The primary response of the cells monitored is the b-wave generated by the Müller's cells. Introduction of hydroxyl radicals with Fe^{2+} and ascorbate considerably shortened the life of the retinas, as measured by loss of the b-wave. This effect was reduced by addition of free radical scavengers.

Example

Leukotriene B_4 (LTB_4) perfused into the isolated retina reduced the ERG amplitude in a dose-dependent manner; LTC_4 and LTD_4 had a similar effect. They may increase Na^+ membrane permeability and have an opposite effect to light on rod outer segment membranes. Platelet activating factor (PAF) and derivatives also were toxic to the ERG; PAF binds to a specific retinal receptor and stimulates phosphatidylinositol breakdown, mobilizing intracellular calcium. The data suggested a role for PAF in visual function.

ALTERNATIVES TO EYE TISSUES

Chemicals that irritate eye tissues will also irritate other sensitive tissues such as egg chorioallantoic membrane, vagina mucous membrane, and ileum (which alters ileum contractility). Therefore, these tissues can also be used as alternatives to eye irritation studies.

Chicken Egg Test

Huhner-Embryonen Test

The Huhner-Embryonen test (HET) can be used to give information on embryolethality, embryonic development and growth, teratogenicity, and systemic toxicity, including immunopathology and metabolic pathways (9). Testing with incubated hen's egg is a borderline case between *in vivo* and *in vitro* systems. The HET has now been extended to include chorioallantoic membrane (CAM) testing as a mucous-membrane irritation test.

Chorioallantoic Membrane Test

Eggs to be treated were first candled in order to discard those that were defective; only fresh, fertile eggs were used. Eggs weighing less than 50 g or more than 60 g were rejected. For CAM testing according to Leighton and coworkers (8), eggs were incubated at 37.5°C ± 0.5°C and a relative humidity of 62.5% ± 7.5%. The eggs were candled on day 5 of incubation and every day thereafter; eggs with nonviable embryos were removed. On day 10 of incubation the egg shell was scratched around the air cell with a dentist's rotary saw and then pared off. After careful removal of the inner egg membranes the vasular CAM was exposed. The test substance, dissolved or suspended, was dropped onto the membrane. Solid test materials were applied directly on the vascular chorioallantois and irrigated with warm water. In every case a series of four eggs was used; two eggs treated with vehicle only served as controls. The CAM, the blood vessels, including the capillary system, and the albumin were examined and scored for irritant effects (hyperemia, hemorrhages, coagulation) at 0.5, 2, and 5 min after treatment.

The CAM can also be used to test for irritation and damage that develop over the course of days rather than minutes. There are two basic procedures for preparing the CAM (Fig. 1). In one procedure, a fertile egg is incubated for a week or more, at which time a window is cut in the shell and a small tear is made in the shell membrane. A small hole is made over the natural airspace at the blunt end of the egg so that the chorioallantoic membrane is dropped below the window. The chemical being tested is applied to the dropped CAM through the window and the aperture is then closed with adhesive tape.

Another procedure for preparing the CAM was developed by Zwilling (54). In the

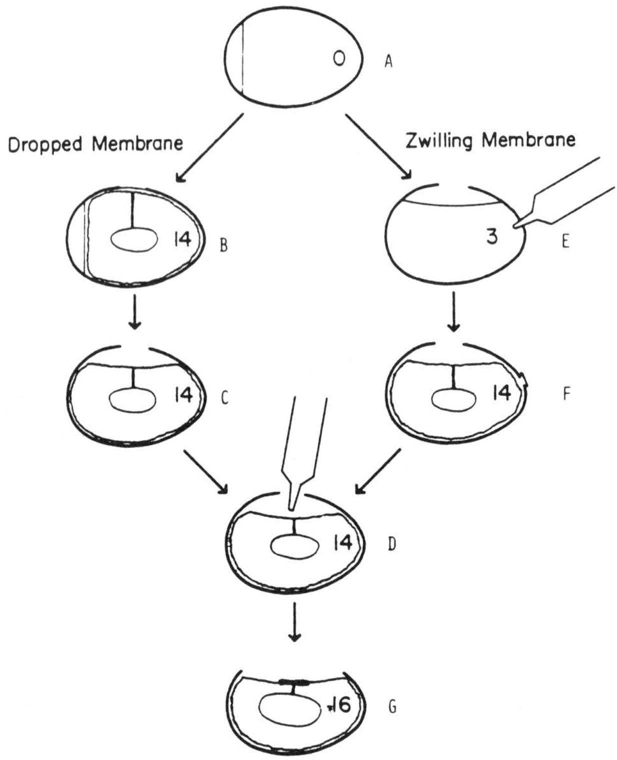

FIG. 4. Two procedures for preparing chicken egg chorioallantoic membrane (CAM). (Reproduced with permission from Leighton et al., ref. 8.)

2- or 3-day-old embryo egg, 2 ml of albumin is removed from the egg near the pointed end, and a window is cut through the shell. In the course of the preparation the airspace shifts; the "floor" of the chamber created now consists of the upper aspect of the liquid contents of the egg. The window is closed with tape and the egg returned to the incubator. The chorioallantois becomes the floor of the chamber. With either technique, a test substance is applied to the CAM and the opening is retaped; 2 or 3 days after application the tape is removed from the window and the adjacent shell removed to enlarge the window and provide a clear macroscopic view of the site of injury on the CAM.

Example

In preliminary experiments with the classically dropped CAM (Figs. 5-7), graded concentrations of a strong acid and strong base were applied to the 14-day-old membrane, with the reaction to injury observed 3 days later (8). The data showed the

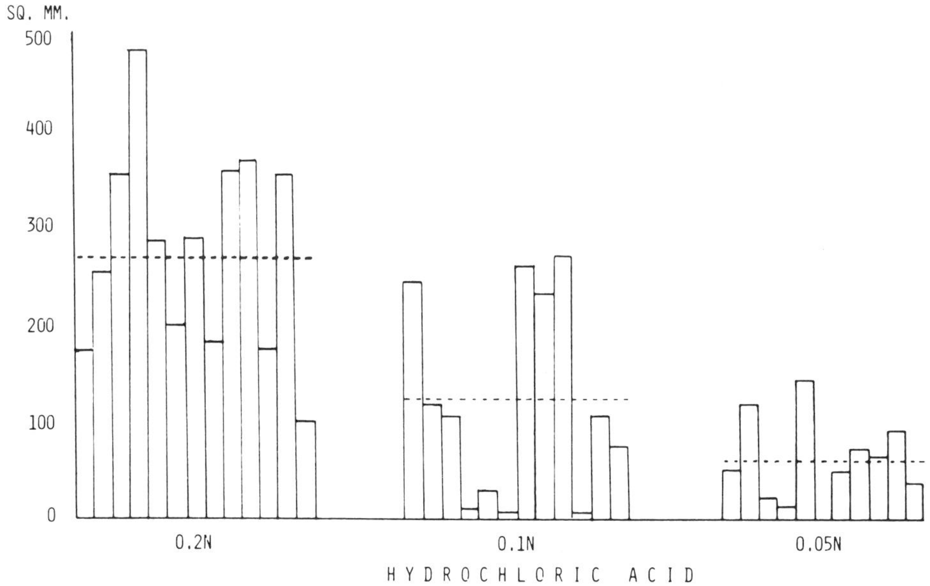

FIG. 5. Acid lesioning of chicken egg chorioallantoic membrane (CAM). (Each bar represents one egg.) (Reproduced with permission from Leighton et al., ref. 8.)

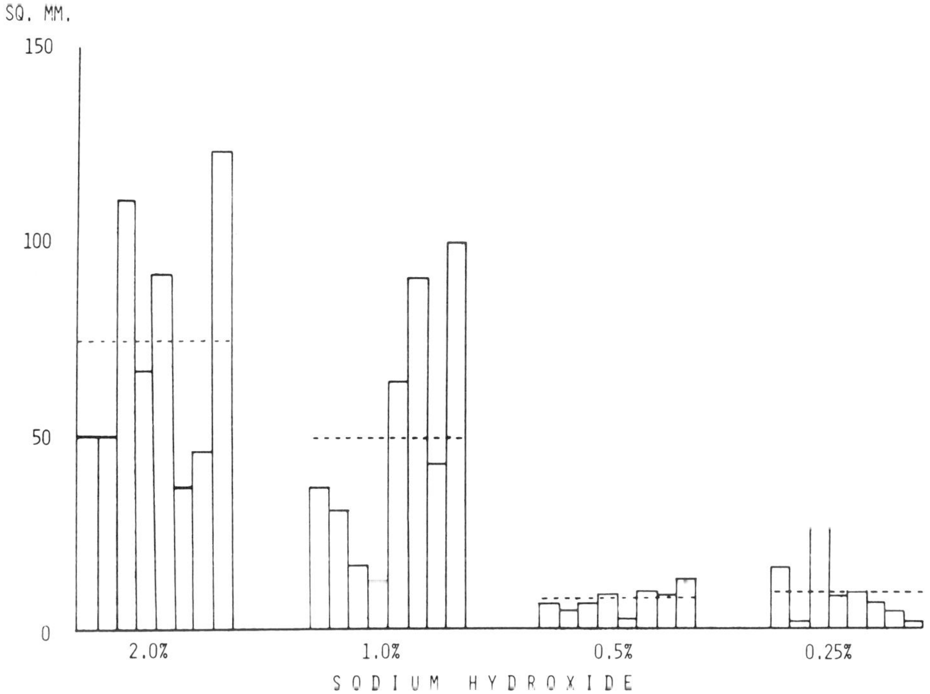

FIG. 6. Sodium hydroxide lesioning of chicken egg chorioallantoic membrane (CAM). (Each bar represents one egg.) (Reproduced with permission from Leighton et al., ref. 8.)

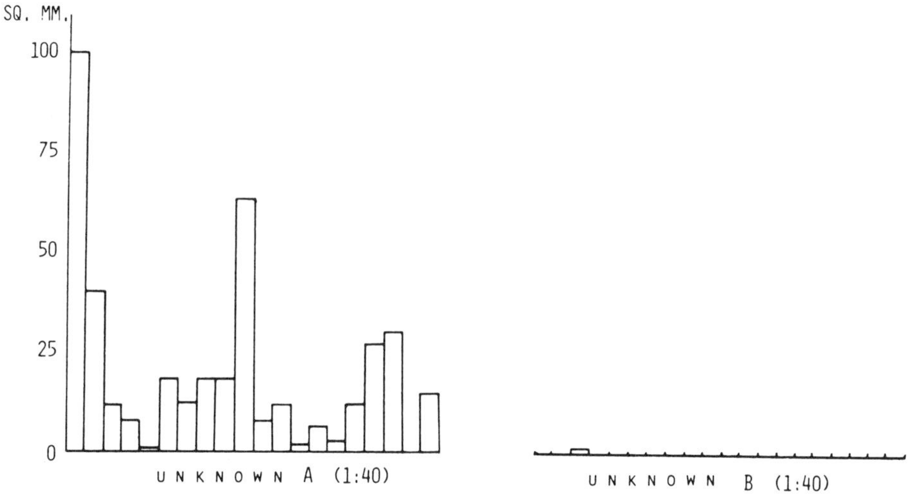

FIG. 7. Lesion of chicken egg chorioallantoic membrane (CAM) with two unknowns, A and B. Unknown A is known to be corrosive to the eyes of rabbits; unknown B is not. (Each bar represents one egg.) (Reproduced with permission from Leighton et al., ref. 8.)

surface areas of lesions in square millimeters, measured as a product of the length of the axes. There was an overall (mean) decrease in size of lesion with decrease in concentration of the acid ($p < 0.001$). A similar correlation of irritant concentration and lesion area was found for NaOH. There was a decrease in the size of the lesion as the concentration of base was lowered ($p < 0.001$).

In other experiments, two substances were used; solution A, which was strongly positive by the Draize test, and solution B, which was negative in the same assay procedure (8). Each solution was diluted 1:40 with normal saline and then applied to Zwilling membranes. There was a clearly significant difference between A and B, despite a fairly large degree of variation between eggs. In these experiments, the numerical time-dependent scores for hyperemia, hemorrhage, and coagulation were summed to give a single numerical value indicating the irritation potential of the test substance on a scale with a maximum value of 21.

Vaginal Mucous Membrane

The vagina and cervix have mucous membranes that are susceptible to a variety of irritants. A general indicator of inflammation and cellular toxicity in these tissues is the release of prostanoids by the affected tissues. Prostanoids are products of arachidonic acid or fatty acid metabolism, released to activate various protective mechanisms for the tissue under attack by noxious stimuli. The type of prostanoid produced depends on the particular cell activated.

Method

Female rats were followed daily with vaginal smears to establish estrus cycles. When cytotoxicity was to be determined using a rat (55), it was anesthetized with pentobarbital and exsanguinated. The reproductive tract was isolated and trimmed of fat and connective tissue. The vagina was divided longitudinally into two or four segments, which were placed in wells containing Krebs' bicarbonate buffer at room temperature. The tissue was then transferred to wells containing either irritant solutions or buffer, which served as a control. After 45 sec the tissues were rinsed with buffer and replaced in wells containing only buffer. The tray containing tissues was placed in a shaking water bath (37°C) in a 95% O_2–5% CO_2 atmosphere. After incubation for 30 min, the medium over the tissue, containing the released prostantoids, was frozen at −70°C and stored until assayed for prostanoids by radioimmunoassay methods.

Example

The concentrations of various prostanoids found in the media of control vaginal tissue were compared to tissues exposed to 70% ethanol. The amounts of PGE_2 produced during different stages of the estrus cycle are slightly different, with the highest production occurring during the estrus. The PGE_2 release is a function of the concentration of ethanol used.

Ileum Contractility

Various surfactants have been shown to inhibit spontaneous drug-induced or electrically induced muscle contractions. When applied to an intact tissue, a surfactant has to penetrate the outer surface layers before reaching the contractile cells. The penetration of superficial cell layers and ability to deactivate contractile fibers determine the overall effect of a surfactant on a muscle preparation; such a preparation might serve as an experimental indicator for ocular irritation. Surfactants are common in household and laboratory products and are common causes of eye irritation. A study (56) has been done to compare the ability of surfactants to hemolyze bovine erythrocytes (chosen as a single cytotoxicity model) and to block spontaneous contractions of mouse and rabbit ileum with the effect of the same surfactants on the rabbit eye *in vivo*.

Methods

Sections of terminal ileum were set up under a resting tension of 0.7 g for mouse and 1.0 g for rabbit in organ baths containing Tyrode-Ringer solution at 35°C and were bubbled with atmospheric air. Spontaneous contractions were recorded via isotonic displacement transducers on Washington 400MD oscillographs. The tissues were allowed 25 min to equilibrate before addition of any surfactant. Surfactants were added at 10-min intervals, so the concentration grew progressively greater. If >50% block of spontaneous activity had not been achieved after six additions the tissue was discarded. Concentration-effect curves were constructed enabling the calculation of the concentration required to produce 50% block of spontaneous activity for mouse ileum (EC_{50} mouse) and rabbit ileum (EC_{50} rabbit).

Examples

The most potent hemolytic action, as previously determined (22), was generally achieved with the longer alkyl chain surfactants. The C-12 (triethanolamine lauryl sulfate, sodium lauryl sulfate) and C-14 (triethanolamine myristyl sulfate) anionics showed greater hemolytic potency than the corresponding C-12 (lauryl trimethyl ammonium bromide) and C-14 (myristyl trimethyl ammonium bromide) cationics. These results are at variance with the *in vivo* results in rabbits, where the cationics were more irritant than the corresponding anionics. Order of potency for EC_{50} mouse or EC_{50} rabbit also differed from the order for EC_{50} hemolysis. There is an apparent trend from EC_{50} hemolysis, in which long alkyl chains were most potent, through EC_{50} mouse to EC_{50} rabbit and finally to *in vivo*, where short chains are most potent. Correlation between EC_{50} rabbit and both corneal and conjunctival irritancy scores *in vivo* is good.

CELL CULTURES

In addition to isolated tissues, cell cultures can also be used as alternatives to the *in vivo* Draize test. Cell cultures are more convenient than isolated tissues and in most cases do not require the sacrifice of animals. Some cell lines are of human origin, eliminating any interspecies differences and the inherent complications these produce in toxicology. However, *in vitro* tests generally have to be used for individual classes of chemicals and to represent a single aspect of the *in vivo* Draize test; this is partly because of the great variation in physicochemical properties and biological activities of the many classes of potentially irritating chemicals. The acceptable cell culture methods must give results that correlate well with human experiences. It is hoped that cell culture *in vitro* methods will eventually replace the Draize test so that eye irritancy tests can be done by more humane methods.

Conjunctiva Cell Culture

Determination of CDT_{50} (50% Cell Damage Time)

Chang's human conjunctival cells were cultured in Eagle's minimal essential medium (pH 7.2) with 10% fetal bovine serum. A sheet of 10 million cells was grown for 3 to 4 days in an incubator at 37°C, trypsinized with 0.25% trypsin and 0.02% ethylenediaminetetraacetic acid (EDTA, pH 7.2), and then suspended in 40 to 50 ml of medium. Two milliliters of cell suspension was transferred to each of 16 to 20 small glass flasks with a counted inoculum cell population of 2 to 3 × 10^5/ml (57,58).

The cultures were sealed and incubated at 37°C for 48 hr to obtain a confluent cell sheet. After decanting of the media from the cultures, a monolayer of cells was exposed to a test solution of 0.5 ml during a given period of time. Controls were exposed to a phosphate buffer solution (PBS). Following exposure to the test agents, the medium was replaced with 2 ml of fresh medium and cells were incubated another 24 hr at 37°C. The sheets of cells were separated by trypsinization and suspended in 2 ml of medium for cell counting. All topical drugs in this study contained benzalkonium chloride (BAC) as a preservative.

Example

The CDT_{50} values of an aminoglycoside preparation with BAC were 3 min 56 sec in micromycin sulfate, 9 min 26 sec in dibekacin sulfate, 17 min 35 sec in sisomycin sulfate, 24 min 24 sec in tobracin, and 77 min 49 sec in amikacin sulfate. Aminoglycosides without BAC, with the exception of micromycin, showed no cytotoxicity. The CDT_{50} of micromycin without BAC was 13 min 20 sec.

Morphological Study

Light Microscopy

After a confluent cell sheet was formed, cells were exposed to test drugs for 30 sec and immediately washed by PBS to completely eliminate the test drug from the medium (57). Cells were examined under the microscope with Giemsa stain. In order to know whether the cells had been restored to their normal appearance, they were examined again under the microscope 48 hr after the passage of cells exposed to 5-fluorouracil (5-FU), a compound causing cell degeneration by interfering with DNA replication.

Scanning Electron Microscope

After the cells had been exposed to test solutions for 30 sec they were washed with PBS and fixed with 2.5% glutaraldehyde for 30 min at 4°C. After being washed with PBS they were fixed with 1% osmium tetroxide and then dehydrated in graded series of ethanol. They were treated in a carbon dioxide critical point drying, coated with gold palladium, and examined under the scanning electron microscope.

Example

When the cells were exposed to 5-FU at concentrations greater than 0.01% for 30 sec, clear signs of cell damage were found. Scanning electron microscopy revealed reduction of microvilli and filopodia.

Quantitative Cytotoxicity Study

Two millimeters of the cell suspension were inoculated into small plastic culture flasks and cultured for 48 hr at 37°C. The cell sheet was then exposed to test solutions for 30 sec. After the test solutions had been excluded by decantation and rinsing with PBS, the cells were cultured for an additional 48 hr. Inhibition of cell growth was evaluated by the Student's t-test with a 5% level of probability being considered significant.

Corneal Cell Culture

Morphology of Human Corneal Epithelium

This part of the book has aimed at presenting a sensitive *in vitro* corneal cell culture model to assess ocular toxicology. Corneal cells are the cells most directly exposed to environmental toxins, and are the cells most affected by the Draize test. It is our hope that corneal cells in culture will replace the Draize test, which has been criticized on several counts (see chapter by Rohde, "*In Vivo* Eye Irritation Test Methods").

The stratified squamous epithelium, characterized by apical tight junctions and superficial microvilli and microplicae, is the primary barrier to penetration of toxic or irritative substances into the eye. Jumblatt and Neufeld (59) have developed a tissue culture system for obtaining sheets of pure rabbit corneal epithelium with morphological features similar to cells *in vivo*. These cultures have been used for corneal wound closure in rabbits. This technique was then applied to human corneal epithelium.

Human corneas with normal epithelium were obtained from donor eyes judged unsuitable for transplantation. The eyes were rinsed with Earle's balanced salt solution (EBSS) containing Garamycin sulfate. The full-thickness cornea was removed to a dish containing EBSS for initiation of tissue culture. Donor human corneal rims were also placed in EBSS containing Garamycin. The scleral portions were trimmed, and the full-thickness corneal rim obtained was 2 to 3 mm in width.

The endothelium was removed from the full-thickness corneas and corneal rims of humans or of rabbits by blunt dissection with forceps, and the stromal-epithelial tissue was used to initiate explant cultures or pure cultures of isolated corneal epithelium. For explant cultures, the posterior lamellae of the stroma were peeled off. The remaining epithelium was minced, drained, placed in a well tissue culture plate, dried for 5 min, and incubated at 37°C in air/CO_2. Pure epithelial cultures were dried for 5 min, and incubated at 37°C in air/CO_2. Pure epithelial cultures were established using cell sheets isolated from the stroma that have undergone digestion with Dipase II. The Descemet's membrane and corneal endothelium were stripped, and remaining cornea was placed in Dipase II in calcium- and magnesium-free Hank's balanced salt solution at 37°C. Cell sheets were peeled and used to initiate cell cultures. The cultures were maintained in medium consisting of equal parts of Dulbecco's modified Eagle medium and Ham's F-12 supplemented with 5% fetal bovine serum, epidermal growth factor, insulin, and cholera toxin.

Using a phase contrast microscope, all cultures were examined for epithelial cell growth. Cultures were fixed using Karnovsky's fixative and processed for microscopy. In the initial cultures in which Dipase II was used to free epithelial cells from the underlying stroma, cultures never grew to confluency. From epithelial/stromal explants, however, extensive epithelial outgrowths could be obtained. Scanning electron microscopy revealed typical epithelial specialization with microvilli and microplicae on the epithelial surface.

Following treatment with Dipase II to digest the proteins anchoring the cells to the culture vessel surface, the cell layers could be released as sheets. These sheets contained columnar basal cells, squamous superficial cells, desmosomes, apical villi, and keratin bundles. Human corneal cell culture was not as successful as rabbit cell culture; human cells treated with Dipase II either failed to attach, or if attached, failed to grow. This lack of success may be due to a difference in enzymatic susceptibility of rabbit and human epithelial-stromal adhesion complexes.

Cytotoxicity

Confluent cultures of rabbit corneal epithelium were grown in complete medium: minimal essential medium with D-valine supplemented with 10% heat-inactivated fetal calf serum, 10 µg/ml crystalline insulin, 20 ng/ml epidermal growth factor, and 0.1 ng/ml cholera toxin (5,6,60). Cultures were inspected daily and the culture medium was changed evey 48 hr. After 7 to 12 days, confluent cultures from the master primary culture plates were reseeded into 24-well Primaria polystyrene tissue culture plates. After 48 hr culture to allow the cells to reattach, the complete medium was removed and fresh complete medium added, either with the drug to be tested in it or with no additions (control). Drugs tested included ophthalmic preservatives, antiviral, and aminoglycoside drugs.

After 5, 30, or 60 min the medium containing the drug (or the control medium) was removed and the culture plates were twice washed with Dulbecco's phosphate buffered saline without calcium or magnesium. Cytotoxicity was determined by measuring DNA synthesis. One-half milliliter of complete medium, containing 1 µCi of sterile ^{3}H-thymidine (specific activity 6.7 mCi/mmol) was added to each well. After 8 to 12 hr of incubation, DNA was extracted. Samples were solubilized in Aquasol and counted in a liquid scintillation counter. Data were expressed as the percentage inhibition of ^{3}H-thymidine incorporation compared to the control.

Example

Increased doses of a variety of cytotoxic agents (60) caused progressive inhibition of ^3H-thymidine incorporation. Cytosine arabinoside produced significant inhibition of ^3H-thymidine incorporation at $10^{-7}M$. Concentrations of methotrexate of 1 mM were required for significant inhibition of ^3H-thymidine incorporation. Melphalan, 5-fluorouracil, and thiotepa significantly inhibited ^3H-thymidine incorporation at $10^{-8}M$, $10^{-6}M$, and $10^{-4}M$, respectively. These are antineoplastic drugs especially sensitive to growing cells. It is not surprising they were toxic to corneal epithelial cells.

Plasminogen Activation Measurement

The enzyme plasminogen activator (PA) is produced and released by a number of cell types in culture; release is correlated with the growth state of the cells. Production and release of PA are also subject to modulations such as hormonal regulation, malignant transformation, mitogenic stimulation, and cellular injury. Chemical injury to cells usually causes them to express lower levels of the enzyme. Therefore, the levels of PA released by cells exposed to chemicals, relative to cells exposed to saline, can be used as an index of chemical injury. Chan (4) used a sensitive photometric method to measure PA in cultured rabbit corneal epithelial cells, and published an initial evaluation of the test's predictability of chemical hazard to the human eye using eight standard toxic chemicals.

Method

Enucleated eyes of rabbits were placed in 0.1 M phosphate-buffered saline at pH 7.3. Sterile saline was injected intrastromally until the whole cornea appeared opaque and swollen. The cornea was dissected along the limbus and separated into anterior and posterior portions. The anterior half, containing epithelium and stroma, was cut into 1-mm squares and treated with Dipase II in serum-free culture medium at room temperature for about 1 hr. The intact epithelium could then be peeled away from the stroma with fine forceps. The epithelial cells were washed twice with serum-free culture medium, minced, and treated with 0.25% trypsin in Puck's saline containing no calcium or magnesium ion. The epithelial cells were dissociated by repeated passage through a hypodermic needle. The cells were washed and collected by centrifugation.

The dissociated epithelial cells were plated in multiwell or microtest plates (Falcon). The cells were maintained as monolayer cultures in Dulbecco's modified Eagle medium supplemented with 2% fetal calf serum and trace substances at 37°C in a humidified atmosphere of 2% CO_2/98% air. Culture in multiwell plates was used to study PA release under normal conditions.

Coleman and Green's (61) two-step coupled assay was used to quantify PA secreted by the cultured corneal epithelial cells. Plasminogen was first activated to plasmin by PA and the resulting plasmin was allowed to react with thiobenzyl benzoxycarbonyl-L-lysinate to form Z-lysin and benzyl mercaptan. Benzyl mercaptan reacts instantly and nonenzymatically with 5,5′-dithiobis (2-nitrobenzoic acid) (DTNB) to form mixed disulfide and colored thiophenolate anion. The resulting color reaction is read at 412 nm using a spectrophotometer. PA was measured by the esterolytic unit (E.U.). One E.U. is equivalent to aproximately 5×10^{-4} Ploug units. In the tests, the percentage inhibition of plasminogen activation (PIPA) was used as an index of the extent of chemical injury.

$$\text{PIPA} = \left(1 - \frac{\text{PA level of culture exposed to chemical}}{\text{PA level of culture exposed to saline}}\right) \times 100\%.$$

Example

Cultures in microtest plates were used for the corneal epithelium plasminogen activator (CEPA) test. The cells were rinsed in normal saline and exposed briefly to a test chemical. Initially, household bleach containing 5% sodium hypochlorite (NaClO) was used to test the response of cells to chemical injury. Then eight test chemicals were used: benzalkonium chloride, triethanolamine, acetic acid, isopropyl alcohol, NaClO, sodium lauryl sulfate, formaldehyde, and sodium hydroxide. Control cultures were exposed to saline alone. After treatment the cells were rinsed in serum-free culture medium and were maintained through a recovery period in which the modulation of PA secretion was initiated. At the end of the recovery period, the culture medium was removed for PA assay. The eight chemicals listed were divided into nonirritant (first four compounds) and irritant (last four compounds) groups. This method has the advantages of requiring only cell culture facilities and a colorimeter, without the need for expensive equipment or hazardous procedures.

To predict chemical hazards to the human eye, CEPA scores can be correlated with the Draize scores. When this was done in this study, only the bleach and the sodium lauryl sulfate were overscored (predicted to be more irritating than they were) and no substance was underscored. The results suggest strongly that the CEPA test can be used to distinguish irritants from nonirritants and will be an effective alternative to the Draize rabbit eye irritancy test.

^{51}Cr-Release Method

The isotopic chromium ^{51}Cr release assay has been widely used to quantitate toxicity in corneal endothelial cell culture systems (11,62). In the present study, the Descemet's membrane and endothelial cells of freshly harvested corneas were cut into 2-mm^2 fragments and placed in 60-mm plastic tissue culture dishes. The explant cultures were maintained in 3 ml of RPMI 1640 tissue culture medium plus 10% calf serum. When the outgrowth extended 10 mm around the explants, then the cells were harvested with 0.1% trypsin and 0.1% EDTA, pelleted by centrifugation, and used in toxicity tests. The cells were preincubated with 0.5 μCi/ml medium with ^{51}Cr (as sodium chromate) for 1 hr during which time the cells took up 60,000 to 200,000 disintegrations per minute (dpm) of the isotope per well. Each monolayer was washed three times to removed unincorporated chromate. When cells are killed, the isotope is released into the culture medium. The isotope in the medium may be measured in a gamma counter or in a liquid scintillation counter.

Three types of cytotoxicity assays have been performed with the ^{51}Cr-release method: (a) a range-finding experiment to identify a maximum no-effect dose of the test substance and a minimum dose resulting in 100% ^{51}Cr release; (b) one assay determining the time course of ^{51}Cr release (indicating how rapidly acting a substance is and defining an appropriate incubation time); and (c) a dose-response study performed by incubating endothelial cells with a range of test substances. From these studies an estimated dose resulting in 50% maximal toxicity (ED_{50}) was derived. The ED_{50}s of different substances allowed these toxins to be ranked or grouped *in vitro* and the order of potency was compared to *in vivo* results.

^{51}Cr-release assays could take several forms. In the ^{51}Cr-release assay, both the amount of the isotope released into the medium and that remaining in the monolayers of cells (^{51}Cr-retention assay) could be measured. Another variation was treating the cells with the test substance first and then measuring the ^{51}Cr uptake of the cells. This latter method was advantageous for long durations of exposure to the test substances.

The assays were conducted in 96-well tissue culture microtiter plates; each well was equivalent to one rabbit. In one typical experiment, adherent cells were labeled for 18 to 24 hr with 1 mCi/1 $\times$ 10^7 cells. The same concentration of ^{51}Cr was used to label suspended cells (for 2 hr). The cells were washed and used for toxicity assay. Using Dulbecco's modified Eagle medium (DMEM) tissue culture buffer, serial tenfold dilutions of test compounds were prepared for preliminary screening. For routine testing, serial twofold dilutions were used.

The radiolabeled cells in microtiter plates were exposed to test compounds for between 0.5 and 4 hr. Then the plates were centrifuged and samples of the supernatants were collected and counted in a gamma counter. The 50% cytotoxic dose (CD_{50}) was calculated by subtracting the number of counts in the supernatants of cells held in control (drug-free) medium from the test results. The results were then calculated as a percent of the maximum.

Example

For the corresponding Draize test, the low-volume eye irritation test described by Griffith et al. (63) was used. Using 0.5 M concentrations of compounds, irritation scores were reported as sums of all scores from the first day when irritation was detected to the last day of irritation. Five of the six surfactants could be ranked, but polysorbate 20 was never ranked correctly in any test. Cytotoxicity data *in vitro* suggested that this compound should rank fifth or sixth in irritancy; the *in vitro* results always suggested the compound was more irritative than the actual *in vivo* tests demonstrated. Despite some variability seen in the cells, data were otherwise quite consistent and the results were reproducible. Some of the variability may have resulted from difficulty in radiolabeling the cells uniformly. The results still suggested that the determination of CD_{50} using these cells yields data appropriate for ranking the relative irritative potential of materials *in vivo* without recourse to the Draize test. The results also indicate that irritating materials are not likely to be classified as nonirritating using this cytotoxicity method.

Lens Cell Cultures

Morphology and Cytotoxicity of Lens Epithelial Cells

Lens epithelial cells derived from 6-day-old rat lenses or from bovine lenses were cultured in medium T 199 (Morgan's medium) supplemented with 20% fetal bovine serum (64,65). Cells were trypsinized weekly, inoculated in fresh petri dishes or cell culture flasks (T-27, T-75), and grown in an incubator under 5% CO_2 at 37.6°C. One day after an inoculation the drugs to be tested were applied at different concentrations in medium. After incubation for specific times, living cells were counted in Fuchs-Rosenthal chambers after trypan blue staining.

Dose-effect curves were established for several compounds by counting viable cells. Three experimental protocols were followed: (a) adding the compound to the cells 1 day after inoculation in order to test the effect of the compound on the proliferation ability of growing cells; (b) adding the compound to densely grown monolayers of cells to study the effect on an already existing (and nonproliferative) monolayer of cells; and (c) adding a compound to cells at each cell transfer over a period of 4 to 6 weeks to detect the effects of long-term treatment.

For detection of cytological alterations, the morphological appearance of cells, after Giemsa staining, was documented by light microscopy using an invertoscope with photographic equipment. Proteins of cells exposed to distinct concentrations of the compounds in question were analyzed by isoelectric focusing on polyacrylamide gels. (These methods are similar to those presented in the section on corneal cell cultures.)

In one study, Rink (64) showed that an organic antioxidant was less toxic than an inorganic one. Antioxidants were tested for safety because they may be useful in preventing cataracts. In another study (65), dexamethasone proved much more toxic than the nonsteroidal anti inflammatory compound indomethacin.

Endocytosis

Endocytosis is believed to play an important role in the transport of macromolecules from the extracellular environment into the cytoplasm of cells. Lo and Zhang (66) studied the vesicular transport (endocytosis) of the protein tracer horseradish peroxidase into the lens epithelium and fiber cells of guinea pig and rabbit.

Freshly isolated adult guinea pig lenses and rabbit lenses were incubated at 34°C in closed vials containing 0.3% horseradish peroxidase (HRP) in TC-199 medium from 5 to 240 min.

All lenses were fixed after incubation in 2.5% glutaraldehyde in 0.1 M cacodylate buffer (pH 7.4) containing 1% tannic acid. Thick tissue slices were cut with a vibrotome for cytochemical demonstration of HRP activity. Thin-section electron microscopy (EM) was also done. Electron micrographs were taken, and quantitative analysis on the number of tracer-carrying endocytic vesicles and secondary lysosomes was done with a computerized digitizer on the electron micrographs. Freeze-fracture EM of lens epithelial cells was done only with rabbit cells.

As shown by thin-section EM, the many endocytic vesicles along the lateral membranes of epithelial cells became filled with the tracer HRP after incubation. Endocytosis was found to occur primarily in the lens epithelial cells, elongating young fiber cells where metabolic activity was the highest. Endocytosis is quite sensitive to ocular toxins, which can abolish endocytosis before causing cytolysis.

Aldose Reductase Activity

The enzyme aldose reductase converts glucose to sorbitol in the lens. When glucose levels are high, as with diabetes, more glucose is reduced to sorbitol. This may lead to development of a sugar cataract. Aldose reductase (AR) inhibition would be advantageous to prevent this. The aldose reductase inhibitors sorbinil, verapamil, AL-1567, and AL-1576 were tested on lenses in culture (67).

Bovine lenses were extracted and placed in TC-199. To imitate metabolic conditions found with diabetes, the culture medium was enriched with glucose. HEPES (*N*-2-hydroxyethylpiperazine-*N*′-2-ethane sulfonic acid) buffer was used with all incubations except verapamil, when sodium bicarbonate was used. One lens of each pair served as control. Lenses were incubated for 8 hr at 37°C, rinsed and dabbed dry, and prepared for analysis. For verapamil, lenses were incubated for 5 hr at 37°C in a pure Ringer solution. Then lenses were placed for 7 hr in TC-199 at 37°C with a higher level of glucose.

After homogenization of lenses in 6% $NaClO_4$ and centrifugation, the substrates were determined in the deproteinized neutralized supernatant. Reduced glutathione (GSH) and oxidized glutathione (GSSG) were measured, and free adenine nucleotides and the metabolites of glycolysis were also analyzed. This work showed how many things could be measured in a lens *in vitro*.

With longer incubation times in glucose, the lenses had elevated levels of the phosphorylated products of glucose and fructose. Verapamil caused a decrease in glucose and fructose concentrations. In fact, verapamil was found to be a relatively poor aldose reductase inhibitor, which impaired lens metabolism to a certain extent. ATP was depleted, whereas AMP rose and glutathione was oxidized to GSSG from GSH. Sorbinil, AL-1567, and AL-1576 all were efficient aldose reductase inhibitors, raising glucose and lowering fructose, and also increasing the ratio of ATP/AMP and

GSH/GSSG. AL-1576 was found to be the most effective AR inhibitor among the four compounds studied.

Cell Elongation and Potassium Efflux

Lens fiber cell differentiation is important for lens growth and is often defective in human cataracts. The most prominent morphological feature of this process is extensive cell elongation. Beebe and Cerrelli (68) studied the mechanism by which cytochalasin D prevents cell elongation.

Explants of chick embryo lenses were cultured in Ham's F-10 medium. Vitreous humor extract was prepared from 15-day-old chicken embryo eyes. Three subprotocols were followed. The vitreous group (a control) was incubated in vitreous humor extract only. The experimental group was incubated with cytochalasin D in vitreous humor for the entire incubation period (up to 6 hr). The reversal group was incubated in the experimental medium for the first 1.5 hr and then rinsed twice with Ham's F-10 medium and incubated in vitreous humor for the remainder of the experiment. Cell lengths for the vitreous and reversal groups were measured at 1.5, 3.0, 4.5, and 6.0 hr using an inverted microscope. The experimental groups were also observed at earlier points. Cell length was measured.

In another protocol, six central epithelial explants from 6-day-old chicken embryo lenses were prepared, and the tissues were treated with chicken vitreous humor or Ham's F-10 medium, with or without cytochalasin D, for 1 hr, and then changed to Ham's F-10 medium for 30 min. Cells were examined as above.

Rubidium 86 was used as a radioactive tracer to follow potassium movement in and out of cells. ^{3}H-labeled mannitol was used to estimate extracellular space of the tissues. Cytochalasin D was prepared in dimethyl sulfoxide (DMSO); control media contained an equivalent amount of DMSO. Eight central lens epithelia were explanted in a 35-mm culture dish, exposed for 30 min to either vitreous extract or Ham's F-10 medium, and later to medium containing ^{86}rubidium and ^{3}H-mannitol. The tissues were then rinsed three times with Ham's medium and placed in an orbital rotator at 10 rpm. The medium was sampled in 100-μl aliquots every minute for 10 min. The tissues were then solubilized with 1% sodium dodecyl sulfate and counted.

Cytochalasin D prevented lens epithelial cell elongation, which normally occurs when 6-day-old lens epithelial cells are exposed to vitreous humor. These epithelial cells remained short for 3 hr. Cytochalasin D also increased the rate of potassium efflux from both vitreous-stimulated and -unstimulated lens epithelia.

^{51}Cr-Release

The cell membrane integrity of lens cells can be determined by the principle provided by ^{51}Cr-release, as was done with corneal epithelium in culture. Stewart-Dettaan and coworkers (69) used this technique on cell monolayers of the lens cell line RLE-R.

Cell Culture

Cell monolayers of the line RLE-R were grown in medium 199 (M199) and exposed to 10 mM hydrogen peroxide for half an hour. Cells were then examined using scanning electron microscopy. Monolayers were photographed using phase contrast microscopy and were placed in Karnovsky's fixative for 1 hr. They were washed with 0.1 M sodium cacodylate-cacodylic acid buffer. After dehydration in an alcohol series the samples were critical-point dried using carbon dioxide. The samples were attached to scanning electron microscopy stubs with high-purity silver daub paint, sputter coated with gold palladium, and examined with a Hitachi scanning electron microscope.

Organ Culture

Lenses were removed from 13-day chick embryos and incubated with ^{51}Cr for 1 hr at 37°C. The labeled lenses were washed three times and incubated in individual tubes in M199 usually containing 10% fetal calf serum, with or without hydrogen peroxide and various protective agents. After 24 hr, lenses and media were counted separately and the percent release of bound chromate was calculated. The ratio was the counts in medium divided by the counts in both the medium and the lens, expressed as a percent. After counting, the lenses were again examined under a dissecting microscope to observe any changes.

Oxidative Stress

Hydrogen peroxide concentrations were assayed using the dianisidine method (70) using horseradish peroxidase in sodium phosphate buffer at pH 7.0. At the end of the experiment the solution was acidified with two drops 6 M HCl and the concentration of colored product estimated at 420 nm with a Beckman spectrophotometer.

When the cells were exposed to 10 mM hydrogen peroxide, the phase contrast micrograph showed globules on the surface of the cells that were much more obvious in the scanning electron micrograph. When labeled control chick lenses were incubated for 24 hr in M199, 63% of the radioactivity was released into the medium. This was increased by hydrogen peroxide. The presence of vitamin C prevented the peroxide-induced increase in ^{51}Cr-release.

Fibroblast Cultures

Cytotoxicity Assayed in Terms of Cell Death

Fibroblasts are nonocular cells but they can be used to assess cytotoxicity of a great variety of substances, including most substances that are potentially toxic to the eyes.

They offer several advantages: (a) there is extensive literature on growth, growth inhibition, and cytotoxicity of compounds to these cells; (b) they are easy to culture, being a naturally proliferative culture; (c) toxicity can be measured in terms of cell death, cell morphology, cell function, and cell detachment, so nonlethal damage can be studied; and (d) they do not require the death of any new animals. Indeed, some lines of fibroblast are of human origin and potential interspecies differences are eliminated from the analysis of the results of the experiments.

At least three cytotoxicity assays are available for fibroblast assays (71,72): (a) the cell detachment assay using detachment of cells after a 4-hr incubation; (b) the growth inhibition assay using a 2-day logarithmic growth period with the test compound present or absent; and (c) cloning efficiency during a 7-day growth and exposure period. In the studies cited here, three types of fibroblasts were used: (a) baby hamster kidney fibroblasts (BHK-21/C13), (b) early (Keller) passage human fibroblasts, and (c) "late late" (MRC-5) passage human fibroblasts.

Method

Solvents used for test compounds were water, Hank's balanced salt solution (HBSS), dimethyl sulfoxide (DMSO), minimal essential medium (MEM), and absolute ethanol. The test compound solutions were filter-sterilized and diluted with MEM immediately before use so that the final concentration of solvent in the medium was 1% for controls and 1% or less for the dilution series. Five concentrations of test compound and one control were placed in a single 24-well dish. Phenol red color changes indicated changes in the pH of the test solutions. BHK-21/C13 cells were cultured in MEM, whereas human Keller and MRC-5 cells were cultured in Dulbecco's MEM under 5% O_2 and 8% CO_2.

Cell Detachment

In the cell detachment assay, BHK cells were placed in 24-well plates, allowed 24 hr to settle and attach, and were exposed to the test substance for 4 hr. Some cells were trypsinized and electrically counted before adding the test substance to get an initial titer. In solvent controls a maximum of 5% of total cells were detached. The lowest concentration of the compound that induced a significant toxic effect (CD_{low}) was determined by measuring the number of detached BHK cells.

Growth Inhibition

Growth inhibition was determined under subconfluent culture conditions. Twenty-four-well plates were seeded with 4,000 cells per well, 24 hr prior to incubation with test substances. Under these conditions the cells will be rapidly dividing after 24 hr. Then cells were exposed to diluted series of test substances in full medium for 48 hr.

Cells were briefly checked for morphological changes and contaminations. The medium was discarded and the cells were washed with phosphate-buffered saline and trypsinized with 0.25% trypsin for 5 to 15 min. The cells were resuspended with fresh medium and electronically counted. The data were expressed as percentage of the initial cell number.

Cloning Efficiency

The cloning efficiency of the BHK cells was determined in 24-well plates. The cells were exposed to test solutions or solvent under conditions identical to the detachment assay cited above. One hundred BHK cells were put into each well with medium and the test compound or solvent. The cells were exposed to test compound for 7 days and then were fixed and stained with Giemsa. This is a test for long-term toxicity.

Example

The ranking order of chemicals tested was similar for all three assays, although the cell detachment assay was up to three orders of magnitude more sensitive than the other two assays. The growth inhibition assay proved to be more reliable than the cloning efficiency assay. The ranking order resulting from the *in vitro* data correlated better with threshold limit values for human workroom air (TLV/TWA) than with LD_{50} values. A crude classification was made of the CD_{low} values into three groups: (a) nonirritant, (b) mild to moderate irritant, and (c) strong irritant or corrosive. When compared with the known irritation potential for skin and mucous membranes derived from human exposure data for the test compounds, the *in vitro* data were more than 80% predictive of the *in vivo* classifications (71). Unfortunately, many of the errors indicated substances were less toxic *in vitro* than they have proven *in vivo*; a bad example is sodium hydroxide. It was hoped that using different thresholds for different classes of chemicals would improve correlation between *in vitro* and *in vivo* results.

Cell Viability Assayed in Terms of Metabolism and Permeability

LS cells derived from NCTC L929 mouse fibroblasts were used in this study (73). Cells were stored under liquid nitrogen in reserve, and then were thawed and grown in 1-liter round-bottom flasks and maintained in suspension at 37°C with a Vibromixer, which utilizes the Bernoulli effect. The culture medium was Eagle's modified MEM (Flow) with 5% (vol/vol) fetal calf serum, 0.859 g/l sodium bicarbonate, 2 mM glutamine, plus penicillin and streptomycin.

Cells were used when the stock culture had reached 1 million cells/ml. Aliquots of 4.9 ml were transferred to 25-ml Erlenmeyer flasks and 0.1 ml of test compounds in the same medium were added. Test compounds in the study cited were detergent-based products labeled by code, diluted from a stock solution of 100 mg/ml. The flasks were gassed with 5% carbon dioxide in air and placed in a shaker at 37°C for 4 hr. The internal standard used to assess the health of the cells was sodium lauryl sulfate, Analar grade (60 mg/ml), which consistently gave a CD_{50} figure of 1.00 ± 0.03 mg/ml.

Viability after 4 hr was assessed in terms of metabolism and permeability, after mixing a combination of the fluorescent dyes, fluorescein diacetate, and ethidium bromide in Eagle's modified MEM with the cell suspension. Esterase activity in living cells causes the formation of fluorescein, whereas the breakdown of the cell permeability barrier of the membrane allows the rapid accumulation of ethidium bromide in dead cells, primarily in the nucleus. Live (green fluorescence) and dead (red fluorescence) cells were counted in a silver-backed modified Fuchs-Rosenthal hemocytometer under a Zeiss fluorescence microscope with epifluorescence condenser.

Cell Viability Assayed in Terms of Intracellular ATP

A sensitive and automated technique was used in this study (74) to estimate the levels of intracellular ATP. ATP is the primary energy donor in the cell and is considered a good indicator of cellular health.

Methods

LS cells derived from NCTC L929 mouse fibroblasts were cultured in Eagle's modified MEM with 5% (vol/vol) fetal calf serum (73). Cells were grown as above in Erlenmeyer flasks in "spinner" culture. Substances truly soluble in culture medium were made up as stock solutions, whereas insoluble and immiscible materials were weighed directly into the Erlenmeyer flasks used for culture; then volumes of medium were added before cells were seeded to give an appropriate range of concentrations. The flasks were gassed with 5% CO_2 in air and incubated in the shaker at 37°C for 24 hr. At the end of the period, the material in the flask was centrifuged to separate phases and the aqueous phase ("extract") was removed. Cells from stock cultures were counted using a silver-backed Fuchs-Rosenthal hemocytometer and placed in centrifuge tubes, 5 million cells per tube, for pelleting by centrifugation. The growth medium was then discarded and the pelleted cells were resuspended in the extracts. Toxicity was determined by the method described above (73), with a 4-hr incubation period.

In a second variation of the procedure, a weighed amount of test material was added to a known volume of growth medium; the concentration of test substance was at least double the approximate CD_{50} from a standard run. The appropriate-sized Erlenmeyer flask was then gassed with 5% CO_2 in air and incubated at 37°C on an orbital shaker for 24 hr. The flask's contents were centrifuged and the aqueous layer (extract) was removed and tested for toxicity.

To check for complete extraction of immiscible organics, sufficient medium was added to an amount of test substance fivefold greater than its CD_{50} to give a total volume of 5 ml. The flask was gassed and shaken to achieve further extraction. The flask contents were centrifuged, the aqueous phase removed, and the oily (nonaqueous) layer resuspended in fresh culture medium. Cells were pelleted as above (5 million cells) and resuspended in the oily medium. The normal protocol described above was used to determine cytotoxicity, using fluorescein diacetate and ethidium bromide.

The assay for ATP utilized the firefly luciferase bioluminescent reaction measured in a Packard Auto Picolite Luminometer charged with Packard luminescence materials, ATP extraction (Picoex B), and luciferase-luciferin (Picozyme F) reagents. Samples from the culture flasks were placed in monitoring tubes that were loaded into the luminometer. The internal standard for which the instrument was programmed was 50 μl of 10^{-7}M ATP (Picochec) in tris-magnesium sulfate buffer, pH 7.75. An ATP standard curve revealed a linear relationship from 10^{-10} 10^{-14} mol ATP in a 19-μl sample.

Example

A lotion formulation was studied by this technique. The complete lotion formulation gave a much higher CD_{50} in the standard test than did the internal standard, sodium lauryl sulfate. The CD_{50} value for lotion obtained using the preincubation technique with variable volumes differed only slightly from that found by the standard method, but there was a marked improvement in standard deviation.

The concentration lowering cellular ATP by 50% (ATP_{50}) value itself did not always give a clear indication of the increased sensitivity of the ATP estimation when compared with the viability dyes technique. Compounds might kill cells without lowering the ATP concentration of the flask proportionally. In no case, however, was the ATP_{50} higher than the CD_{50}.

Cell Viability Assayed in Terms of Neutral Red Uptake

The neutral red (NR) assay developed by Borenfreund and Puerner (75) is based on the inability of dead and damaged mouse fibroblast 3T3 cells to take up the dye neutral red. If dye-treated cells are lysed, the color is released and can be measured photometrically. Toxic effects of test substances are manifested as a reduction in the intensity of the extracted color compared with the untreated controls. Applying this assay to monolayer cultures is particularly advantageous. The test consists of two parts: (a) screening of cells under an inverted phase contrast microscope for the detection of morphological alterations, and (b) a quantitative spectrophotometric procedure, based on the incorporation of neutral red, a supravital dye, into the lysosomes of viable cells (75,76). Both of these assays were carried out, in the study cited, in the same culture in a 96-well test plate.

Cell Culture

Mouse embryo fibroblast 3T3 cells were grown in Dulbecco's modified Eagle medium (DMEM) containing calf serum and antibiotics. To subculture, the growth medium was discarded and the cells were rinsed with trypsin in serum-free DMEM and incubated until the cells became rounded and could be detached from the plastic surface. The cells were resuspended in fresh growth medium and dispensed into tissue culture flasks.

Assay Procedure

The 3T3 cells were harvested from 75%-confluent cultures by trypsin treatment and were resuspended in fresh growth medium and incubated for 6 hr to allow the cells to become firmly attached to the plastic. A constant plate format was maintained for all assays using eight replicates for each treatment as follows: column 1, blanks (no compound or NR); columns 2 and 12, controls (NR only); columns 3 to 11, dilutions of test substances. Test substances were diluted in growth medium. The original growth medium was decanted from plated cells and replaced with control DMEM or with medium containing the diluted test substance. The plates were returned to the incubator for 17 hr. The medium was then removed, each well was rinsed, and growth medium containing NR was added to all except the blank wells. After 3-hr incubation, the NR medium was removed and the wells were rinsed. Plates were inverted and allowed to drain before the addition of extraction medium. After 30-min extraction, plates were shaken briefly and the optical density of the solutions in the wells was determined using a Kontro SL/T210 automatic plate reader. The more dye present, the healthier the cells were in that well.

This method is a rapid, reliable, inexpensive, and reproducible *in vitro* assay for screening potentially toxic agents. If it is adopted, the number of animals used to determine ocular toxicity could be greatly reduced.

Cell Viability Assayed in Terms of Uridine Uptake

This toxicity system measures the ability of xenobiotics to inhibit the uptake of uridine into cultured cells (6,10). Uridine uptake is a much more sensitive indicator of the toxic action of compounds than is cell death. The concentration of the test substance required to produce a 50% inhibition in uridine uptake (UI_{50}) provides a measure of toxicity. The uridine uptake inhibition test is also readily applicable to the assessment of toxicity of mixtures of compounds. Cells treated simultaneously with irritants bearing different chemical functional groups may show additive uridine uptake inhibition effects. In addition, because this procedure can quantitatively indicate nonlethal cytotoxicity, it can be used to determine the ability of cells to recover from toxic insult.

Balb/c 3T3 mouse fibroblasts were plated into 35-mm dishes at 50,000 cells/dish.

After 8 hr the medium was removed and replaced with fresh growth medium (for control dishes) or medium containing various concentrations of test agents. Freshly plated cells will be rapidly growing and multiplying and synthesizing DNA and RNA. After 4 hr of incubation the media were removed, the cells were washed with buffered saline, allowed to take up ^{3}H-uridine for 15 min, and then were dissolved in 0.5 N NaOH. Aliquots were taken for the determination of cell protein/dish and uridine uptake. Changes in cell protein/dish (an indication of cell death) and in uridine uptake relative to control cultures were plotted against the concentration of toxicant.

Examples

Screening of groups of compounds previously ranked for toxicity *in vivo* indicated that UI_{50} values formed an excellent rank correlation with published Draize test results. Cells treated simultaneously with irritants bearing different chemical functional groups showed additive uridine uptake inhibition effects. This effect is very relevant to human eye irritation; humans are as likely to come into contact with preparations that are combinations of many substances as they are to encounter a pure irritant substance. The effects were generally reversible: cultures treated with levels of irritants that reduced uridine uptake capacity by 40% to 80% were able to recover most of their uridine uptake capacity within 20 hr.

Cell Viability Assayed in Terms of DNA Synthesis

Guinea pig fibroblasts, prepared by trypsinization of guinea pig kidneys, were cultured in Eagle's medium and grown to confluency in plastic Falcon flasks (77). The cells were harvested and reseeded in culture tubes at uniform titers. The reseeded cells will start to multiply immediately and synthesize DNA. The medium in the tubes contained graded concentrations of compounds to be tested (Ferguson and Prottey (77) used surfactants) or control medium. Labeled [6-^{3}H] thymidine was added to all tubes and the cells were incubated overnight. Then the cells were collected by centrifugation and resuspended in medium fortified with unlabeled thymidine to wash out residual radioactive thymidine in the cytosol; only thymidine in the DNA remains. After centrifugation again the medium was removed and cell pellets were extracted three times with ice-cold 5% (wt/vol) trichloroacetic acid, followed by a single extraction with absolute ethanol. These extracts were discarded. Finally, the cell pellet residues were extracted three times with trichloroacetic acid at 70°C to stabilize the labeled DNA. Aliquots of the combined radioactive trichloroacetic acid extracts were then counted in a Packard 4000 liquid scintillation counter to determine the level of thymidine uptake into DNA.

Peritoneal Cell Cultures

Measurement of Serotonin (5-HT) Release

Peritoneal mast cells can be harvested and cultured; they are another model system for studying cytotoxicity. Rat peritoneal mast cells release serotonin (5-HT) under certain conditions. This release can be affected by toxic compounds. An *in vitro* experimental system for measuring cytotoxicity by measuring 5-HT release was developed by Chasin and coworkers (78). This assay was distinguished by the cells needing to be exposed to hormones. It was found that low concentrations (1 μg/ml) of an active compound, compound 48/80, consistently produced a six- to eightfold increase in serotonin release. Disodium chromoglycate (DSCG), a standard inhibitor of histamine release, effectively inhibited compound 48/80-stimulated serotonin release.

Methods

Rat peritoneal mast cells were obtained from female Sprague-Dawley rats (180 to 250 g). After sacrificing by carbon dioxide inhalation, 10 to 15 ml of Tyrode's buffer and heparin were injected i.p. followed by 25 to 30 ml more of Tyrode's buffer. After massaging 1 min, a midline incision was made in the abdominal wall and the fluid was removed with a Pasteur pipette. Cell washings, containing about 10% mast cells, were pooled. The cells were washed by centrifugation and then incubated to preload them with radioactive 5-hydroxytryptophan (the precursor of 5-HT) for 3 hr in a Gyrotary water-bath shaker at 37°C. The cells were then washed three times by centrifugation followed by suspension in fresh medium. The final pellet of cells was reconstituted so that each assay tube held about 4 million cells/ml. The assay was run in triplicate in disposable 12 × 75 mm plastic test tubes. Drugs were added in 100-μl aliquots to the tubes before the addition of cells. After cells were added, the tubes were incubated at 37°C in a shaking water bath. Then tubes were cooled and the cells and supernatant were separated by centrifugation at 4°C. Supernatant fractions were decanted into Aquasol (scintillation counting fluid) and counted by a liquid scintillation counter. Cell pellets were resuspended, boiled to release radioactivity, and decanted into Aquasol.

Example

It was found that significant [^{3}H]-serotonin release could be stimulated by only 1 μg/ml of compound 48/80; these cells are sensitive to toxicants. DSCG inhibited the release of serotonin effectively.

The major limitation of the serotonin release assay is that only peritoneal mast cells that release serotonin can be used. Human mast cells produce little or no serotonin so human systems cannot be studied.

Measurement of Histamine Release

Peritoneal mast cells also may release histamine; this property has been used in an *in vitro* alternative to *in vivo* tests (79,80). Using mixed rat peritoneal cells, a technique was developed to assess the ability of test substances to cause histamine release, which was determined fluorometrically. The assay allowed test materials to be ranked in terms of irritation potential (ocular and dermal). Histamine is an important mediator of primary-irritant type responses through its ability to increase vascular permeability, which thereby allows edema and inflammatory cell infiltration. It is reasonable to assume that materials promoting membrane permeability could result in nonspecific histamine release and thereby elicit a primary irritant response.

Methods

Male Wistar rats (400 to 500 g) were used as a source of mast cells. Cells were collected, pooled, washed in Hank's balanced salt solution containing 1% bovine serum albumin (HBSS-BSA), and resuspended in HBSS-BSA. The final suspension contained 4% to 6% mast cells. The rest consisted mostly of macrophages, leukocytes, and erythrocytes.

Cells were exposed to test materials for 10 min at 37°C. Exposures were terminated by the addition of ice cold saline, and cells were collected by centrifugation. The supernatant was decanted and stored at −15°C until assayed.

Spontaneous release of histamine was assessed using the method of Shore et al. (81). The supernatants from the test aliquots were compared to aliquots of cell suspensions exposed only to HBSS-BSA. The pellets obtained were resuspended in saline and incubated for 5 min at 100°C to release all histamine. The total histamine release was expressed as a percentage of the average total histamine content of similar aliquots of pooled cells. Acid was added to stop the condensation reaction between fluorophore and histamine; albumin was included to minimize spontaneous degradation. Reacted samples were also centrifuged prior to detection of condensation product fluorescence at 450 nm.

Example

The observations recorded agree with *in vivo* studies and with data assessing the effects of materials upon membrane integrity of cultured rabbit corneal cells. Three materials tested were propylene glycol, triethanolamine, and triethanolamine lauryl sulfate. The histamine release was dependent upon the concentrations of these substances. The order of potency was based upon determinations of the lowest concentration causing significant histamine release.

Chemotaxis of Macrophages

Chemotaxis is a specific characteristic of the inflammation reaction. Agents released from cells at the site of inflammation or irritation cause macrophages to migrate to the inflamed area. A Boyden chemotactic chamber can be used to measure the movement of macrophages toward an area of inflammation (82).

Methods

The Boyden chemotactic chamber is a perspex chamber that consists essentially of two compartments that are separated during the course of an experiment by a Millipore filter membrane. Mouse peritoneal macrophages placed on one side of a permeable membrane are attracted to fibroblast-conditioned medium obtained from cultured cells that have been exposed to an irritant (82). The movement of the macrophages from their source on one side of the membrane toward the other side can be easily quantitated by staining and counting a specified area of the membrane after 4 hr of chemotaxis.

Measurement of Lysosomal Enzyme Release

The release of lysosomal enzyme *in vivo* is widely believed to be a contributing factor to inflammation; thus it might be expected that primary cutaneous inflammation caused by surfactants involves lysosomal membrane damage. This study was undertaken to examine the major structural factors influencing lysosomal lysis by surfactants (83).

Methods

Rabbits were injected intraperitoneally with 200 ml of 0.1% glycogen in pyrogen-free saline. Four hours later 100 ml of heparinized saline were introduced into the peritoneal cavity and exudate was withdrawn by gravity drainage. The peritoneal exudate was centrifuged and the supernatant discarded. The cell pellet was washed by resuspension in isotonic saline containing 50 IU heparin/ml, and was again centrifuged. The washed pellet was then resuspended in ice-cold 0.34 M sucrose to yield a suitable cell concentration. The cells were homogenized by forcing the suspension through a Millipore filter grid, and the homogenate was centrifuged. The opaque supernatant (granule-rich suspension) was decanted, and the pellet taken up in a small voluem of ice-cold sucrose and rehomogenized. This suspension was diluted and recentrifuged. The supernatant from this step was combined with that obtained from the first centrifugation, and the pooled fraction constituted the granule rich suspension used in the lysis test.

Example

The lysis of granules by surfactants was measured by the method of Lowe and Turner (84). The granule-rich suspension was diluted with 0.34 M sucrose to an optical density (OD) of about 0.5. One-half milliliter of the suspension was incubated in a semimicro glass cuvette in a Unicam SP 800 photometer (Pye-Unicam, Cambridge, England) and the OD at 400 nm was recorded for 1 min. Then 0.01 to 0.05 ml of surfactant solution was mixed in and the decrease in OD over 20 sec was measured. The maximum decrease in OD possible was determined by adding the detergent Triton X-100.

A variety of detergents were tested. The ranking of detergents was found to be independent of concentration so a standard concentration of 0.5 mM was used. It was found that detergents were more potent at cell lysis in proportion to the polarity of the head group, and activity increased with carbon chain length. Unlike Prottey and Ferguson (79), Gibson (83) reported that nonionic detergents were less potent than anionic ones. Although there was some correlation between irritancy of detergents and their ability to lyse membranes, there were some noted exceptions, particularly sodium lauryl isothionate, which is very mild *in vivo* and very potent on the lysis test.

HeLa Cell Cultures

Cytotoxicity

HeLa cells are another kind of cell that can be cultured *in vitro* and used to test for cytotoxicity (85,86). HeLa cells were continously subcultured in Sani glass flasks nourished by Parker 199 medium with 10% (vol/vol) calf serum. Before use in tests, cells were harvested by using Versene (0.2 mg EDTA/liter PBS; SBL, Solna, Sweden) and then made round by suspension in a spinner culture for 2 hr. The cells were counted by the Buerker technique and the cell density of the spinner culture adjusted to 100,000 cells/ml. Compounds were dissolved in sterile saline or directly in the medium. Test solutions were diluted in steps of 1:5 in the test areas of 5 × 8 cups of a 96-cup flat-bottomed microtiter tray. Each test area thus consisted of five identical dilution series. Then the cups were inoculated with cells from the spinner culture, so each cup contained 50,000 cells/ml in 0.2 ml Parker's medium 199, including 5% (vol/vol) calf serum, 3 mg/ml glucose, 20 mg/ml phenol red, 200 IU benzylpenicillin/ml, 0.1 mg/ml streptomycin sulfate, and a varying concentration of the test substance. Cultures were sealed with sterile liquid paraffin and plastic film and incubated at 37°C for 7 days. This system is a model for long-term toxicity.

After 24 hr, and at later time points, cell viability was determined by microscopy on an inverted microscope. Cultures with the same percentage of spindle-shaped and fusiform cells as reference cultures were considered not inhibited, whereas cultures with 100% round cells, like the original inoculum, were considered totally inhibited. Partially inhibited cultures, with less outgrowth of fusiform cells, could also be recognized. After 7 days the pH of each culture was determined with the color indicator phenol red. Violet cultures (pH 8.0) were considered totally inhibited, whereas orange-yellow cultures (pH 6.0 to 6.5) were considered fully viable; the fall in pH was produced by acid metabolites of the cells. Red cultures were judged to be partially inhibited. Approximated IC_{50} (50% inhibitory concentration) values could be calculated from the geometric mean value between the minimal total inhibitory and the maximal noninhibitory concentrations.

Example

Selling and Erwall (86) compared Draize scores for 18 compounds with cytotoxicity to HeLa cells and found good correlation for most compounds. However, HeLa cells were not greatly affected by 1-heptanol or allyl alcohol, which are severe irritants and are toxic to other lines of cells in culture.

Cell Viability Assayed with RNA and DNA

This technique (22) utilizes the ability of relatively intact cells to liberate fluorescein from its precursor fluorescein diacetate and then retain it. Ethidium bromide is a red fluorescent compound that intercalates with RNA and DNA, staining them red. Damaged cells lose the green fluorochromasia that fluorescein gives them and appear red when treated with ethidium bromide. Ethidium bromide also stains nuclear material of intact cells but the green fluorescein fluorescence masks the red fluorescence.

Methods

Hep2 and HeLa cells were grown in medium of the following constitution: tissue culture medium 199 (TC-199) with Hank's salts but without sodium bicarbonate; 20 mM HEPES buffer (*N*-2-hydroxyethylpiperazine-*N'*-2-ethane sulfonic acid); 20 μg/ml streptomycin sulfate; 100 IU benzylpenicillin potassium salt; 100 μg/ml kanamycin; and 5 mM sodium bicarbonate.

The pH of the medium at 37°C was adjusted to 7.35 with 0.1 N NaOH. The medium was sterilized by filtration into sterile bottles. Heat inactivated newborn calf serum was transferred into the medium to a final concentration of 10% (vol/vol). Cells were grown in this medium in sterile plastic tissue culture flasks at 37°C. Stock cultures were grown to confluence and subcultured by pouring in a small volume of phosphate-buffered saline (PBS) with 200 μg/ml EDTA. Shaking the flasks resulted in cell detachment. Approximately 60,000 to 100,000 cells/ml in TC-199 medium were transferred into polystyrene tissue culture dishes containing plastic tissue culture coverslips. The cells were maintained for at least 17 hr in a humidified incubator at 37°C to allow for cell detachment.

A stock solution of 5 mg/ml fluorescein diacetate in acetone was prepared and stored at −20°C. One-tenth milliliter of this solution was added to 100 ml PBS with 0.03 g ethidium bromide. The growth medium was decanted and cells adherent to the coverslip were washed three times with PBS. A test solution (in the example, a detergent), prepared in TC-199 medium without serum, was placed on the cells and they were incubated in the humidified incubator for set periods of time. After incubation the treatment solution was poured off and the cells were washed three times with PBS. The dye solution was placed on the cells and 3 min later cell fluorochromasia was observable when the cells were examined with a Vickers M41 Photoplan fluorescence microscope. A calibration control of sodium lauryl sulfate was included. Cells were considered to exhibit green fluorochromasia if any fluorescein was visible in the cell. About 300 cells were counted randomly per coverslip using an eyepiece graticule.

In vivo data on ocular toxicity of the same detergent was provided by studying New Zealand white female albino rabbits. The test material was instilled directly onto the cornea of the right eye only of each animal, six animals per test group. The lids were held together for 1 sec and the conjunctival, corneal, and iridial responses were recorded.

Example

The results were expressed graphically as the percentage of red cells per slide on the ordinate against the detergent concentration on the abscissa. The concentration of detergent required to produce 50% red cells after a 1 hr exposure (ED_{50}) and the time taken to result in 50% red cells using a fixed detergent concentration over varying intervals of time (ET_{50}) were calculated and compared to the *in vivo* results. It was found that some potent agents *in vitro* were not highly irritating *in vivo*, whereas some mild agents *in vitro* were very irritating. The results *in vitro* agreed more with Gibson (83) *in vitro* than with *in vivo* data. Cationic detergents in general were more irritating whereas anionic detergents were more cytotoxic. The author felt that the technique showed promise as a simple method of detecting irritancy *in vitro* but felt the anomalies need to be resolved.

Madin-Darby Canine Kidney Cell Culture

An initial physiological event in the development of eye irritancy may be a change in the permeability of the corneal epithelium; an increase in permeability allows the irritant access to the underlying stroma. Normally there are tight junctions and desmosomes between corneal epithelial cells. A cell line in culture that also develops tight junctions between cells is the Madin-Darby canine kidney (MDCK) cell line (12). These cells have been used as a model system for determining ocular irritancy and compared to *in vivo* irritancy potential for series of chemicals.

Cells were cultured in Dulbecco's modified Eagle medium combined with Ham's F-12 medium containing 10% fetal calf serum, and supplemented with antiobiotics. The cells were subcultured into 96-well flat-bottomed plates for the FRAME neutral red release (NRR) assay and onto Anocell 10 porous tissue culture plate inserts in multiwell plates for fluorescein leakage testing (87).

Neutral Red Release Assay

Cells were grown to confluence in the wells of the plate. The medium was then replaced with medium containing neutral red (50 μg/ml) for 3 hr. Viable cells take up neutral red, a vital dye. Then the normal medium was replaced. For assay, the cells were decanted and washed with 200 μl calcium-free Dulbecco's phosphate-buffered saline (PBS), and then were treated with 50 μl of the test sample (eight concentrations, three wells/concentration). Test chemicals were either added neat or dissolved in PBS. The test reagent was removed after 1 min and the cells were washed with PBS. Healthy cells take up and retain neutral red; damaged cells release it.

A neutral red destain solution (1% acetic acid, 50% ethanol, and 49% distilled water) was added to each well (0.1 ml) to fix the cells and release the neutral red they contained. The optical density of the destain solution in each well was read using an Anthos 2001 plate reader. The plate reader was zeroed on a blank well containing no cells. From the optical density values obtained, the concentration of the test substance was calculated that would cause loss of 50% of the preloaded neutral red relative to the PBS-treated control cultures.

Fluorescein Leakage Assay

Anocell 10 inserts were placed in the wells of a 24-well plate with 0.5 ml medium. Twenty of the inserts were seeded with cells and grown to confluence over 4 days. Then the cells were washed with water and treated with the test reagents (four concentrations, two inserts per concentration). Controls were treated with distilled water. After 1 min the test reagent was removed and the cells were washed again with distilled water. The inserts were removed to fresh wells containing PBS plus calcium. Into each insert, 500 μl 0.02% fluorescein in calcium-containing PBS was added. The plates were incubated for 1 hr; if the cells were intact they would form a tight sheet that did not allow fluorescein to pass from inside the insert into the well outside. Then the inserts were removed and the optical density of the solution remaining in each well was measured using an Anthos 2001 plate reader. The concentrations of test samples were calculated, which caused 20% (FL_{20}) or 50% (FL_{50}) leakage of fluorescein across the filter, compared to inserts containing no cells (i.e., maximum leakage).

Example

In general, the NRR assay showed a good correlation with eye irritancy, as potent eye irritants caused loss of neutral red from cells at low concentrations, whereas mild or nonirritating compounds caused little or no loss of neutral red except at extremely high concentrations. Exceptions to the rule were the corrosives mercuric chloride and silver nitrate, which failed to cause significant neutral red release. Similar results were observed using the fluorescein leakage assay. Compounds that were potent irritants caused substantial leakage of fluorescein, whereas mild or nonirritants caused fluorescein leakage only at high concentrations. However, silver nitrate and mercuric chloride were the most potent compounds at causing fluorescein leakage. The discrepancies in the sensitivities of the two methods to silver nitrate and mercuric chloride are currently under investigation.

TOXICITY PREDICTION

Drug efficacy and safety are two parameters that have to be studied before the Food and Drug Administration (FDA) can approve the human clinical trial with investigative new drugs (IND). Reasonable prediction of drug toxicity on humans has to be made depending on the laboratory data obtained from animal experiments. Prediction from laboratory animal data to humans in the real world, however, has always been controversial and dangerous because of species and environmental differences between animals in the controlled lab and humans in the noncontrolled environment (88). Extrapolation of *in vitro* data to *in vivo* systems does not necessarily deal with metabolism, excretion, compartmentalization, and blood circulation, which are common factors needed to be considered in *in vivo* experiments.

Traditionally, prediction of drug toxicity from *in vitro* to *in vivo* or from animal data to human systems was one by using a straight line predictive technique and by discarding insignificant parameters. Obviously, this method is too simplistic and unreasonable. The real world is much more complicated and requires alternative non-straight-line predictive techniques.

The alternative nonlinear predictive technique is designed to cope with random events that occur mostly in the real world. Therefore, it should be able to incorporate historically stored data, to take inputs from diversified scientific disciplines, and to consider simultaneously the host factors, external influences, and physiochemical characteristics of the chemical in question.

The chemical toxicity can be considered as a particulate entity traversing through time and space in a random order driven by internal and external forces. Therefore, the brownian equation could be used to describe its random movement through time and space. With this equation, various parameters can be fed into the equation including molecular weights of the chemicals, eye irritation of chemicals on man, external factors of the chemicals on functional systems, and so forth.

Another major problem in predicting toxicity is in the use of animal experimental data on humans. The reason could be due largely to the lack of continuity in time and space on animal and human data. Historical data are based to some degree on a posteriori data and are required to make a priori probability judgments on future time phase. Bayes' equation could be used properly to deal with these two entities.

The denominator of Bayes' equation defines historical data experiments, case reports, and data banks. It also includes the long-term memory of reports in physiochemistry, toxicology, and medical practice of agents. The numerator represents the projection and prediction of brownian motion by the intuitive force of experts in the field. With Bayes' equation, an extremely large number of parameters can be dealt with simultaneously, including interactions of organisms, tissue cultures, toxic chemicals, and so forth. The data bank in our expert's long-term memory is equivalent to the denominator of Bayes' equation and is complimentary to the data banks of a computerized information system. The short-term memory of the expert is equal to the numerator in Bayes' equation but is far superior over the computerized information data because the speed of using recent information by the expert to weigh probabilities is almost instantaneous in comparison to batching operations.

A nonlinear approach for predicting chemical toxicity is now workable. It allows a multidisciplinary approach to incorporate a large number of inputs for simultaneous assessment. With the assistance of a computer, it can predict chemical toxicity in humans efficiently. Most importantly, the prediction can be accomplished without dependence solely on animal data but on the large mass of historical data, tissue culture data, invertebrate data, exposure data, and long- and short-term memories of man. For more details, the readers are advised to read Tamura's article in *Product Safety Evaluation* (88).

ACKNOWLEDGMENT

This chapter was written with the assistance of Feng Zhao, who performed the literature searches and made copies of the papers.

REFERENCES

1. Code of Federal Regulations. *Title 16, Subchapter C, Federal Hazardous Substances Act, Part 1500.42 (Test for eye irritants)*. Revised Jan. 1, 1981. Washington, DC: U.S. Government Printing Office, 1982.
2. OECD. Guidelines for testing of chemicals, acute eye irritation/corrosion, Guideline 405. Adopted 24 Feb., 1987, Organization for Economic and Cooperative Development, Paris.
3. Dooman KA, Cascieri TM, Demetrulius J, Driedyer A, Griffith JF, Grochocki, GT, Kong B, McCormick WC, North-Root H, Rozen MG, Sedlak RI. In vitro methods for estimating eye irritancy of cleaning products. Phase I: prelimary assessment. *J Toxicol Cutan Ocular Toxicol* 1988;7:173–185.
4. Chan KY. An in vitro alternative to the Draize test. In: Goldbert AM, ed. *Alternative methods in toxicology, vol 3: In vitro toxicology*. New York: Mary Ann Liebert, 1985;403–422.
5. North-Root H, Yackowvich F, Demetrulius J, Gacula M, Heinz JE. Evaluation of an in vitro cell toxicity test using rabbit corneal cells to predict the eye irritation potential of surfactants. *Toxicol Lett* 1982;14:207–212.
6. Shopsis C, Borenfreund E, Walberg J, Stark DM. In vitro cytotoxicity assays: a potential alternative

to the Draize ocular irritancy test. In: Goldberg AM, ed. *Alternative methods in toxicology, vol 2: Acute toxicity testing: alternative approaches.* New York: Mary Ann Liebert, 1984;101-114.
7. Lazarus HM, Imperia PS, Botti RE, Mack RJ, Lazz JH. An vitro method which assesses corneal epithelial toxicity due to antineoplastic, preservative and antimicrobial agents. *Lens Eye Toxi Res* 1989;6:59-85.
8. Leighton J, Nassauer J, Tchao R, Verdone J. Development of a procedure using the chick egg as an alternative to the Draize rabbit test. In: Goldberg AM, ed. *Alternative methods in toxicology, vol 1: Product safety evaluation.* New York: Mary Ann Liebert, 1983;163-177.
9. Luepke NP. Hen's egg chorioallantoic membrane test for irritation potential. *Food Chem Toxical* 1985;23:287-291.
10. Shopsis C, Sathe S. In vitro uridine uptake inhibition as a cytotoxicity test. *Toxicology* 1984;29:195-206.
11. Shadduck JA, Everitt J, Bay P. Use of in vitro cytotoxicity to rank ocular irritation of six surfactants. In: Goldberg AM, ed. *Alternative methods in Toxicology, vol 3: In vitro toxicology.* New York: Mary Ann Liebert, 1985;643-649.
12. Shaw AJ, Clothier RH, Balls M. Loss of trans-epithelial impermeability of a confluent monolayer of Madin-Darby canine kidney (MDCK) cells as a determinant of ocular irritancy potential. *ATLA* 1990;18:145-151.
13. Burton ABG, York M, Laurence RS. The in vitro assessment of severe eye irritants. *Food Cosmet Toxicol* 1981;19:471-480.
14. York M. An isolated rabbit eye technique. In: Balls M, Riddell P, Worden J, eds. *Animals and alternatives in toxicology testing.* New York: Academic Press, 1983;309-371.
15. Gordon VC, Kelly CP. An *in vitro* method for determining ocular irritation. *Cosmet Toilet* 1989:104:69-73.
16. Gordon VC, Kelly CP. Validation of an in vitro method for determining ocular irritation of cosmetic ingredients and products. *Cosmet Toilet* 1989;104:67-69.
17. Gordon VA, Bergman HC. External evaluation of the Eytex system in twelve labs to determine the correlation of results with in vivo results. In: Goldberg AM, ed. *Progress in in vitro toxicology.* New York: Mary Ann Liebert, 1989:99-112.
18. Griffith JF. Dose-response studies with chemical irritants for predicting hazards to the human eye. *Toxicol Appl Pharmacol* 1980;55:501.
19. Dickens MS, Kruszewski FH, Hearn LH, Smith KT, Teal JJ, Gordon VA. Application of the EYTEX system to the evaluation of cosmetic products. In Regnier M, Imbart IK, eds. Validation of the Eytex system as a screen for predicting the ocular irritancy potential of chemical products. 1990. Unpublished.
20. Muir CK. A simple method to assess surfactant-induced bovine corneal opacity *in vitro*: preliminary findings. *Toxicol Lett* 1984;22:199.
21. Igarashi H. In vitro—opacity of the isolated cornea produced by NaLS. *Toxicol Lett* 1986;32:249.
22. Scaife MC. An investigation of detergent action on cells *in vitro* and possible correlation with *in vivo* data. *Int J Cosmet Sci* 1982;4:179.
23. Elgebaly SA, Gillies C, Forouhar F, Hashem M, Baddour M, O'Rourke J, Kreutzer DL. An in vitro model of leucocyte mediated injury to the corneal epithelium. *Curr Eye Res* 1985;4:31-41.
24. Elgebaly SA, Downes RT, Bohr M, Forouhar F, O'Rourke J, Kreutzer DL. Inflammatory mediators in alkali-burned corneas; preliminary characterization. *Curr Eye Res* 1987;6:1263-1273.
25. Kreutzer DL, O'Flaherty JT, Orr W, Showell HJ, Ward PA, Becker EL. Quantitative comparison of various biological responses of neutrophils to different active and inactive chemotactic factors. *Immunopharmacology* 1978;1:39-49.
26. Boyum A. Separation of blood leucocytes, granulocytes and lymphocytes. *Tissue Antigens* 1974;4:269-274.
27. Elgebaly SA, Forouhar F, Gillies C, Williams S, O'Rourke J, Kreutzer DL. Leucocyte-mediated injury to corneal endothelial cells: a mode of tissue injury. *Am J Pathol* 1984;116:407-416.
28. Elgebaly SA, Herbert N, O'Rourke J, Kreutzer DL. Characterization of neutrophil and monocyte-specific chemotactic factors derived from the cornea in response to hydrogen peroxide injury. *Am J Pathol* 1987;126:22-32.
29. Maurice DM. Influence on corneal permeability of bathing with solutions of different reaction and tonicity. *Br J Ophthalmol* 1955;39:463-473.
30. Maurice DM, Singh T. A permeability test for acute corneal toxicity. *Toxicol Lett* 1986;31:125-130.

31. Schleich T, Matson GB, Willis JA, Acosta G, Serdahl C, Campbell P, Garwood M. Surface coil phosphorus-31 nmr studies of the intact eye. *Exp Eye Res* 1985;40:343-355.
32. Lerman S, Moran M. NMR pulse relaxation studies on the normal aging and cataractous lens. *Exp Eye Res* 1989;48:451-459.
33. Lerman S, Ashley DL, Long RC, Goldstein JH, Megaw JM, Gardner K. Nuclear magnetic resonance analyses of the cold cataract: whole lens studies: *Invest Ophthalmol Vis Sci* 1982;23:218-226.
34. Lauterbur PC. Image formation by induced local interactions: examples employing nuclear magnetic resonance. *Nature* 1973;242:190-191.
35. Weisman IO, Bennett LH, Maxwell LR Sr, Woods MW, Burk D. Recognition of cancer in vivo by nuclear magnetic resonance. *Science* 1972;178:1288-1290.
36. Aguayo JB, Blackband SJ, Schoenigar J, Mattingly MA, Hintermann M. Nuclear magnetic resonance imaging of a single cell. *Nature* 1986;322:190-191.
37. Lerman S. Moran M. Acrylamide and iodide fluorescence quenching studies on whole human lenses and their protein extracts. *Curr Eye Res* 1988;7:403-410.
38. Mitton KP, Dzialoszynski T, Weerheim J, Trevithick JR, Sivak JG. Modeling cortical cataractogenesis x evaluation of lens optical function by computer based image analysis using *in vitro* rat lens elevated glucose model. In: Lerman S, Tripathi RC, eds. *Ocular toxicology.* New York: Marcel Dekker, 1990;211-228.
39. Korte I, Ohrloff C, Hockwin O. Influence of drugs on lens metabolism in vitro. *Concepts Toxicol* 1987;4:326-332.
40. Muller A, Moller B, Dragomirescu V, Hockwin O. Profiles of enzyme activities in bovine lenses. *Concepts Toxicol* 1987;4:343-349.
41. Kuck JFR, Kuck KD. In vitro—the emory mouse cataract: increased accumulation of calcium during cataractogenesis. *Lens Eye Toxi Res* 1989;6:853-862.
42. Smith PK, Krohn RI, Hermanson GT, et al. Measurement of protein using bicinchoninic acid. *Anal Biochem* 1985;150:76.
43. Wallach JFR, Steck TL. Properties of the metal derivatives of calcein: determination of aluminum, alkaline earths, cobalt, copper, nickel and zinc. *Anal Chem* 1963;35:1035.
44. Kuck JFR, Kuck KD. The Emory mouse cataract: the effects on cataractogenesis of alpha-tocopherol, penicillamine, triethylenetetramine and mercaptopropionylglycine. *J Ocular Pharmacol* 1988;4:243.
45. Rae JL, Cooper KE. Potassium channels in chick lens epithelium change with maturation. *Lens Eye Toxic Res* 1989;6:833-843.
46. Beebe D, Feagans D. A tissue culture system for studying lens cell differentiation. *Vision Res* 1981;21:113-118.
47. Jain MK. Role of cholesterol in biomembranes and related systems. In: Kleinyeller A, ed. *Membranes and transport.* New York: Academic Press, 1977;1-77.
48. Borchman D, Delamere NA, McCauley LA, Paterson CA. Studies on the distribution of cholesterol phospholipid and protein in the human and bovine lens. *Lens Eye Toxic Res* 1989;6:703-724.
49. Peterson GL. A simplication of the protein assay method of Lowry et al. which is more generally applicable. *Ann Biochem* 1977;83:346.
50. Bartlett GR. Phosphorus assay in column chromatography. *J Biol Chem* 1959;234:446.
51. Huang TC, Chen CP, Wefler V, Raftery A. A stable reagent for the Liebermann-Bruchaud reaction. Application to rapid serum cholesterol determination. *Anal Chem* 1961;33:1405.
52. Doly M, Gaillard G, Braquent P. Electroretinogram and mediators of inflammation. In: Bazan NG, ed. *Lipid mediators in eye inflammation.* New York: Basel Karger, 1990;149-167.
53. Tseng MT, Liu KN, Radtke ND. Isolated perfused bovine eye—a model for acute retinal toxicity screening. In: Lerman S, Tripathi RC, eds. *Ocular toxicology.* New York: Marcel Dekker, 1990;369-371.
54. Zwilling E. A modified chorioallantoic grafting procedure. *Transplant Bull* 1959;6:115-116.
55. Dubkin NH, DiBlasi MC, Thomas CL, Wolff MC. Development of an *in vitro* test for cytotoxicity in vaginal tissues: effect of ethanol on prostanoid release. In: Goldberg AM, ed. *Alternative methods in toxicology, vol 2: Acute toxicity testing: alternative approaches.* New York: Mary Ann Liebert, 1984;127-138.
56. Muir CK, Flower C, Van Abbé NJ. A novel approach to the search for in vitro alternatives to in vivo eye irritancy testing. *Toxicol Lett* 1983;18:1-5.
57. Takahashi N, Ikowa N. The cytotoxic effect of 5-FU on cultured human conjunctival cells. In: Lerman S, Tripathi RC, eds. *Ocular toxicology.* New York: Marcel Dekker, 1990;315-330.
58. Takahashi N, Mukai Y, Nakaizumi H, Sasaki K. An evaluation of the cytotoxicity of ophthalmic

solutions on cell culture: aminoglycosides and dexamethasone sodium phosphate. *Concepts Toxicol* 1987;4:383-389.
59. Jumblatt MM, Neufeld AH. A tissue culture model of the human corneal epithelium. In: Goldberg AM, ed. *Alternative methods in toxicology, vol 3: In vitro toxicology*. New York: Mary Ann Liebert, 1985;393-404.
60. Lazarus HM, Imperia PS, Botti RE, Mack RJ, Lass JH. An in vitro method which assesses corneal epithelial toxicity due to antineoplastic, preservative and antimicrobial agents. In: Lerman S, Tripathi RC, eds. *Ocular toxicology*. New York: Marcel Dekker, 1990;59-85.
61. Coleman PL, Green GDJ. A sensitive coupled assay for plasminogen activator using a thiol ester substrate for plasmin. *Ann NY Acad Sci* 1981;370:617.
62. Douglas HJ, Spilman SD. In vitro ocular irritancy testing. In: Goldbeg AM, ed. *Alternative methods in toxicology, vol 1: Product safety evaluations*. New York: Mary Ann Liebert, 1983;205-230.
63. Griffith JF, Nixon GA, Bruce RD, Reer PJ, Bannan EA. Dose-response studies with chemical irritants in the albino rabbit eye as a basis for selecting optimum testing conditions for predicting hazard to the human eye. *Toxicol Appl Pharmacol* 1980;55:501-513.
65. Rink H, Seifert R, Bauer K. Effects of hydrocortisone, dexamethasone and indomethacin in lens epithelial cells growing in vitro. *Concepts Toxicol* 1986;4:397-406.
66. Lo WK, Zhang W. In vitro. Endocytosis of macromolecules in the lenses of guinea pig and rabbit. *Lens Eye Toxic Res* 1989;6:603-612.
67. Hockwin O, Korte I, Noll E, Schwarz B. The effect of aldose reductase inhibitors on bovine lens metabolism in vitro. *Lens Res* 1984;2:243-262.
68. Beebe DC, Cerrelli S. Cytochalasin prevents cell elongation and increases potassium efflux from embryonic lens epithelial cells: implications for the mechanism of lens fiber cell elongation. *Lens Eye Toxic Res* 1989;6:589-601.
69. Stewart-Dettaan PJ, Sanval M, Creighton MO, Inch WR, Trevithick JR. ^{51}Cr release and oxidative stress in the lens. In: Lerman S, Tripathi RC, eds. *Ocular toxicity*. New York: Marcel Dekker, 1990;183-202.
70. Trevithick JR, Metzenberg RL. Kinetics of the inhibition of *Neurospora* invertase by products and oxidative stress. *Arch Biochem Biophys* 1964;107:260.
71. Reinhardt CA, Pelli DA, Zbinden G. Interpretation of cell toxicity data for the estimation of potential irritation. *Food Chem Toxicol* 1985;23:247-257.
72. Kennah HE, Albulesen D, Hignet S, Barrow CS. A critical evaluation of predicting ocular irritancy potential from an in vitro cytotoxicity assay. *Fundam Appl Toxicol* 1989;12:281-290.
73. Kemp RB, Meredith RWJ, Gamble S, Frost M. A rapid cell culture technique for assessing the toxicity of detergent-based products *in vitro* as a possible screen for eye irritancy *in vivo*. *Cytobios* 1983;36:155-159.
74. Kemp RB, Meredith RWJ, Gamble SH. Toxicity of commercial products on cells in suspension culture: a possible screen for the Draize eye irritation test. *Food Chem Toxicol* 1985;23:267-270.
75. Borenfreund E, Puerner JA. A simple quantitative procedure using monolayer cultures for cytotoxicity assays (HTD/NR-90). *J Tiss Cult Methods* 1984;9:7-9.
76. Hockley K, Baxter D. In vitro: use of the 3T3 cell-neutral red uptake assay for irritants. *Food Chem Toxicol* 1986;24:473-475.
77. Ferguson TFM, Prottey C. The effect of surfactants upon mammalian cells. *Food Cosmet Toxicol* 1976;14:431-434.
78. Chasin M, Scott C, Shaw C, Persico F. A new assay for the measurement of mediator release from rat peritoneal mast cells. *Int Arch Allergy Appl Immunol* 1979;58:1-10.
79. Prottey C, Ferguson TFM. The effect of surfactants upon rat peritoneal mast cell in vitro. *Food Cosmet Toxicol* 1976;14:425-430.
80. Jacaruso RB, Barletta MA, Carson S, Trombetta LD. Release of histamine from rat peritoneal cells in vitro as an index of irritation potential. *J Toxicol Cutan Ocular Toxicol* 1985;4:39-48.
81. Shore PA, Burkhalter A, Cohn VH. A method for the fluorometric assay of histamine in tissues. *J Pharmacol Exp Ther* 1959;127:182-186.
82. Stark DM, Shopsis C, Borenfreund E, Walberg J. Alternative approaches to the Draize assay: chemotaxis, cytology, differentiation and membrane transport studies. In: Goldberg AM, ed. *Alternative methods in toxicology, vol 1: Product safety evaluation*. New York: Mary Ann Liebert, 1983;179-203.
83. Gibson WT. Lysis of rabbit polymorphonuclear leucocyte granules by surfactants of differing structure and irritancy. *Food Cosmet Toxicol* 1980;88:511-515.

84. Lowe JS, Turner EH. The effect of adjuvant arthritis and drugs on the ability of rat plasma to inhibit the Triton X-100-induced lysis of rabbit polymorphonuclear leucocyte granules. *Biochem Pharmacol* 1973;22:2069.
85. Ernst R, Arditti J. Biological effects of surfactants. IV. Effects of non-ionics and amphoterics on HeLa cells. *Toxicology* 1980;15:233-242.
86. Selling J, Erwall B. Screening for eye irritancy using cultured HeLa cells. *Xenobiotica* 1985;15:713-717.
87. Shaw AJ, Clothier RH, Balls M. Loss of trans-epithelial impermeability of a confluent monolayer of Madin-Darby canine kidney (MDCD) cells as a determinant of ocular irritancy potential. *ATLA* 1990;18:145-151.
88. Tamura RM. A model for toxicological prediction. In: Goldberg AM, ed. *Alternative methods in toxicology, vol 1: Product safety evaluation*. New York: Mary Ann Liebert, 1983;315-330.

Ophthalmic Toxicology, edited by
George C. Y. Chiou. Raven Press, Ltd.,
New York © 1992.

6

Ophthalmic Toxicity by Systemic Drugs

Jimmy D. Bartlett

Department of Optometry, University of Alabama at Birmingham School of Optometry Birmingham, Alabama 35294

During the past several decades considerable attention has been devoted to how systemic drug therapy can affect ocular tissues or visual functions. Various monographs and major reviews have addressed this subject (1,2), and mechanisms have been devised that encourage reporting of possible cause-and-effect relationships between systemic drug use and ocular effects (3,4). By encouraging the reporting of such relationships, it is hoped that our understanding of ocular toxicity associated with systemic drugs will be improved and that, ultimately, patient care will be enhanced by preventing such adverse reactions or by finding better methods of treating such effects once they occur.

The eye has an extremely rich blood supply but a relatively small total mass, and thus exhibits an unusually high susceptibility to toxic substances. Drug molecules present in systemic circulation can reach the ocular structures by way of the uveal or retinal vasculatures. Once they reach the eye, systemic drugs can be deposited in several locations acting as drug depots, such as the cornea, crystalline lens, and retina. Moreover, systemic medications can affect numerous ocular and visual functions, including pupil size and reactivity, accommodation, intraocular pressure, and lid position. Thus, many systemically administered drugs have the potential to cause adverse ocular effects, and nearly all ocular structures can be vulnerable. This picture is complicated even more by the fact that multiple drug therapy can influence the eye through mechanisms that are currently not well understood (5,6).

This chapter considers the clinically important ocular or visual responses attributable to systemic drug therapy. Innumerable anecdotal reports exist in the literature describing the presumed ocular effects of various systemic medications or dosage formulations. This chapter, however, emphasizes only those clinical responses that, over time, have become well documented, and only the most common drugs that affect the eye are considered. The ocular toxicity associated with each drug class is considered in terms of its pathogenesis, specific ocular manifestations, and appropriate patient management strategies.

ANTICHOLINERGIC DRUGS

Drugs with anticholinergic properties can commonly affect the eye by inhibiting the cholinergic innervation to lacrimal gland tissues, iris sphincter muscle, or ciliary muscle. Clinically important effects can be induced in the lacrimal system, pupil, intraocular pressure, or accommodation. Among the most important drugs capable of causing clinically significant ocular effects include atropine, scopolamine, antihistamines, anxiolytic agents, and tricyclic antidepressants.

Ocular Manifestations

Atropine and related drugs inhibit glandular secretions in a dose-dependent manner. Thus, dryness of mucous membranes, including dry eye, is a common side effect of anticholinergic drug use (7,8). In one study (9) oral administration of atropine caused tear secretion to fall from 15 µl/min to 3 µl/min. A similar dose of atropine given subcutaneously gave a nearly 50% reduction in lacrimal secretion (10). Scopolamine 1 to 2 mg orally caused a reduction in tear secretion from 5 µl/min to 0.8 µl/min (9).

In addition to their receptor-blocking effects, H_1 antihistamines have varying degrees of atropine-like actions, including the ability to alter tear film integrity (10–12). Both aqueous and mucin production have been reported to decrease with antihistamine use (9). Koeffler and Lemp (13) administered 4 mg/day of chlorpheniramine maleate to a 20-year-old age group of volunteers. Tear secretion was measured by use of the standard Schirmer's test. A significant reduction in tear flow was observed on the days when chlorpheniramine was taken.

Drugs with anticholinergic effects, such as atropine or related compounds, can cause significant mydriasis. Systemic administration of 2 mg or more of atropine can result in pupillary dilation and cycloplegia (14).

Since patients with extremely narrow anterior chamber angles are at risk for the development of angle-closure glaucoma, drugs that can potentially dilate the pupil may induce acute or subacute angle-closure glaucoma (15,16). This includes any medication with anticholinergic or strong adrenergic agonist properties (17). Hiatt and associates (18) have shown, however, that the risk of elevating intraocular pressure with systemically administered anticholinergic agents is small, even in patients with narrow angles.

Patient Management

In most instances drug-induced effects on the eye are self-limited once the anticholinergic medication is reduced or discontinued. Symptoms of dry eye, dilated pupil, or cycloplegia may be annoying but are rarely incapacitating. During drug therapy annoying symptoms can be relieved using appropriate artificial tear formulations or ocular lubricants for dry eye, or by employing appropriate reading lenses for symptoms induced by cycloplegia. In rare cases of angle-closure glaucoma induced by anticholinergic medication, treatment should be instituted following the usual guidelines.

ANTIADRENERGIC DRUGS

Drugs classified as β-adrenergic receptor antagonists have become the mainstay in the treatment of systemic hypertension, ischemic heart disease, cardiac arrhythmias, and migraine headache. When systemically administered, these drugs can cause dry eye syndrome and can reduce intraocular pressure.

Pathogenesis

The mechanism responsible for reduced aqueous tear secretion is unknown. It has been documented, however, that ß-adrenergic antagonists reduce tear lysozyme levels, with a reduction of IgA (19,20).

Most studies (21-28) indicate that ß-antagonists exert their primary ocular hypotensive action by inhibiting aqueous formation. Of the commercially available ß-antagonists, timolol is the most widely investigated ocular hypotensive agent, but all ß-antagonists may act by a similar mechanism. Neufeld (28) has postulated that timolol can act on secretion, ultrafiltration, or both. Since aqueous formation depends on blood flow and perfusion pressure within the ciliary vasculature, timolol may induce a net vasoconstriction by preventing ß-receptor-mediated vasodilation of the afferent vessels in the ciliary processes. This vascular action of timolol, however, has not been confirmed experimentally. It has also been suggested (28) that timolol reduces aqueous formation through a direct action on the ciliary epithelium. The intracellular effects of ß-receptor blockade at the level of the nonpigmented ciliary epithelium are still unclear.

Ocular Manifestations

Reduced aqueous tear secretion is a reported side effect of orally administered ß-adrenergic antagonists. Although most of the reported cases deal with practolol (29), other ß-blockers, such as propranolol and timolol have also been implicated in dry eye syndrome (19,30). Ocular side effects of practolol have been described as an oculomucocutaneous syndrome, in which patients suffer from symptomatic lesions of the conjunctival and lid tissues (29). Atenolol, metoprolol, oxyprenolol, and pindolol have all been implicated in patients with dry eye symptoms and in reduction of tear lysozyme (19,20).

Systemically administered ß-adrenergic antagonists are well known to reduce intraocular pressure (31-33). This occurs both in patients with normal pressure as well as in those with glaucoma. The ocular hypotensive action observed after systemic administration may be beneficial in patients with ocular hypertension or in the glaucoma patient controlled with antiglaucoma drugs other than epinephrine. The reduction of intraocular pressure induced by systemic ß-receptor antagonists ranges from 20% to 41%. Intraocular pressure decreases following systemic administration of atenolol (34), metroprolol (35), nadolol (36), propranolol (37), or timolol (38).

Patient Management

Patients who incur dry eye syndrome associated with systemically administered ß-adrenergic antagonists should be treated symptomatically using artificial tear solutions and ointment formulations as required. Reduction of intraocular pressure associated with systemic ß-adrenergic antagonists may actually prove beneficial if the patient has ocular hypertension or glaucoma. However, since systemic ß-blockers also reduce blood pressure, this route of administration may be detrimental in certain glaucomatous patients. The reduction of perfusion pressure to the optic nerve produced by decreased systemic blood pressure may offset the benefit derived from reducing intraocular pressure. Conversely, when the systemic ß-blocker is discontinued, intraocular pressure may increase to levels that increase the risk of optic nerve damage and visual field loss associated with glaucoma. Thus, patients should be monitored carefully if ß-blocker therapy is discontinued.

CARDIOVASCULAR DRUGS

A benzofuran derivative, amiodarone, has been used for several decades to treat a variety of cardiac abnormalities. This drug is highly effective in the treatment of atrial and ventricular arrhythmias as well as in the treatment of Wolff-Parkinson-White syndrome (39). Following its introduction into clinical practice, however, amiodarone was observed to cause keratopathy early in the course of treatment, and ultrastructural changes can also occur in the conjunctiva and eyelids.

Digitoxin and digoxin have been widely used for the treatment of congestive heart disease and certain cardiac arrhythmias. Visual symptoms associated with digitalis have been recognized for several centuries and include symptoms of dimness of vision, flickering or flashing scotomas, as well as disturbances of color vision.

Pathogenesis

Amiodarone belongs to a group of drugs having the physical and chemical properties of cationic amphiphilia (40). Amphiphilic drugs bind to polar lipids and accumulate within lysosomes. Several investigators (39,41–43) have performed electron microscopy on ocular tissues of patients who had taken amiodarone, and these studies have consistently revealed intracytoplasmic membrane-bound lamellar bodies similar to myelin. These changes have been noted not only in the corneal epithelium, conjunctiva, and crystalline lens, but have also been found in the corneal endothelium, the iris, ciliary body, choroid, and retina (39,41). The presence of such complex lipid deposits within these tissues has led recent investigators to conclude that amiodarone keratopathy is probably a drug-induced lipid storage disease. The whorl-like pattern of the keratopathy may result from an effect at the limbus on the epithelial cells that are migrating centripetally (44). Exposure to light may have an important role since the lenticular changes are largely limited to the pupillary aperture (45).

The retina, rather than optic nerve, appears to be the site of digitalis toxicity (46). Binnion and Frazer (47) have demonstrated in dogs that the highest concentrations of digoxin are found in the choroid and retina, and electrodiagnostic studies have confirmed cone dysfunction in patients with digitalis intoxication (48). The precise mechanism underlying digoxin's toxicity may involve inhibition of Na^+-K^+-activated adenosine triphosphatase (ATPase), an enzyme that plays an important role in the maintenance of normal cone function.

Ocular Manifestations

Keratopathy occurs as early as 6 days following initial amiodarone therapy (49), but it more commonly appears after 1 to 3 months of treatment (50). Virtually all patients will demonstrate corneal changes after 3 months of therapy (49,51). These corneal deposits are bilateral, but are often asymmetric, and they are easily observed with the slit lamp. The keratopathy can be divided into several stages (41,49,50). In grade I, a faint horizontal line, similar to a Hudson-Stähli line, appears in the interpalpebral fissure at the junction of the middle and lower third of the cornea. It consists of golden-brown microdeposits in the epithelium just anterior to Bowman's layer. Transition to grade II occurs by 6 months, during which the deposits become aligned in a more linear pattern and extend toward the limbus. (The grade II pattern does not necessarily proceed to grade III.) In grade III, the deposits increase in number and density, and the lines extend superiorly to produce a whorl-like pattern within the visual axis. Grade IV keratopathy is characterized by irregular, round clumps of deposits. The development of the first three stages of keratopathy is shown in Fig. 1, and a clinical representation of amiodarone keratopathy is shown in Fig. 2. Upon discontinuing drug therapy, the keratopathy gradually resolves within 6 to 18 months (50).

The severity of the keratopathy appears to be significantly correlated with total drug dosage as well as with duration of treatment (41,52,53). It is possible, however, for patients taking lower doses of amiodarone to demonstrate marked keratopathy, whereas other patients taking high doses of drug show minimal corneal changes (41). In general, patients taking low dosages of drug (100 to 200 mg daily) retain clear corneas or demonstrate only mild keratopathy regardless of duration of treatment or cumulative dosage. Patients taking higher dosages (400 to 1,400 mg daily) demonstrate more advanced keratopathy depending on the duration of treatment (52). Once

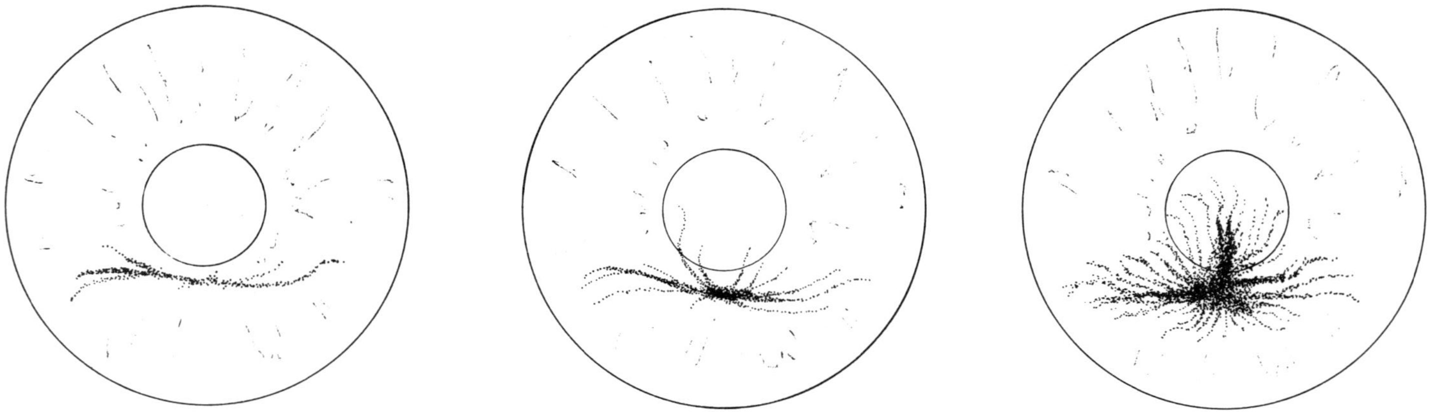

FIG. 1. Stages of amiodarone keratopathy. *Left*, grade I; *center*, grade II; *right*, grade III. (Modified from Klingele et al, ref. 273.)

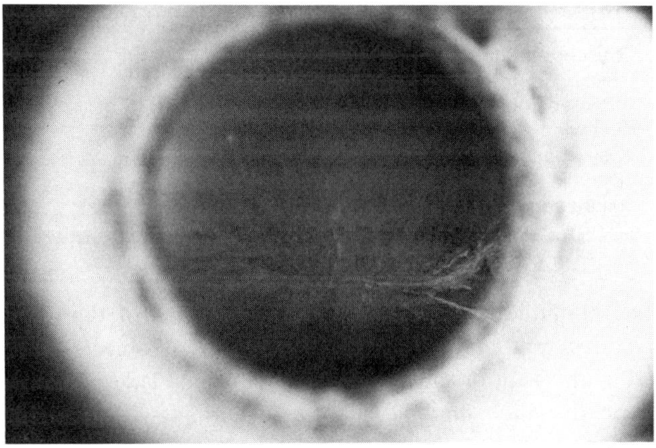

FIG. 2. Clinical photograph of grade III amiodarone keratopathy. (From Bartlett and Jaanus, ref. 2, with permission.)

the keratopathy becomes fully developed, it remains relatively stationary until the drug dosage is reduced or discontinued (41).

Amiodarone-induced lenticular opacities have also been reported (41,50,54). Fine anterior subcapsular lens deposits occur in about half of patients taking amiodarone in moderate to high doses (600 to 800 mg daily) (54) after a duration of treatment of 6 to 18 months. The deposits first appear as small, golden-brown or white-yellow punctate opacities located just below the anterior lens capsule. They are loosely packed and cover an area greater than 2 mm in diameter within the pupillary aperture (54). Unlike the lenticular deposits associated with chlorpromazine therapy, which develop prior to corneal changes, the lens opacities associated with amiodarone develop in the presence of marked keratopathy.

Symptoms associated with amiodarone induced corneal and lenticular changes are minimal or absent (41,50,51). Lenticular opacities generally cause no visual symptoms, but moderate to severe keratopathy can lead to complaints of blurred vision, glare, halos around lights, or light sensitivity. Visual acuity is usually normal but may be slightly decreased if the keratopathy is severe.

Although chronic administration of this antiarrhythmic agent has produced no visible biomicroscopic changes in the conjunctiva, electron microscopic studies of human material have indicated that some ultrastructural changes may occur during therapy (41,55). Intracytoplasmic membrane-bound deposits similar to myelin have been demonstrated in the cytoplasm of nearly all ocular structures, including the conjunctival epithelium (55). Amiodarone has also been reported to concentrate within a chalazion that developed in a patient who had been taking the drug for 2 years (56).

The most common symptoms induced by the cardiac glycosides are changes in color vision and various visual phenomena (Table 1). These symptoms often

TABLE 1. *Visual symptoms in cardiac glycoside intoxication*

Dyschromatopsia
Flickering or flashes of light
Colored spots
Snowing vision
Disturbances of visual acuity
Dimming of vision
Glare sensitivity

precede cardiac abnormalities as the earliest symptoms of digitoxin intoxication (57). A common symptom is snowy vision, wherein objects of regard appear to be covered with frost or snow (48,58). Elevated dark adaptation thresholds have been reported, which gradually return to normal within 2 to 3 weeks after digitalis is discontinued (59).

Complaints of color vision disturbances are common with both digoxin and digitoxin, but color vision impairment can often be detected even in patients without symptoms (60). Both the incidence and severity of color vision impairment tend to correlate with the plasma glycoside level (60). About 80% of patients with digoxin intoxication will demonstrate generalized color vision deficiencies (60), but detectable color vision impairment occurs even at therapeutic drug levels. In contrast, patients treated with digitoxin in therapeutic concentrations usually show no significant color vision abnormality (61).

The onset of visual symptoms following drug administration may be as soon as 1 day but is often within 2 weeks of initial therapy. Occasionally ocular toxicity is not shown until several years of treatment (58). Once digitalis therapy is discontinued, however, visual symptoms usually subside within several weeks.

Patient Management

Since the corneal and lenticular changes associated with amiodarone therapy are benign, special follow-up of affected patients is not required unless the opacities have caused visual symptoms. In the rare cases in which visual symptoms are annoying or incapacitating, reducing or discontinuing drug therapy usually results in resolution of the corneal findings. It is unusual for ocular side effects to necessitate discontinuation of drug therapy, but occasionally treatment must be discontinued because of drug intolerance or other side effects such as diarrhea, vomiting, pulmonary fibrosis, or liver damage (41,50). Because the early stages of amiodarone keratopathy can mimic a Hudson-Stähli line, a careful drug history relative to amiodarone use should be carefully elicited. More advanced stages of amiodarone keratopathy may resemble the corneal changes of Fabry's disease or chloroquine toxicity. Because of the systemic implications of Fabry's disease, patients with no history of amiodarone or chloroquine use should be evaluated by an internist.

Patients taking cardiac glycosides should be monitored carefully for visual symptoms, including color vision changes, flashing or flickering lights, and other entoptic phenomena. Color vision evaluation, especially during the first several weeks of therapy, can be especially helpful in detecting signs of early intoxication. Periodic color vision testing should be performed as long as the patient continues taking the medication, and detectable changes in color vision should warrant consultation with the prescribing physician with regard to potential digitalis intoxication.

PHENOTHIAZINES AND ETHANOL

Chlorpromazine and thioridazine, both phenothiazine derivatives, are commonly used for their antipsychotic effects. Often high, prolonged dosages are required, and these have led to well-documented pigmentary changes in the cornea, crystalline lens, and retina. It is now generally accepted that chlorpromazine is the only phenothiazine to cause toxic changes in the cornea and lens, and it is recognized that only thioridazine produces retinal toxicity. Although most of the current literature describes the toxic effects on the cornea, lens, and retina, phenothiazines have also been reported to affect the conjunctiva, sclera, eyelids, pupils, and lacrimal system, and to have the potential to induce cycloplegia.

Ethyl alcohol is widely consumed in the form of beer, whiskey, and other alcoholic beverages. This drug can lower intraocular pressure and can induce changes in extraocular muscle motility.

Pathogenesis

The precise nature of chlorpromazine-induced pigmentary granules observed in the cornea and crystalline lens is unknown. A common hypothesis, however, is that the pigmentary changes are a result of drug interaction with ultraviolet light as it passes through the cornea and lens, causing exposed proteins to denature, opacify, and accumulate in the anterior subcapsular region of the lens as well as in corneal stroma (62).

It is known that the phenothiazines bind to melanin in the uveal tract, especially the choroid (63,64). Drug uptake by the choroid occurs even in patients whose serum levels of thioridazine are in the nontoxic range (65). It has been proposed that such drug binding is retinotoxic by damaging the choriocapillaris, thus leading to changes in the retinal pigment epithelium (63,66). It is also possible that thioridazine may alter retinal enzyme kinetics, inhibiting the oxidation of retinol. Alterations in the enzyme systems of Müller cells and photoreceptors may lead to atrophy and disorganization of the rods and cones as one of the initial degenerative changes, followed later by loss of the retinal pigment epithelium and choriocapillaries (66).

The effect of the phenothiazines on pupil size, the lacrimal system, and accommodation is related to the anticholinergic properties of these drugs. Thus, the phenothiazines can cause pupillary dilation, cycloplegia, and dry eye associated with decreased aqueous tear secretion.

Ethyl alcohol is distributed in total body water and penetrates the eye very rapidly. However, penetration of the vitreous is somewhat slower than penetration of the aqueous. This lag results in a sufficient osmotic gradient between plasma and vitreous to draw fluid from the eye (67). Ethyl alcohol also inhibits secretion of antidiuretic hormone (ADH) (68). A hypotonic diuresis is produced following its administration, and it has been suggested that this also contributes to the increase of serum osmolality induced by ethyl alcohol.

Ocular Manifestations

Both corneal and lenticular changes are associated with chlorpromazine therapy (69–73). Thaler and associates (69) have divided the lenticular pigmentation into five stages. The earliest sign of lenticular toxicity (grade I) is fine dot-like opacities on the anterior lens surface. At this stage the pigmentary deposits are small and tend to assume a disciform distribution within the pupillary area. Grade II lenticular changes consist of dot-like opacities that are more opaque and denser than in grade I. The pigmentary granules may begin to assume a stellate pattern. As the condition progresses, grade III changes are characterized by larger granules of pigment within an anterior subcapsular stellate pattern that is easily recognized. At this stage the opacity can range in color from white to yellow to tan. The stellate pattern has a dense central area with radiating branches (Fig. 3). A readily visible stellate pattern with three to nine star points characterizes grade IV lenticular pigmentation. The lens changes at this stage can be recognized with a penlight, and diagnosis does not necessarily require slit lamp examination. Grade V lenticular changes are characterized by a central, lightly pigmented, opaque mass surrounded by smaller clumps of pigment.

Corneal pigmentary changes almost invariably occur only in patients who have concomitant lens opacities in the higher grades (69,72). There is often little or no corneal involvement with lens grades I and II, but grades III and higher have detectable corneal pigmentation ranging from light to heavy (69). The pigmentation is white, yellow-white, brown, or black, and occurs at the level of the endothelium and Descemet's membrane primarily in the interpalpebral fissure (Fig. 4).

Although patients may occasionally report glare, halos around lights, or hazy vision, both the corneal and lenticular changes only rarely reduce visual acuity. The keratopathy and lenticular pigmentary changes usually progress to a point beyond which no further changes are observed (73). Upon reducing or discontinuing drug therapy, the pigmentary deposits are generally irreversible (70,72,73). This is not surprising given that the deposits associated with chlorpromazine are located in avascular tissues. In rare instances the lenticular pigmentation can begin after chlorpromazine therapy is discontinued (71).

The corneal and lenticular changes associated with chlorpromazine are dose-related. Lenticular pigmentation is rarely observed when the total dosage is less than 500 g, and the prevalence of pigmentary changes increases with total dosages between 1,000 and 2,000 g, until 90% of patients demonstrate pigmentation when the

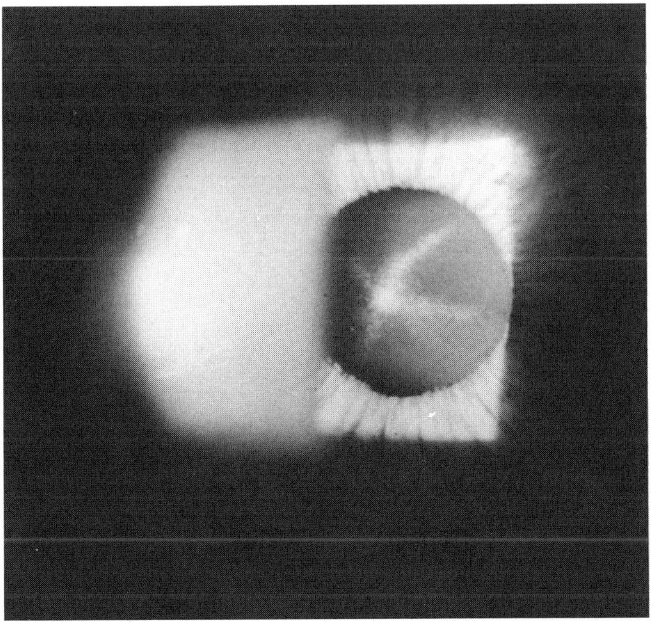

FIG. 3. Stellate pattern of anterior subcapsular cataract associated with chlorpromazine. (From Bartlett and Jaanus, ref. 2, with permission.)

total dosage exceeds 2,500 g (69,74). Since some psychiatric conditions may require daily dosages exceeding 800 mg, lenticular pigmentation can appear as early as 14 to 20 months of therapy (69). Dosages consisting of 200 mg daily have been reported to cause lenticular changes in as early as 6 months of therapy (72). Corneal toxicity has been reported to occur within 6 months of therapy in 12% of patients receiving 2,000 mg of chlorpromazine daily but in only 1% of patients receiving 300 mg of chlorpromazine daily (72).

Thioridazine can cause significant retinal toxicity, leading to reduced visual acuity, changes in color vision, and disturbances of dark adaptation. These symptoms typically occur 30 to 90 days after treatment is begun (66,75). Visual field changes consist of concentric contractions or irregular paracentral or ring scotomas (66). The fundus appearance is often normal during the early stages of symptoms, but within several weeks or months a pigmentary retinopathy develops, characterized by fine clumps of pigment developing first in the periphery and progressing toward the posterior pole (Fig. 5) (63,75). In milder cases the pigment remains fine and peppery, but in more severe cases the pigment can form plaque-like lesions with multiple confluent areas of hypopigmentation and choroidal atrophy (66). Retinal edema can also occur (75), but the optic discs and retinal vasculature are usually normal.

The electroretinogram (ERG) and electro oculogram (EOG) are often normal during the early stages of toxicity, but as the retinal pigmented epithelium (RPE)

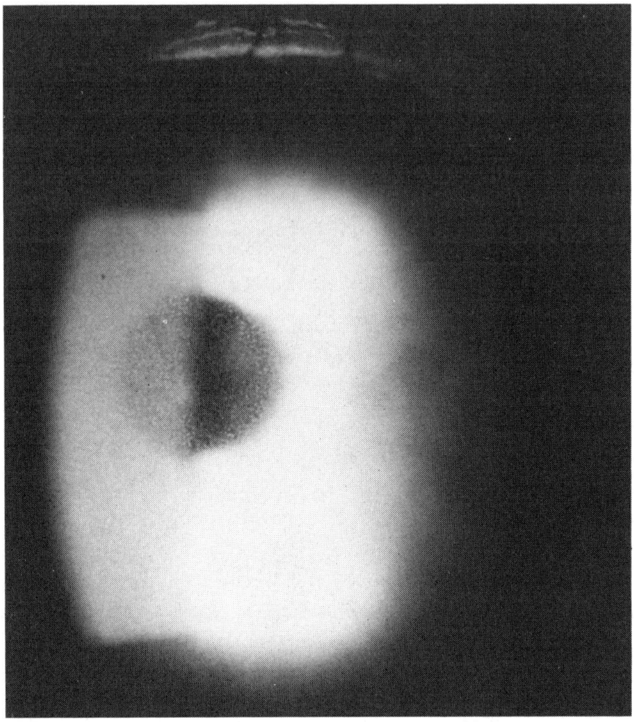

FIG. 4. Heavy pigment deposits on corneal endothelium associated with chlorpromazine. (From Bartlett and Jaanus, ref. 2, with permission.)

becomes diffusely abnormal, the EOG becomes attenuated (76). The amplitude of the oscillatory potential of the ERG decreases in proportion to the daily dosage of thioridazine, but the a- and b-waves as well as the latencies are normal (77). Godel and associates (78) have suggested that the ERG will be diminished to red stimuli in the initial stages of retinal toxicity.

It is now recognized that the primary clinical factor associated with thioridazine retinopathy is the daily drug dosage (63). Before the dose-related retinal toxicity was recognized, dosages exceeding 1,600 mg per day were commonly used. Few cases of pigmentary retinopathy have been reported, however, with daily dosages of less than 800 mg (79). Thus, thioridazine therapy appears to be safe with regard to retinal toxicity as long as daily dosages of less than 800 mg are employed (63,71,80).

Although it is possible for thioridazine retinopathy to resolve despite continued drug therapy, this usually occurs only in patients taking low dosages (75). If significant resolution is to occur, drug therapy must generally be reduced or discontinued. Depending on the severity of toxicity, retinal function can return to normal, but the pigmentary changes are often permanent. In severe cases there may be permanent

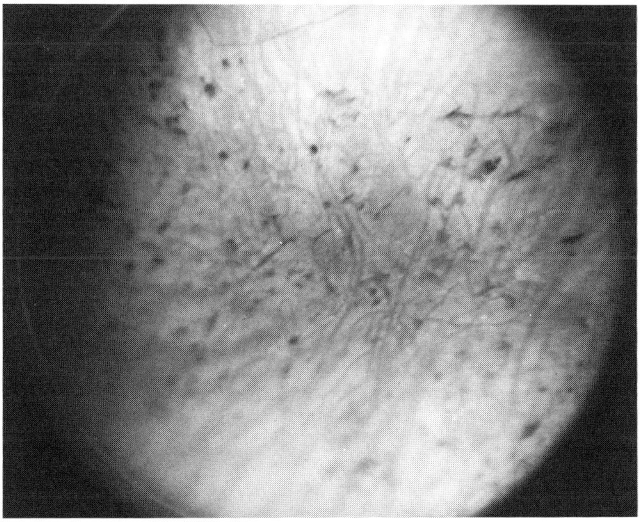

FIG. 5. Retinal pigment epithelial hyperplasia and atrophy in a 33-year-old man with thioridazine retinopathy. (From Bartlett and Jaanus, ref. 2, with permission.)

impairment of visual acuity, visual field, and dark adaptation (63,71). The pigmentary retinopathy may even progress after thioridazine therapy has been discontinued (81), and some cases of progressive retinopathy can have a late onset, occurring from 4 to 10 years following discontinuation of thioridazine (63,76).

Discoloration of the conjunctiva, sclera, and exposed skin of the eyelid has been reported with administration of phenothiazine derivatives (82–85). The skin of the face and lids can be equally pigmented, whereas the palpebral folds contain an area of nonpigmented skin deep within the creases. The discoloration is usually slate-blue. Melanin-like granules have been observed in the superficial dermis of the skin, (82,83). This oculodermatologic syndrome is usually associated with pigmentary deposits in the exposed interpalpebral area of the bulbar conjunctiva, especially near the limbus (82–85). The palpebral conjunctiva does not appear to be involved. Patients exposed to dosages of chlorpromazine ranging from 500 to 3,000 mg per day for 1 to 6 years may develop discoloration of the exposed skin, lids, and bulbar conjunctiva (84,85). There have been sporadic reports of allergic conjunctivitis and edema of the eyelids associated with phenothiazine use (86).

Transient disturbances of accommodation often occur in patients taking chlorpromazine and other phenothiazines (87,88). These effects are most likely due to the anticholinergic properties of the medication and are most pronounced when benztropine is administered along with the phenothiazine (89,90). The visual symptoms may also be ascribed to reduced tearing and drying of the cornea, causing blurred vision. In patients with narrow anterior chamber angles, acute or subacute angle-closure glaucoma secondary to dilated pupils could also contribute to symptoms of blurred vision (87).

Oral administration of ethyl alcohol can reduce intraocular pressure in both normal and glaucomatous eyes (67,91). Normal individuals demonstrate only a minimal reduction of pressure following consumption of 50 ml of 43% ethyl alcohol in the form of whiskey (92). Patients with open-angle glaucoma, however, have a much greater reduction of pressure lasting for 3 to 5 hr. Although the ocular hypotensive effect is slower in onset than with other commercially available hyperosmotic agents, the maximum effect occurs in 1 to 2 hr (67).

Alcohol is well documented to affect eye movement ability (93–96). Both smooth pursuits and saccades are impaired when blood ethanol concentrations reach the range of 60 to 100 mg/dl. Bittencourt and associates (94) have reported a direct linear relationship between blood alcohol concentration and reduction in smooth pursuit velocity. Their results indicate that at a blood ethanol concentration of 80 mg/dl, the capacity of the eyes to track objects moving across the visual field is impaired by 25%.

Patient Management

Patients receiving high-dosage or long-term, low-dosage chlorpromazine therapy should be monitored annually by careful slit lamp examination. Since lenticular pigmentation is the most frequent ocular change observed, slit lamp examination of the lens with the pupil dilated is the most direct method for detecting early chlorpromazine toxicity. It may be possible to delay ocular pigmentary changes by avoiding long-term, high-dosage therapy, or by employing intervals of treatment with nonphenothiazine drugs such as haloperidol (70,72). If the corneal and lenticular changes occur but visual acuity is not affected and the patient is asymptomatic, the drug dosage can generally be continued without modification. If the patient becomes symptomatic, however, the dosage should be reduced or therapy should be changed to a different drug.

Since the danger of retinal toxicity with thioridazine is significantly correlated with daily dosage, patients should generally be placed on dosages less than 800 mg per day (63,66). Patients should receive careful fundus examinations during the first 2 to 4 months of therapy and every 6 months thereafter (63). Electrodiagnostic tests such as the ERG and EOG may be of limited value in detecting early retinopathy (78,97). If symptoms or objective signs of retinal toxicity are observed, the medication should be discontinued to improve the chances of resolution. Since the pigmentary retinopathy may be progressive even after thioridazine has been discontinued, patients should receive follow-up examinations on an annual basis.

Management of drug-induced cycloplegia entails the use of appropriate spectacle lenses to correct for accommodative insufficiency, and the use of artificial tears and lubricants for the relief of symptoms associated with dry eye. These management strategies are usually sufficient without modifying the drug therapy.

It is important for the practitioner to be cognizant of the ability of ethyl alcohol to reduce intraocular pressure. Patients presenting for routine eye examination following consumption of ethyl alcohol may be found to have borderline "normal" intraocular pressures that may increase once the effects of the alcohol have subsided. These patients perhaps should be monitored for development of glaucomatous optic nerve damage and visual field loss.

The fact that alcohol can affect eye movement ability has been employed to devise a test known as the alcohol gaze nystagmus test. This procedure was developed to augment the traditional field evaluation of suspected drunk drivers by law enforcement officials. The test involves the observation of ocular version movements, end-point nystagmus, and angle of lateral deviation at which the nystagmoid movements begin. When properly administered and evaluated, the test can help to correctly identify about 80% of drivers with blood alcohol levels of 0.10% or higher (98,99).

CHEMOTHERAPEUTIC AGENTS

Systemically administered antimicrobial agents usually present no risk to the eye or vision. Some of these drugs, however, can cause a variety of ocular complications, ranging from discoloration of contact lenses to transient myopia or optic neuropathy.

Ocular Manifestations

Drug penetration into tears has been reported with certain antimicrobial agents. Sulfonamides, tetracyclines, erythromycin, and rifampin have been assayed in tears of human subjects (100). Ampicillin and penicillin penetrate into the tears very poorly, but in contrast, erythromycin levels in tears have been found to be higher than the serum concentration, implying active transport of this antibiotic into tears following systemic administration (100). Following its oral administration, 36% to 88% of the daily erythromycin dosage is present in tears. An interesting observation is that the preocular tear film can become discolored after the use of systemic rifampin (101). The tears usually become orange but may also be pink or red. Contact lenses may become stained, leading to the recommendation that soft contact lens wear be discontinued during rifampin therapy (102).

Eyelid edema, conjunctivitis, and chemosis have been reported with high dose administration of sulfanilamide (103). These reactions appear to be analogous to systemic hypersensitivity reactions such as urticaria and edema seen in some patients who are allergic to sulfonamides. Tilden and associates (104) reported bilateral anterior uveitis associated with systemic administration of sulfamethoxazole.

Mattsson (105) described two cases of transient myopia associated with oral sulfonamides in which there was reduced accommodation, shallow anterior chamber angles, and moderate mydriasis. Vaginal absorption of sulfonamides can also lead to myopia. Chirls and Norris (106) reported a patient with myopia following use of a vaginal sulfonamide suppository, and Maddallena (107) described a patient with 7 D (diopter) of induced myopia following use of a sulfonamide vaginal cream.

Conjunctival deposits similar to those seen in epinephrine-treated glaucoma patients have been observed in patients treated orally with tetracyclines (108,109). Dosages range from 250 to 1,500 mg per day of tetracycline and at least 100 mg per day of minocycline. The deposits appear as dark brown to black granules in the palpebral conjunctiva (108). The granules vary in size and are located in conjunctival cysts, surrounded by minute, gray-white, noncrystalline soft spots. Under ultraviolet light microscopy the brown pigment concentrations give a yellow fluorescence characteristic of tetracycline (109).

Optic neuropathy as a consequence of chloramphenicol therapy is well known, especially when the drug is used to treat cystic fibrosis in children. This drug causes both optic neuritis and retrobulbar neuritis (110). Severe, bilateral reduction of visual acuity accompanied by dense central scotomas is characteristic of most cases (110–112). Although there may be no fundus changes, the optic discs are usually edematous and hyperemic, the retinal veins are engorged and tortuous, and hemorrhages are often seen in the parapapillary area (113). Optic atrophy is a late sign. Peripheral neuritis characterized by numbness and cramping of the feet often precedes the visual complaints by 1 to 2 weeks and may therefore serve as an early warning sign of impending ocular toxicity (110).

Visual impairment associated with chloramphenicol therapy usually recovers after the drug is discontinued, but pretreatment visual acuity is often not regained and visual field defects may persist (113). Some patients may tolerate further prolonged treatment with chloramphenicol without recurrent optic neuritis, and occasionally patients can demonstrate improvement of visual function despite continued treatment (113). Most cases of optic neuritis associated with chloramphenicol therapy have occurred in children with cystic fibrosis who were treated with large daily dosages of drug, 1 to 6 g daily. Although the onset of visual symptoms can be as early as 10 days after therapy has begun, ocular toxicity commonly occurs after several months or years of treatment (111,114). Harley and associates (111) have reported a dosage-dependent relationship between chloramphenicol therapy and optic neuritis. The incidence of optic neuritis varied from 5% of patients treated with a daily dosage of 10 to 25 mg/kg body weight, to 38% of patients treated with a daily dosage exceeding 50 mg/kg body weight. There was no vision loss among patients treated for less than 3 months, but the incidence of optic neuritis increased to 16% in patients treated longer than 12 months.

Pathogenesis

Transient myopia caused by systemically administered drugs is produced by ciliary body edema, resulting in relaxation of the zonules, which causes thickening and anterior movement of the crystalline lens (115). Drug-induced myopia associated with sulfonamides has been documented by ultrasonographic A-scan measurements and refraction to be due to edema of the ciliary body (116). The ciliary body edema, occasionally associated with retinal edema, has led to the speculation that sulfonamide-induced myopia may be related to hypersensitivity reactions (105).

It has been hypothesized that either tetracycline or its metabolites form an insoluble chelation complex that results in pigmentation of the palpebral conjunctiva (109).

The precise mechanism by which chloramphenicol produces optic neuritis is unknown, but visual evoked potentials have confirmed optic nerve involvement in patients taking chloramphenicol (117). Although not substantiated, several authors have proposed that chloramphenicol may induce optic neuropathy by causing a vitamin deficiency (118). Genetic factors may be involved, and it has also been suggested that chloramphenicol may be metabolized to degradation products that are potentially toxic to the optic nerve (113). Histopathologic studies have found bilateral optic atrophy with primary involvement of the papillomacular bundle, loss of the retinal ganglion cells, and gliosis of the nerve fiber layer (111). The presence of peripheral visual field defects in some patients is evidence that there is also involvement of the peripheral portion of the visual pathway (112).

Patient Management

Most of the ocular effects of systemically administered antimicrobial agents are benign and will usually subside quickly once drug therapy is reduced or discontinued. It is important, however, that patients who are to receive long-term chloramphenicol therapy undergo a comprehensive baseline examination consisting of visual acuity, visual fields, color vision, and fundus examination. The risk of optic neuropathy is minimized if the daily dosage of drug is limited to 25 mg/kg body weight or less for a period of time not exceeding 3 months (111). Patients or their parents should be encouraged to be alert to the development of peripheral neuritis, which might indicate impending vision loss. Once signs or symptoms of optic neuropathy are detected, drug therapy should be promptly discontinued.

ANTITUBERCULOSIS

Ethambutol was introduced in 1961 for the treatment of tuberculosis. Severe toxic side effects were initially reported, but these were linked to use of the racemic mixture of the drug. The dextroisomer was consequently selected as the most therapeutically useful and has been found to have a lower incidence of ocular toxicity than the racemic form (119).

Pathogenesis

Although the mechanism by which ethambutol causes retrobulbar neuritis is largely unknown, van Dijk and Spekreijse (120) and Kakisu and associates (121) have suggested that ethambutol may affect the amacrine and bipolar cells of the retina since color vision can be affected without altering visual acuity.

Ocular Manifestations

Ethambutol is well documented to cause ocular symptoms of reduced visual acuity, changes in color vision, and visual field loss (122). Signs of ocular toxicity can appear as early as several weeks following initial therapy, but the onset of ocular complications usually occurs several months after therapy is begun (123–125). Although various forms of optic neuritis have been described, the primary ocular manifestation of ethambutol toxicity is retrobulbar neuritis. This commonly occurs in several forms (Table 2): (a) The most common form involves the loss of visual acuity associated with a central or pericentral scotoma along with color vision disturbances. This type is caused by compromise of the central optic nerve fibers. (b) Less commonly, ethambutol can affect the peripheral optic nerve fibers, causing defects in the peripheral visual field. (c) In rare cases ethambutol can cause visible retinal manifestations, including hyperemia and swelling of the optic discs, flame-shaped hemorrhages on the optic disc and in the retina, and macular edema. After several weeks these signs can be followed by primary optic atrophy (126,127).

Color vision disturbances are probably the most sensitive indicator of early ethambutol optic neuropathy (128). When the patient is examined with sensitive tests such as the Farnsworth Munsell 100-Hue or desaturated Panel D-15, both red-green or blue-yellow defects may be observed in early stages of toxicity (128). These changes in color vision can occur even before visual acuity and visual fields are affected.

Contrast sensitivity function can also be affected, in some cases before visual acuity or color vision become impaired (129). Salmon and associates (129) have suggested that testing using Arden contrast sensitivity plates may be effective in detecting subclinical toxic optic neuropathy associated with ethambutol.

Once changes have occurred in visual acuity, visual field, or color vision, these functional disturbances may continue to deteriorate even after ethambutol has been discontinued (127). More often, however, there is recovery of pretreatment visual acuity and visual field several months or years following discontinuation of drug treatment (122). The degree of recovery depends largely on the extent to which

TABLE 2. *Characteristics of ethambutol optic neuropathy*

Characteristic	Central (axial)	Peripheral
Toxic dosage	Low	High
Visual acuity	Reduced	Normal
Visual field	Central scotoma	Peripheral constriction
Color vision	Red-green deficiency	Normal

Modified from Garrett CR, ref. 134.

ethambutol has compromised optic nerve function, and if the ocular toxicity is not recognized early, the drug can cause permanent loss of vision (130).

There is considerable evidence that ocular toxicity associated with ethambutol therapy is dose-related (199). It is now recognized that ethambutol rarely causes ocular changes at a dosage of 15 to 20 mg/kg body weight/day (125), and this has led to the current recommendation that ethambutol dosages should not generally exceed 15 mg/kg body weight/day. Some clinicians employ the drug in dosages of 25 mg/kg/day for a period of time not exceeding 2 months, followed by a maintenance dose of 15 mg/kg/day, and this has been shown to cause virtually no ocular complications (123,131).

Patient Management

Patients beginning treatment with ethambutol should have baseline examinations and frequent monitoring of visual acuity, visual fields, color vision, and fundus appearance. Since it is rare for ocular toxicity to occur with dosages as low as 15 mg/kg/day, patients taking such dosages can be monitored every 3 to 6 months (128). Patients with renal insufficiency, however, have impaired ability to excrete the drug and therefore may be at greater risk for developing ocular changes. These patients should be monitored on a monthly basis (126,132). Patients with low plasma zinc levels should also be monitored more carefully (133). Periodic evaluations must include color vision, static threshold visual fields, visual acuity, and ophthalmoscopy. Use of the desaturated Panel D-15 test or the Farnsworth Munsell 100-Hue is effective for the detection of subtle color vision changes associated with early ethambutol toxicity (128). Several authors have recommended use of visual evoked potentials for the routine monitoring of patients taking ethambutol (130,134). This procedure has been shown to be effective for the detection of subclinical optic nerve disease that can precede changes in visual acuity and color vision.

Ethambutol therapy must be discontinued in patients who develop reduced visual acuity, color vision deficiency, or visual field defects characteristic of optic neuropathy (135). If discontinuation of drug therapy alone does not result in improvement of visual function, consideration can be given to treatment with hydroxycobalamin. Guerra and Casu (136) have reported recovery of visual acuity in four patients treated with hydroxycobalamin several months after the discontinuation of ethambutol had failed to improve visual acuity. Although the mechanism of action of hydroxycobalamin in the treatment of ethambutol-induced optic neuropathy is uncertain, this vitamin may act by neutralizing the chelating action of ethambutol on the optic nerve.

ANTIMALARIAL COMPOUNDS

Chloroquine and hydroxychloroquine are used for the treatment of malaria, rheumatoid arthritis, discoid and systemic lupus erythematosus, and other collagen diseases. These quinoline drugs have been employed for these purposes since the early 1950s.

These drugs are well known to cause changes in the cornea and retina, and to induce clinically significant cycloplegia.

Quinine has been employed for the treatment of malaria, but it is now used primarily for the management of leg cramps, myotonia congenita, and eyelid myokymia. Quinine toxicity has been recognized for many years, and overdosage of quinine is still encountered in patients who attempt abortion or suicide. Accidental ingestion of quinine can also lead to serious side effects. Acute vision loss is one of the most significant reactions associated with quinine use.

Pathogenesis

The origin of chloroquine-induced corneal opacities is somewhat obscure but appears to represent reversible binding of the drug to intracellular nucleoproteins (137). The changes induced by the quinolines are limited to the corneal epithelium, which the drug may reach by deposition in the tear film or by the limbal vasculature (138). Individual susceptibility probably plays an important role in the development of chloroquine keratopathy since, at lower dosages (e.g., 250 mg chloroquine or 200 mg hydroxychloroquine daily), there appears to be no relationship between the occurrence of keratopathy and total dosage and duration of therapy (139). Patients receiving chloroquine doses exceeding 750 mg daily or hydroxychloroquine doses exceeding 800 mg daily appear to develop keratopathy earlier in the course of treatment (140,141).

Although the precise mechanism by which chloroquine and hydroxychloroquine cause retinal toxicity is unknown, it is widely recognized that these drugs bind tenaciously to melanin within the eye (142,143). It is understood, moreover, that the pigmented tissues of the eye will continue to hold the drug for prolonged periods of time after drug therapy is discontinued (142). This can lead to degenerative changes of the retinal pigmented epithelium (RPE). Rosenthal and associates (142), however, have shown that chloroquine also accumulates in the retina itself, suggesting that the neurosensory retina may also have the ability to bind the drug. Investigations in monkeys have shown that chloroquine initially causes degenerative effects in the ganglion cells, followed by disruption of the photoreceptors and finally of the RPE and choroid (142). Ramsey and Fine (144) have confirmed in humans that the initial pathologic change occurs in the ganglion cells and that the changes within the RPE and photoreceptors occur late in the disease process. The destructive process within the RPE leads to migration of pigment-laden cells from the RPE to the outer nuclear and outer plexiform layers (137,145). There is frequently sparing of the foveal cones, which explains the ophthalmoscopic appearance seen in cases of "bull's-eye" maculopathy (143). Attenuation of the retinal arterioles is thought to be secondary to the extensive retinal damage (143).

The precise mechanism underlying the cycloplegic effect of chloroquine is unknown. However, the fact that the accommodative insufficiency is rapid in both its onset and reversibility suggests that the effect is related to melanin binding (137). The change in amplitude of accommodation might also be explained by a drug effect on the central nervous system (146).

Our current understanding of the pathogenesis of quinine ocular toxicity is largely derived from various electrodiagnostic studies demonstrating that quinine has a direct toxic effect on the retinal photoreceptors and ganglion cells (147–149). There is also damage to the retinal pigment epithelium (148). Visual evoked potentials confirm the conduction abnormality in the nerve fiber layer associated with secondary optic atrophy (150).

Ocular Manifestations

The pattern of chloroquine keratopathy can be divided into three stages (151). In the early stage diffuse punctate deposits appear in the corneal epithelium. Later the deposits aggregate into curved lines that converge and coalesce just below the central cornea. Finally, green-yellow pigmented lines appear in the center of the cornea as a whorl-like opacity.

Less than half of affected patients with corneal changes have visual symptoms (152), but the most common complaints relate to halos around lights, glare, and photophobia. Visual acuity usually remains unchanged (137,152). Upon discontinuation of drug therapy, both subjective symptoms and objective corneal signs invariably disappear (153–155).

Keratopathy occurs in 30% to 75% of patients treated with either chloroquine or hydroxychloroquine (139,157), but the corneal changes are much less frequently observed in patients treated with hydroxychloroquine (152,154). Although Calkins (140) reported that the corneal findings are related to total (cumulative) drug dosage or duration of therapy, more recent studies (139,158) have found no correlation between severity of keratopathy and the dosage or duration of drug therapy (140,152), and there is no relationship between the development of corneal deposits and the occurrence of retinopathy (158). In about half of patients treated with chloroquine there is decreased or absent corneal sensitivity unrelated to the development of corneal opacity (137).

During the past decade hydroxychloroquine has become the preferred quinoline for the treatment of collagen diseases because of fewer side effects, and its ocular toxicity is considerably less than that of chloroquine (141,155). Tobin and associates (159) monitored 99 patients treated with hydroxychloroquine during a 7-year period. All patients received the drug for at least 1 year, and most patients received a daily dosage of 400 mg. No keratopathy was observed in any patient. At higher dosage levels, however, a higher incidence of keratopathy has been reported (141). In a group of patients receiving an average daily dosage of 800 mg, 6% developed keratopathy within 6 months of beginning therapy, and the incidence increased to 32% during the second 6 months. Corneal changes were present in all patients after 4 years of hydroxychloroquine treatment. Shearer and Dubois (141) have reported a rapid rise in the incidence of keratopathy when the total drug dosage exceeds 150 g.

Upon reducing or discontinuing drug therapy, the corneal opacities decreased or disappeared during an average of 8 months.

The first visible evidence of chloroquine retinopathy is a fine, pigmentary mottling within the macular area with or without loss of the foveal reflex (160,161). However, even before visible ophthalmoscopic changes are detectable, a "premaculopathy" state can exist in which the drug interferes with metabolism of the macular tissues, causing subtle relative visual field defects in patients with ophthalmoscopically normal maculas (162,163). As the macular pigmentary change progresses, a classic pattern develops consisting of a granular hyperpigmentation surrounded by a zone of depigmentation, which, in turn, is surrounded by another ring of pigment. Although this clinical picture can vary in intensity, it is pathognomonic of chloroquine retinopathy and is referred to as a "bull's-eye" lesion (Fig. 6) (137,160,161). Variations of retinal pigment epithelial disturbances can occur and are commonly observed as a well-circumscribed area of RPE atrophy in the macular area, which can resemble a macular hole (Fig. 7) (137,160). In moderate to advanced cases of retinal toxicity, the arterioles may become attenuated, and the optic disc can become pale (137,164,165). Occasionally there may be signs of macular edema (137,165). There usually is a high degree of bilateral symmetry between the eyes, but occasionally the toxicity can affect one eye more than the other.

Some patients with chloroquine retinopathy may have retinal changes that resemble retinitis pigmentosa (137,166,167). There is peripheral RPE hyperplasia, but, in contrast to retinitis pigmentosa, the pigment does not tend to accumulate around the retinal veins (168). These peripheral lesions can occur with or without simultaneous macular involvement (Fig. 8). Other changes include attenuated retinal vessels, optic

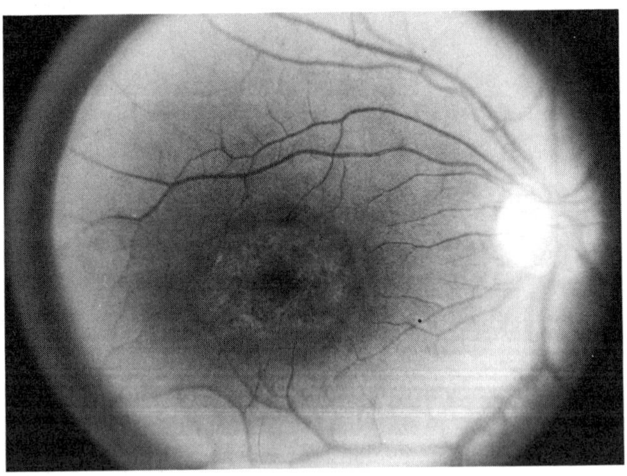

FIG. 6. Characteristic "bull's-eye" maculopathy associated with chloroquine toxicity. (From Bartlett and Jaanus, ref. 2, with permission.)

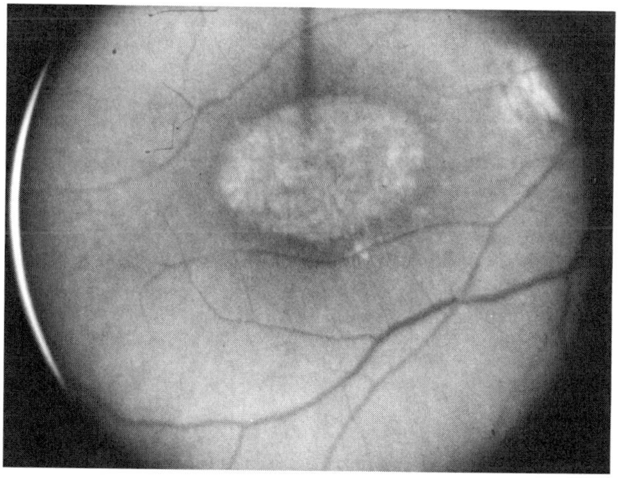

FIG. 7. Retinal pigment epithelial atrophy in macular area as a consequence of chloroquine therapy. (From Bartlett and Jaanus, ref. 2, with permission.)

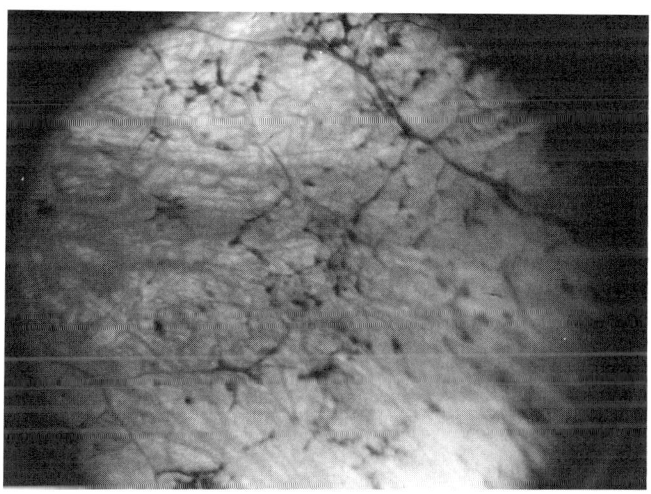

FIG. 8. Peripheral retinal pigment epithelial hyperplasia characteristic of pseudoretinitis pigmentosa in a 42-year-old man with chloroquine toxicity. (From Bartlett and Jaanus, ref. 2, with permission.)

atrophy, peripheral visual field loss, and a subnormal electroretinogram. The fact that the dark adaptation threshold is normal or only minimally abnormal further differentiates this condition from true retinitis pigmentosa (196).

Although the visual fields may be normal even in the presence of definite macular pigmentary changes (158), visual field loss generally correlates well with the degree of retinal damage. The typical visual field defects in chloroquine retinopathy consist of central, paracentral, or pericentral scotomas (153,170). The paracentral scotomas may be confluent and form a complete ring scotoma.

In the early stages of retinopathy electrodiagnostic studies are usually of little value in detecting early chloroquine toxicity (137,161). Both the ERG and EOG can be normal or abnormal. Advanced cases of chloroquine retinopathy, however, are generally characterized by markedly abnormal or even extinguished ERGs (170,171). This is especially true in cases involving the retinal periphery.

Although it is possible for patients with chloroquine maculopathy to be asymptomatic, extensive macular damage will often lead to symptoms of decreased visual acuity, metamorphopsia, and visual field disturbances (137,162). Paracentral ring scotomas can cause reading difficulty. Although color vision is normal in the early stages of chloroquine toxicity, more extensive macular damage can lead to severe impairment of color vision. Dark adaptation is typically normal, an important feature distinguishing the peripheral retinal changes from those seen in retinitis pigmentosa (137).

Risk factors for the development of chloroquine retinopathy include daily dosage, duration of treatment, serum drug levels, and patient age. The incidence of retinopathy increases with patient age, and in older patients retinal toxicity appears to correlate with total drug dosage (158,172,173). Ehrenfeld and associates (173) contend that daily dosage is the most critical risk factor. Most cases of chloroquine retinopathy occur in patients taking 500 mg daily, but dosages as low as 250 mg or less daily can also be retinotoxic (137,152,166,174). Retinopathy can develop when the total cumulative dosage is as little as 100 g (the equivalent of 250 mg daily for 1 year), but the risk increases significantly when the total dosage exceeds 300 g (157). The duration of therapy required to produce chloroquine retinopathy can be as little as 6 months, but most patients require 2 to 4 years of therapy before retinal changes develop (139,164).

Chloroquine retinopathy tends to remain stable once therapy is discontinued (166). Some patients, however, may demonstrate regression of macular changes if the retinal involvement is mild and if the visual acuity is normal (166). Although some patients with the classic "bull's-eye" maculopathy may have reversible macular changes (158), patients with moderately advanced retinopathy may show progression even after drug therapy is discontinued (166,175). Progressive impairment of visual acuity can occur for up to 5 years following discontinuation of chloroquine therapy (176).

The risk of retinopathy associated with hydroxychloroquine appears to be considerably less than that associated with chloroquine (177). Tobin and associates (159) reported retinal toxicity in only 4 of 99 patients receiving hydroxychloroquine in a daily dosage of 400 mg for at least 1 year. No patient, however, sustained significant vision loss, and the abnormalities were reversible after the medication was discontinued. In some cases the macular changes may be reversible without recurrence even if the medication is reinstituted (178). As little as 73 g of hydroxychloroquine taken over 6 months has been reported to cause retinopathy (178), and the incidence of retinopathy may be as high as 30% if the cumulative dosage exceeds 800 g (179). Several investigators (159,180), however, have discounted the role of cumulative dosage and believe that the risk of maculopathy associated with hydroxychloroquine therapy is more closely related to daily dosage. Johnson and Vine (180) found no evidence of retinopathy in nine patients treated with massive total dosages of hydroxychloroquine ranging from 1,054 to 3,923 g. These authors suggest that patients who take prudent daily dosages of hydroxychloroquine (400 mg/day or 6.5 mg/kg body weight/day, whichever is less) are at little risk for developing retinopathy even when therapy is prolonged.

Accommodative insufficiency, with its associated reading difficulty, is a common side effect of long-term chloroquine therapy (137,146,152). This usually begins within several weeks after treatment is begun, and the effect appears to be dose related (137,146,163). As many as 40% of patients taking 500 to 750 mg daily will have impairment of accommodation (181). The accommodative insufficiency is often rapid in onset but is quickly reversible upon reduction or discontinuation of drug therapy (137).

Mild toxic reactions from quinine are characterized by slight reduction of visual acuity or "flickering" of vision. In more severe cases symptoms consist of sudden complete loss of vision, dizziness, and even deafness. Patients with acute quinine overdose frequently have no light perception in both eyes, and pupils are often dilated and nonreactive (147,148). Patients may complain of impairment of night vision, but color vision is usually normal. The visual fields usually demonstrate concentric contraction, and improvement of the visual fields following the acute episode may require days or months, but the field loss may show no recovery and become permanent (150).

Ophthalmoscopic examination of the fundus soon after acute quinine overdose may reveal a normal fundus (148), but constriction of the arterioles, optic disc pallor, venous dilatation, or retinal edema can also be observed.

The visual prognosis for patients with acute quinine toxicity is guarded. Visual acuity can improve from no light perception to 20/20 within days to several weeks (148,150). Sometimes vision does not improve to normal for several months. As vision recovers there is progressive constriction of the retinal vessels, and the optic disc becomes pale. Although central vision often returns to normal levels, the visual fields can remain constricted (150).

Patient Management

Patients taking chloroquine or hydroxychloroquine should receive careful baseline and periodic slit lamp examinations. Early identification of the corneal changes is facilitated by using retroillumination (140). It is important for the ophthalmic practitioner to distinguish early chloroquine keratopathy from the normal development of Hudson-Stähli lines, which it can resemble. Fabry's keratopathy is another important condition in the differential diagnosis. The verticillate corneal findings are similar to those induced by chloroquine, but the systemic implications in Fabry's disease warrant consultation with an internist. Since the drug-induced corneal condition is relatively benign and only rarely results in significant visual symptoms, the development of chloroquine keratopathy does not contraindicate continued use of the medication (152,154). If, however, symptoms of glare, halos, or reduced vision are bothersome to the patient, consideration can be given to decreasing or changing drug therapy.

Since early chloroquine or hydroxychloroquine retinopathy is frequently reversible if drug dosage is reduced or discontinued, patients should be monitored carefully after receiving baseline evaluations. Baseline examinations of the fundus and using Amsler charts are especially important since chloroquine and hydroxychloroquine maculopathy can resemble age-related macular disease. Once drug treatment has started, it is prudent to monitor patients every 6 months, especially if the patient is over 65 years of age (173,174). Elderly patients should be monitored more carefully since chloroquine and hydroxychloroquine are detoxified and eliminated from the body by the liver and kidney, respectively, which might be impaired in these patients (155). As the patient is monitored over time, careful ophthalmoscopic examination of the fundus, including retinal periphery, is one of the most sensitive indicators of early retinopathy (179,182). Testing of contrast sensitivity function is also useful to detect early macular dysfunction (183). Visual field assessment using static threshold techniques is of value in detecting the early stages of visual field loss (184). Patients should be encouraged to self-evaluate using the Amsler charts every 2 weeks (174). Electrodiagnostic testing, however, as well as fluorescein angiography are less sensitive than routine ophthalmoscopy or color photography in the detection of early retinal toxicity (185). Since the clinical signs and symptoms of retinal toxicity may not appear until after drug therapy is discontinued, it is important to monitor patients for several years after drug therapy has been stopped, especially for patients who have received at least 300 g of chloroquine or the equivalent of hydroxychloroquine (173,186).

Because the cycloplegic effects of chloroquine are transient and are related to drug dosage, symptoms of accommodative insufficiency can be managed by prescribing appropriate reading lenses during long-term drug therapy, or drug dosage may be reduced or discontinued. The cycloplegic effects of chloroquine will often abate when the dosage is reduced, and accommodation will completely return to pretreatment levels after drug therapy is discontinued (146).

The maximum daily dosage of quinine should generally not exceed 2 g, and quinine toxicity is common in dosages over 4 g (148). Toxic reactions to relatively small doses of quinine are probably idiosyncratic in nature but can result in a clinical picture similar to that caused by higher doses. Since central vision tends to spontaneously recover even without treatment, patients with acute quinine toxicity should be managed by immediate gastric emptying, administration of activated charcoal, and other supportive measures. Following the acute episode, patients should be monitored carefully for improvement in visual acuity, visual fields, and fundus appearance.

ANTINEOPLASTICS

Of the commonly used antineoplastic agents, tamoxifen citrate and carmustine (BCNU) are most likely to adversely affect ocular tissues. Tamoxifen is an orally administered nonsteroidal antiestrogen and is one of the most effective antitumor agents for the palliative treatment of metastatic breast carcinoma in postmenopausal women. This drug has been in clinical use since 1970 and is used both alone and in combination with other agents usually without serious side effects. Carmustine is used for the treatment of various malignant neoplasms, including metastatic malignant melanoma, malignant gliomas of the central nervous system, metastatic breast cancer, and leukemia.

Pathogenesis

The first clinicopathologic correlation of tamoxifen retinopathy was provided by Kaiser-Kupfer and associates (187). These investigators have shown that high-dosage tamoxifen treatment causes widespread axonal degeneration, primarily in the perimacular area. The yellow-white lesions seen on fundus examination appear to represent products of the axonal degeneration. They are 3 to 10 μm in diameter in the macular area, from 30 to 35 μm in diameter in the perimacular area, and they are confined to the nerve fiber and inner plexiform layers.

The retinal toxicity resulting from intracarotid infusion of carmustine is probably related to the increased flow of drug into the ophthalmic artery. The precise mechanism whereby carmustine causes retinal toxicity is unknown, but several investigators (188,189) have suggested that the drug may be toxic to the retinal and choroidal vasculature, causing segmental intraretinal vasculitis with or without vascular obstruction. This process leads to nerve fiber infarcts and retinal hemorrhage.

Ocular Manifestations

Tamoxifen retinopathy has been well documented, and the retinal findings include white or yellow refractile opacities in the macular and perimacular area, with or without macular edema (Fig. 9) (190,191). Although the lesions are usually more numerous in the macular area, they can also extend to the ora. The lesions occur in the sensory retina, and many appear superficial to the retinal vessels. The affected patient may experience a reduction of visual acuity associated with the macular lesions, and the visual fields can show abnormalities corresponding to the retinal lesions. At

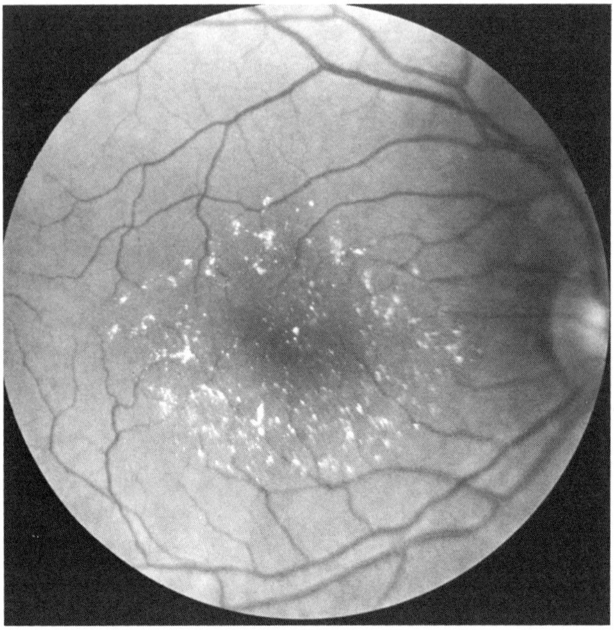

FIG. 9. Tamoxifen maculopathy in a 66-year-old woman administered 120 mg of tamoxifen twice daily for 2 years. Note macular edema with yellow-white crystalline deposition. (From Bartlett and Jaanus, ref. 2, with permission.)

normal dosage levels tamoxifen rarely causes retinal toxicity (192,193), but when taken in high dosages (e.g., 90 to 100 mg twice daily) the toxic effects can be observed within 17 to 27 months as the total cumulative dosage exceeds 90 g (187,190,191). In rare cases, however, tamoxifen can be retinotoxic in low dosages. Griffiths (194) reported a patient with tamoxifen retinopathy who had received less than 8 g of drug. Once tamoxifen therapy is discontinued, the number and size of the retinal lesions generally remain unchanged, and the degenerative changes are irreversible (187).

Retinal toxicity associated with carmustine usually begins within 2 to 14 weeks following intraarterial infusion of the drug (188). Approximately 65% of patients develop retinal complications consisting of retinal infarction, periarteritis, periphlebitis, nerve fiber layer hemorrhage, or macular edema (189). Loss of vision commonly occurs, and visual acuity can be reduced to 20/60 to light perception or even no light perception (188). Ischemic optic neuropathy has also been reported (195). Although a definite relationship between dosage of carmustine and retinopathy has not been established, retinal complications can be avoided using intracarotid administration by passing the infusion catheter beyond the origin of the ophthalmic artery (196).

Patient Management

Since tamoxifen retinopathy can occur at relatively low total dosages of drug, it is important to obtain a baseline examination before therapy is begun. This should include best corrected visual acuity, visual fields, Amsler chart evaluation, and fundus photography. The patient should be monitored carefully during therapy since macular compromise can result in irreversible vision loss. Annual examinations are sufficient if normal drug dosages are administered. Patients receiving higher than normal doses, however, should be monitored every 6 months.

The retinotoxic effects of intracarotid carmustine can be minimized or avoided by employing an infusion catheter that is advanced beyond the origin of the ophthalmic artery (196,197).

ISOTRETINOIN

An analogue of vitamin A, 13-*cis*-retinoic acid is used to treat severe recalcitrant cystic acne and other keratinizing dermatoses. Oral administration of 1 to 2 mg/kg body weight/day causes suppression of sebaceous gland activity and inhibition of keratinization. Ocular complications include blepharoconjunctivitis, dry eye symptoms, contact lens intolerance, and subepithelial corneal opacities. Impairment of dark adaptation can also occur (198).

Pathogenesis

The meibomian glands are important modified sebaceous glands of the eyelids, and when sebaceous gland activity is suppressed by isotretinoin, the normal lipid layer of the preocular tear film becomes deficient, thus promoting evaporation of the underlying aqueous layer, leading to dry eye or blepharoconjunctivitis.

Although the precise mechanism explaining isotretinoin's effect on dark adaptation is unclear, it has been suggested that the drug may become incorporated into the rod photoreceptor elements during the process of outer disk shedding and renewal (199). Weleber and associates (200) have hypothesized that isotretinoin may compete for normal retinol binding sites on cell surfaces or transport molecules, accounting for the reduction in retinal sensitivity.

Ocular Manifestations

Milson and associates (201) observed a dose-dependent relationship between isotretinoin therapy and blepharoconjunctivitis. Dosages of 2 mg/kg body weight/day of isotretinoin resulted in blepharoconjunctivitis in 43% of patients, whereas dosages of 1 mg/kg body weight/day showed a 20% incidence of blepharoconjunctivitis. A retrospective study (202) of 237 patients showed the most common ocular side effect was blepharoconjunctivitis, occurring in 37% of patients.

The incidence of dry eye symptoms has been estimated to be as high as 20%, with about 8% of patients experiencing contact lens intolerance (202). Isotretinoin has been observed to decrease tear breakup time (202,203). Analysis of lacrimal gland fluid of rabbits and human tears of subjects treated with isotretinoin has shown the presence of this compound in tears. Thus, the actual presence of isotretinoin in tear fluid could decrease stability of the lipid layer of the tear film, which would enhance tear film rupture and the formation of dry spots. This effect could be responsible, in turn, for the dry eye symptoms, contact lens intolerance, and conjunctival irritation accompanying isotretinoin therapy (204).

Impairment of dark adaptation with or without excessive glare sensitivity has been reported with isotretinoin therapy in dosages of 1 mg/kg body weight/day (200). These complaints may be associated with an abnormal ERG or EOG. Once therapy is discontinued, both the abnormal dark adaptation and abnormal ERG usually resolve within several months.

Patient Management

Decreasing the dosage or discontinuing the drug will usually alleviate the side effects, although several months may be required in some patients before significant relief is obtained. In the meantime, treatment of dry eye symptoms or blepharoconjunctivitis using artificial tear preparations and ocular lubricants is usually satisfactory. Symptoms of contact lens intolerance can be managed with artificial tear preparations or reduction of wearing schedules (205).

Patients taking isotretinoin should be monitored for changes in night vision. A history of night vision impairment should suggest more definitive evaluation procedures such as visual fields, dark adaptometry, and electroretinography. If retinal function is documented to be abnormal, the drug should be withdrawn. Once drug therapy has been discontinued, retinal function should be monitored for improvement.

CORTICOSTEROIDS

Corticosteroids are sometimes used to treat collagen diseases such as rheumatoid arthritis and systemic lupus, and they are also used for the treatment of sarcoidosis. However, because of their potential for systemic side effects, steroids are limited to conditions for which less conservative therapy is inadequate. The association between steroid use and cataracts has been well known for several decades, but direct interpretation of published reports of patients with steroid-induced cataracts is often subject to error because of variations in duration of treatment and in the steroid dosages used. In 1960, Black and associates (206) were the first to suggest that systemic steroid therapy could lead to posterior subcapsular (PSC) cataracts. They had observed PSC cataracts in 39% of a group of patients with rheumatoid arthritis who had undergone prolonged systemic steroid therapy. Although several authors subsequently refuted the relationship between systemic steroids and PSC cataracts, it is now widely accepted that under certain circumstances oral steroid therapy can induce cataract formation. Recently PSC cataracts have been reported to be associated with nasal or inhalation steroids (207). Steroids are also widely known to elevate intraocular pressure in patients with open anterior chamber angles.

Pathogenesis

Although the precise mechanism whereby steroids lead to cataract formation is unknown, Urban and Cotlier (208) have proposed that steroids gain entry into the fiber cells of the crystalline lens and then react with specific amino groups of the lens crystallins. This alteration frees protein sulfhydryl groups to form disulfide bonds, which subsequently lead to protein aggregation and ultimately to complexes that refract light. Other mechanisms have also been proposed (209–211).

The pathogenesis of steroid-induced pressure elevation is less well understood. As with topically applied steroids, steroids administered systemically may reduce aqueous outflow facility in susceptible patients (212), but there is substantial evidence that systemically administered steroids may also increase aqueous formation, leading to elevated pressure (213–215). Diotallevi and Bocci (216) have shown that systemically administered steroids can increase aqueous production without elevating intraocular pressure, implying a concomitant increase in aqueous outflow. Compared with topical steroids, systemic steroids may evoke different changes in the ocular fluid dynamics because of the distinctly different routes of administration (214). Patients on long-term systemic steroids may accumulate excessive amounts of mucopolysaccharide in the trabecular meshwork, causing obstruction of aqueous outflow by hydrating the trabeculum (217).

Ocular Manifestations

Systemic steroids can produce PSC cataracts (Fig. 10) that are clinically indistinguishable from complicated cataract and cataracts caused by exposure to ionizing radiation (206). They often cannot be distinguished from age related PSC cataracts except that the latter frequently have other associated findings such as anterior capsular or subcapsular vacuoles, cortical opacities, or nuclear sclerosis. Even if the steroid dosage is reduced or discontinued, the cataract usually remains unchanged and will neither progress in size nor become smaller or less dense (218,219). On rare occasions, however, the size of the opacity may decrease following reduction of steroid therapy. It has been suggested that spontaneous regression of steroid-induced PSC cataract might occur in cases associated with relatively low doses of steroid or when the duration of treatment is less than

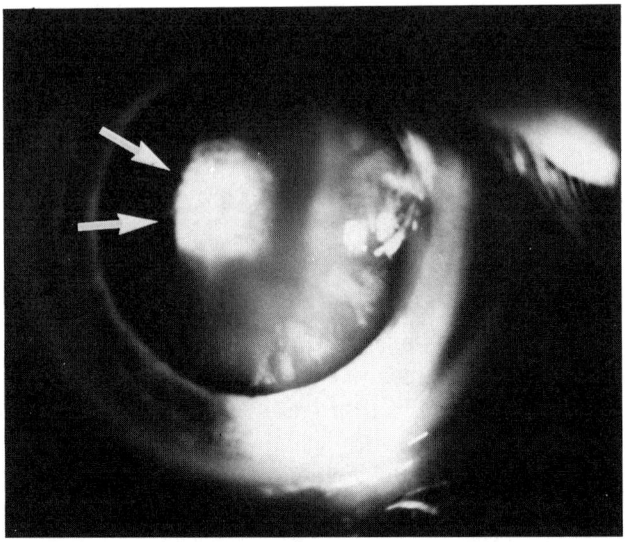

FIG. 10. Posterior subcapsular (PSC) cataract (*arrows*) in a 48-year-old man who had taken oral prednisone 7.5 mg daily for 13 years for treatment of rheumatoid arthritis. Visual acuity was 20/30 (6/9). (From Jaanus, ref. 274, with permission.)

2 years (218). In other cases progressive changes may occasionally occur when the steroid dosage is reduced or discontinued (218).

Several of the earliest studies on the relationship between systemic steroids and cataracts suggested that the dosage or duration of treatment was significantly correlated with the development of cataract (219–221). Furst and associates (219), however, proposed that it is possible for patients to develop steroid-induced cataract even when taking very low doses of steroid. In 1961, Oglesby and associates (220) provided data to suggest that no patient taking steroids for less than 1 year or longer would develop lens opacities. The relationship of dosage and duration of therapy was further defined by Crews (222), who suggested that steroids could cause cataracts with short-term therapy only if the dosage was extremely high.

Because of considerable variation in the numbers of patients studied, dosage and duration of treatment, criteria for cataract diagnosis, route of drug administration, and the underlying disease process itself, attention has focused more recently on the possibility that PSC cataract formation may be related more to factors of individual susceptibility than to drug-related factors of dosage or duration of therapy (223–225). Shalka and Prchal (224) found no statistically significant correlation between PSC opacities and total steroid dosage, weekly dosage, duration of therapy, or patient age. There may also be special susceptibility among various ethnic groups. Hispanics are apparently more predisposed to steroid-induced PSC cataracts than are either Caucasians or blacks (226,227).

It has been suggested that children are more susceptible than adults to the development of steroid-induced cataracts (218), developing them at a lower dosage and in a shorter period of time than do adult patients (219). This can be attributed to the relatively massive doses of steroid, in relation to body weight, sometimes prescribed in children (208).

Visual impairment is rare in patients with steroid-induced PSC cataracts (208,218,221,225). Astle and Ellis (228) reported that 88% of a group of patients with steroid-induced cataracts had visual acuity of 20/40 or better in each eye. Although severe reduction in visual acuity is uncommon, patients may nevertheless report light sensitivity, frank photophobia, reading difficulty, or glare.

In addition to their systemic effects, steroids administered orally can cause elevated intraocular pressure, although the prevalence of elevated pressure is less than that occurring with topical steroids (113). This is probably due to the lower concentration of steroid within the anterior chamber when steroids are administered systemically. Nevertheless, it is possible for systemic steroids to elevate pressure enough to cause glaucomatous damage to the optic disc and visual field (229).

The long-term administration of systemic steroids typically produces a relatively small increase in pressure (228), and the elevated pressure is self-limiting as the drug therapy is reduced or discontinued. In one study (214) about 34% of the patients on systemic steroids had ocular pressures of 29 mm Hg or higher, whereas only 6% of the control group had similar pressure elevations.

As with topically applied steroids, the degree of response to systemic steroids is not related to dosage or duration of treatment, but is due, instead, to factors of individual susceptibility or responsiveness to the effects of steroids (214,215). In patients who are steroid responders, pressure elevations with systemic steroids average about 60% of those produced by topically applied steroids (212). Thus, patients with glaucoma would be expected to be particularly sensitive to the pressure-elevating effects of systemic steroids.

Patient Management

Patients taking systemic steroids should have careful slit lamp examinations performed through a dilated pupil every 6 months. Since it is possible for patients to develop cataracts even when taking very low doses of steroid (230), every patient, regardless of dosage or duration of treatment, must be carefully evaluated for the presence of drug-induced cataracts. When drug-induced cataracts are discovered, the prescribing practitioner should be notified so that the dosage can be reduced, if possible, to a minimum that will control the disease process. Alternatively, alternate-day therapy can be considered, or a nonsteroidal anti inflammatory drug may be substituted. Episodes of renal transplant rejection can often be equally well controlled by lower doses of steroid, and these reduced dosages may help to prevent cataracts following transplantation (231).

Ocular hypertension or open-angle glaucoma associated with systemic steroid therapy should be managed according to the usual guidelines governing treatment of these conditions. A reduction of steroid dosage, if possible, almost always results in reduction of intraocular pressure. If continuation of steroid therapy is deemed necessary, the ocular pressure can often be controlled with topical antiglaucoma therapy despite continuation of systemic steroids (232).

NONSTEROIDAL ANTI-INFLAMMATORY DRUGS

Nonsteroidal anti-inflammatory agents are commonly used for their analgesic, anti-inflammatory, and antipyretic actions in the treatment of arthritis, musculoskeletal disorders, dysmenorrhea, and acute gout. Although these drugs are widely used and are often employed for prolonged periods of time, ocular side effects occur very rarely (233). They can occasionally be toxic to the cornea or retina.

Pathogenesis

Controlled, prospective clinical trials are needed to further establish and clarify the association between nonsteroidal anti-inflammatory agents and corneal opacities. The mechanism of such ocular changes is unknown. With regard to retinal effects, most investigators have speculated that indomethacin may have a direct or indirect effect on the retinal pigment epithelium, but the precise mechanism has not been established (233–235). Localization of the retinotoxic effect to the retinal pigment epithelium is supported by changes observed in the ERG and EOG in patients with indomethacin retinopathy (233).

Ocular Manifestations

The incidence of corneal toxicity associated with indomethacin therapy has been reported to be 11% to 16% (234,235). The corneal lesions appear either as fine stromal, speckled opacities or have a whorl-like distribution resembling that seen in chloroquine keratopathy. The corneal changes diminish or disappear within 6 months of discontinuing indomethacin therapy (234,235). Although no definite relationship has been established between dosage of drug and corneal changes (235), Palimeris and associates (234) found corneal opacities in patients who had taken indomethacin for 12 to 18 months with the daily dosage ranging from 75 to 200 mg and the total dosage ranged from 20 to 70 g. Symptoms associated with the corneal opacities can include mild light sensitivity or even photophobia. Corneal sensitivity, however, is normal (234).

Salicylates are well known to have anticoagulant properties, and in high dosages or prolonged use these drugs can cause conjunctival or retinal hemorrhage (236–238). However, most of the reported cases of retinopathy associated with nonsteroidal anti-inflammatory agents have involved indomethacin therapy. Although there have been no prospective, controlled clinical trials investigating the relationship between indomethacin and retinopathy, there is evidence that the drug can induce pigmentary changes of the macula and other areas of the retina (233–235,239). The lesions usually consist of discrete pigment scattering of the retinal pigment epithelium perifoveally as well as fine areas of depigmentation around the macula. In some cases the pigmentary changes can be more marked in the periphery of the retina (233). Depending on the amount of retinal involvement, the ERG and EOG can be normal or abnormal (233–235). Likewise, the amount of retinopathy will dictate whether or not changes occur in visual acuity, dark adaptation, and visual fields. Acquired color vision deficiencies of the blue-yellow type have been reported (234,240). No definite relationship has been established between the dosage of indomethacin and retinal toxicity. When drug therapy is discontinued, however, most of the functional disturbances associated with the retinopathy will usually improve although the pigmentary changes of the retina are generally irreversible (233–235,240). Significant improvement of color vision, visual acuity, dark adaptation, and visual fields may require at least 6 to 12 months following discontinuation of drug therapy.

Patient Management

Since the corneal opacities associated with nonsteroidal anti-inflammatory drugs are benign and represent no significant threat to vision, patients taking these drugs can be monitored annually for evidence of corneal toxicity. Patients who develop evidence of keratotoxicity should be reassured regarding the benign nature of these changes. The benign corneal opacities do not warrant reducing or discontinuing drug therapy except in unusual circumstances in which severe corneal changes cause visual symptoms that are annoying or incapacitating.

Patients taking high or prolonged doses of salicylates or indomethacin should be monitored carefully for evidence or retinal hemorrhage or pigmentary changes, especially in the macular area. Evaluation of color vision may be helpful to identify patients with early retinotoxic effects associated with indomethacin (240). Consideration should also be given to other functional disturbances, and these can be monitored by performing serial visual acuity, visual fields, and dark adaptation. Once retinal toxicity is documented, the prognosis for improved retinal function is good provided indomethacin therapy is decreased or discontinued.

GOLD COMPOUNDS

Both parenteral and oral gold salts are used in the treatment of rheumatoid arthritis After prolonged administration, gold can be deposited in various tissues of the body, a condition known as chrysiasis. Ocular chrysiasis can involve the conjunctiva, cornea, crystalline lens, and eyelids.

Pathogenesis

The available evidence suggests that gold is deposited in the cornea and crystallin lens by circulation in the aqueous fluid in the anterior chamber (241). The mechanism of gold deposition in the conjunctiva and eyelids has not been established but presumably occurs by direct transfer from systemic circulation.

Ocular Manifestations

Corneal chrysiasis consists of numerous, minute gold particles appearing as yellowish-brown to violet or red particles distributed irregularly in the stroma (241–243). The deposition of gold generally spares the peripheral 1 to 3 mm as well as the superior one-fourth to one-half of cornea (241), and the deposits tend to localize to the posterior one-third of the stroma (241,244). There is typically no involvement of the epithelium, Descemet's membrane, or endothelium. Figure 11 shows the general distribution of gold deposits in a typical case of corneal chrysiasis.

Corneal chrysiasis is a common finding in patients on long-term maintenance gold therapy for rheumatoid arthritis. McCormick and associates (241) found gold deposits in 97% of patients receiving continuous gold therapy consisting of a cumulative dosage of at least 1,000 mg. Gottlieb and Major (242) reported corneal chrysiasis in 45% of patients who had received a mean cumulative dosage greater than 7 g during a mean 6-year period. Although no correlation exists between the density of corneal deposits and the cumulative dose, there is a positive correlation between the duration of gold therapy and the density of corneal deposits (241).

Lenticular chrysiasis appears as fine, dust-like, yellowish, glistening deposits in the anterior capsule or in the anterior suture lines (242). Deposition of oral auranofin occurs in the anterior subcapsular region (Fig. 12) (245).

Various studies (241,242) have established the prevalence of lenticular chrysiasis from parenteral gold to be from 36% to 55%. Although there is no correlation between the dosage of gold and the presence of lenticular deposits (242), the deposi-

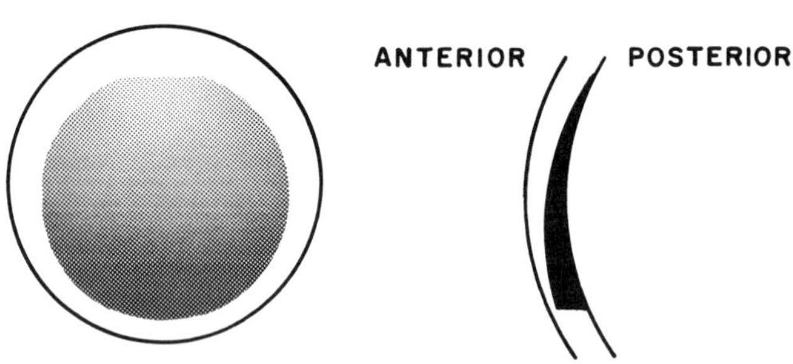

FIG. 11. Distribution of gold deposits in corneal chrysiasis. The deposits spare the peripheral and superior cornea and are more dense inferiorly. (Modified from McCormick et al., ref 275.)

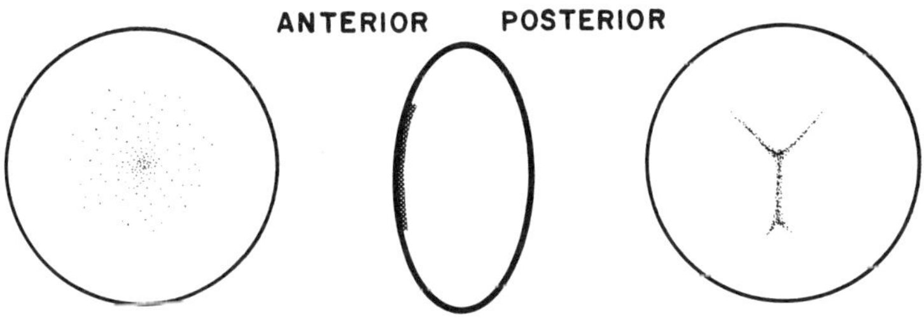

FIG. 12. Lenticular chrysiasis. Gold deposits can diffusely involve the anterior capsule and concentrate within the axial region, or can involve the anterior suture line. (Modified from McCormick et al., ref. 275.)

tion of gold in the lens generally requires at least 3 years of parenteral chrysotherapy (241). The lowest cumulative dosage to produce such lenticular deposits is about 2,500 mg (241). Weidle (245) reported lenticular chrysiasis in a 72-year-old woman who had received 960 mg of oral auranofin during a 5-month period.

There is no significant correlation between corneal chrysiasis and lenticular chrysiasis, and there is no evidence that gold therapy leads to true cataract formation (242). Deposits of gold in the cornea or lens do not cause visual disturbances or other symptoms.

Patient Management

Since ocular chrysiasis does not lead to visual impairment, inflammation, or corneal endothelial changes, gold therapy does not need to be reduced or discontinued (241,245). This benign process requires only routine monitoring. The deposits often disappear within 3 to 6 months following cessation of therapy, but they may occasionally be found years after chrysotherapy has been discontinued.

ORAL CONTRACEPTIVES

Although ocular side effects have been widely reported with oral contraceptive use, most of these effects have been based primarily on isolated, anecdotal case reports. Animal studies as well as prospective clinical trials in humans have failed to document any significant relationship between use of oral contraceptives and ocular side effects (246). Various authors have speculated that oral contraceptives may influence contact lens wear or cause cataracts, but there is no firm evidence to suggest that such a relationship actually exists (246–253)

Nevertheless, there is circumstantial evidence that retinal vascular disease may have an association with oral contraceptives because patients have been reported with retinal lesions that disappeared when the drug was discontinued, promptly reappearing when the drug was resumed, and then regressing when treatment was again discontinued (254,255). Furthermore, the retinal vascular disturbances occur at an unusually young age when vascular damage associated with arteriosclerosis is rare.

Pathogenesis

The mechanism underlying retinal vascular complications associated with oral contraceptives is unknown. Schenker and associates (256) have shown that oral contraceptives may cause changes in the retinal microvasculature. Fluorescein angiography was used to demonstrate narrowing of the capillary arterioles and postcapillary venules. Women who complained of headache while taking oral contraceptives demonstrated dilation of perimacular vessels several weeks after the drug was discontinued. Retinal vascular occlusive episodes might also occur as a consequence of marked intimal proliferation, or as a result of contraceptive-enhanced platelet adhesiveness. Fibrinogen and clotting factors may also be increased (246,257).

Ocular Manifestations

The most common retinal findings reportedly associated with oral contraceptive use are retinal vascular occlusions. These may present as typical branch or central retinal vein occlusion (258), branch or central retinal artery occlusion (259), or may involve atypical presentations such as tortuosity of the perimacular venules (260) or combined central retinal artery and vein occlusion (257). Acquired color vision deficiencies have also been reported. Marre and associates (261) found acquired tritanomaly in 28% of women using oral contraceptives when tested with the Panel D-15 test. Table 3 lists other retinotoxic effects reported with use of oral contraceptives (254,262).

Patient Management

The risk of retinal vascular disease associated with oral contraceptive use in women of childbearing age is generally considered to be minimal. Certain predisposing factors, however, may increase the risks of retinal vascular episodes. Women who

TABLE 3. *Retinotoxic effects reported with oral contraceptive use*

Central or branch retinal vein occlusion
Central or branch retinal artery occlusion
Perivasculitis
Impending central retinal vein occlusion
Retinal artery attenuation
Macular hemorrhage
Retinal edema

TABLE 4. *Risk factors for vascular complications associated with oral contraceptives*

Migraine headache
Phlebitis
Inclination to varicosity
Systemic hypertension
Hyperlipidemia or hypercholesterolemia
Diabetes
Cigarette smoking
Obesity

experience migraine headache, phlebitis, diabetes, or those who are obese may be at increased risk for vascular complications (246,254,262). Other risk factors are listed in Table 4. These patients should therefore be monitored more carefully for evidence of retinal disease. If the patient develops retinal vascular complications that are suspected to be associated with the oral contraceptive, consideration can be given to changing the mode of contraception.

PHOTOSENSITIZING DRUGS

Photosensitizing drugs are compounds that absorb optical radiation (ultraviolet [UV] and visible) and undergo a photochemical reaction resulting in chemical modifications in nearby molecules of the tissue (263). The psoralen compounds are photosensitizing drugs widely used by dermatologists to treat psoriasis and vitiligo. This treatment is commonly referred to as PUVA therapy and involves the administration of 8-methoxypsoralen (8-MOP) or related compounds, followed by exposure to UVA radiation (320 to 400 nm) for short periods of time (199). The most common photosensitizing reactions involve the skin and eye. Cataract formation is now well documented in patients undergoing PUVA therapy (263).

Pathogenesis

The eye and the skin are the only tissues of the body that are particularly susceptible to damage from nonionizing wavelengths of optical radiation (280 to 1,400 nm) (199). The crystalline lens has the ability to absorb varying amounts of UV radiation and thus photobind susceptible drugs present in that tissue. Most ocular damage from photosensitizing drugs occurs on exposure to UV radiation (263). Because the adult crystalline lens effectively filters most UV radiation, there is minimal risk of photobinding susceptible drugs in the retina. UV radiation, however, can penetrate to the retina in aphakic and pseudophakic individuals and in young eyes, thus causing potential photosensitizing damage to the retina (199).

Ocular Manifestations

Lerman and associates (264) have demonstrated psoralens in the crystalline lens following oral administration and have further shown that the psoralens may photobind to lens protein if subsequently exposed to UVA radiation. Stern and associates (265) have shown that there is a slightly greater prevalence of nuclear sclerosis and PSC opacities, but without decreased visual acuity, in patients treated on over 100 occasions than in patients treated on fewer occasions. The incidence of symptomatic cataract, however, is not significantly increased if patients wear UVA-blocking lenses following each treatment.

Patient Management

If the eye is protected from UV radiation during PUVA therapy, free 8-MOP can be found in the lens for only 24 hr (263). Thus, to prevent permanent photobinding of this drug, dermatologists usually provide UV filtering lenses to patients undergoing PUVA therapy. The patient should wear the lenses for at least 24 hr beginning when the drug is first taken. These filters must be worn both indoors as well as outdoors since there is sufficient UV radiation in ordinary fluorescent lighting to photobind the 8-MOP (263). These measures are generally effective in preventing development of cataracts associated with PUVA therapy (265,266).

TALC

Tablets of medication intended for oral use contain inert filler materials such as talc (magnesium silicate), corn starch, cotton fibers, and other substances (267). Chronic drug abusers are known to prepare a suspension of medication for injection by dissolving in water the crushed tablets of cocaine, heroin, or other narcotic. They then boil the solution and filter it through a crude cigarette or cotton filter prior to injecting the solution. The talc particles eventually embolize to the retinal circulation and produce a characteristic retinopathy.

Pathogenesis

As the talc, corn starch, and other insoluble tablet fillers embolize to the lungs, they become trapped within the pulmonary tissues and eventually cause pulmonary hypertension. This leads to the development of collateral vessels that allow part of the venous return to bypass the lungs and enter the left side of the heart, where the particles are allowed to further embolize to the eye (268). The presence of talc particles in the eye is an indication that substantial foreign body damage has occurred in the lungs (269).

The particles lodge in the walls of the precapillary arterioles and capillaries, producing focal occlusion of these vessels in the retina and choroid. The occlusions are caused primarily by the cellular reaction to the emboli (270). The neovascular lesions of talc retinopathy are thought to be associated with peripheral arteriolar nonperfusion, which leads to retinal ischemia and secondary neovascularization (268).

Ocular Manifestations

Fundus examination reveals multiple, tiny, yellow-white, glistening particles scattered throughout the posterior pole, but they are more numerous in the capillary bed and small arterioles of the perimacular area (Fig. 13) (269). Some patients can also have macular edema, dot-like and flame-shaped hemorrhages, as well as arterial occlusion.

Retinal neovascularization can appear in the retinal periphery as neovascular tufts in the shape of sea fans at the junction of the perfused and nonperfused retina. This is a potentially serious complication of talc injection because it can lead to retinal detachment, vitreal hemorrhage, and optic disc neovascularization (271).

Most patients have no significant visual symptoms (271). Some patients, however, may report blurred vision, blind spots in the visual fields, and occasionally have severe reduction of vision.

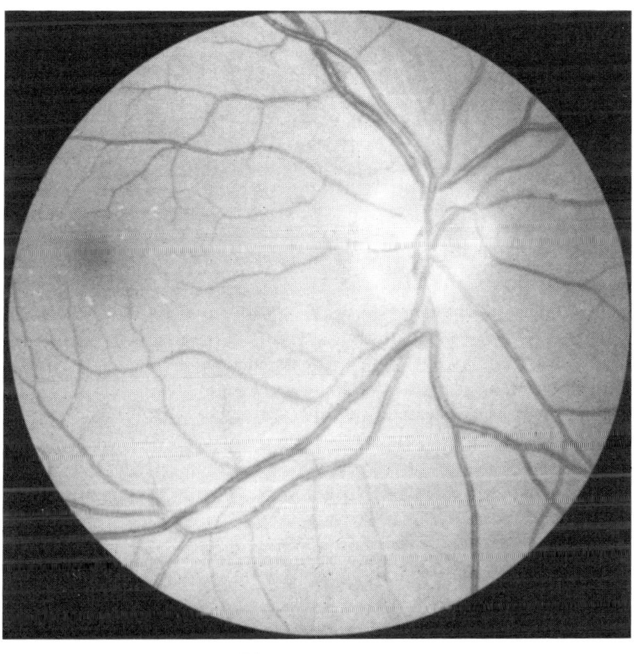

FIG. 13. Talc retinopathy characterized by numerous yellow-white intraarteriolar particles scattered throughout the perimacular area. (From Bartlett and Jaanus, ref. 2, with permission.)

Patient Management

Because of the psychological and emotional implications involved in the diagnosis, the practitioner must rule out other conditions that may have a similar clinical appearance. The differential diagnosis includes Gunn's dots, multiple cholesterol emboli, drusen, and Stargardt's disease. Once the diagnosis has been established, appropriate drug abuse counseling should be offered to prevent further risk of severe pulmonary or ocular complications. Consideration should also be given to pulmonary consultation since patients with eye findings usually have acute or chronic impairment of pulmonary function (272). Proliferative retinopathy can be treated with the use of laser photocoagulation, and vitreal hemorrhage may require vitrectomy (268).

REFERENCES

1. Fraunfelder FT. *Drug induced ocular side effects and drug interactions.* Philadelphia: Lea & Febiger, 1982.
2. Bartlett JD, Jaanus SD. Ocular effects of systemic drugs. In: Bartlett JD, Jaanus SD, eds. *Clinical ocular pharmacology.* Stoneham, MA: Butterworth, 1989;801-842.
3. Fraunfelder FT, Meyer SM. The national registry of drug-induced ocular side effects. *J Toxicol Cutan Ocular Toxicol* 1982;1:65-70.
4. Applebaum M, Jaanus SD. A study of utilization of diagnostic pharmaceutical agents and the incidence of adverse effects. *Am J Optom Physiol Opt* 1983;60:384-388.
5. McQueen EG. Pharmacological basis of adverse drug reactions. In: Avery GS, ed. *Drug treatment.* New York: Adis Press, 1980;Chap. 7.
6. Koneru PB, Lien EJ, Koda RT. Oculotoxicities of systemically administered drugs. *J Ocul Pharmacol* 1986;2:385-404.
7. Peters NL. Snipping the thread of life. Antimuscarinic side effects of medications in the elderly. *Arch Intern Med* 1989;149:2414-2420.
8. Mader TH, Stulting RD. Keratoconjunctivitis sicca caused by diphenoxylate hydrochloride with atropine sulfate (Lomotil). *Am J Ophthalmol* 1991;111:377-378.
9. Balik J. Effect of atropine and pilocarpine on the secretion of chloride ion into the tears. *Cesk Oftalmol* 1958;14:28-33.
10. Erickson OF. Drug influences on lacrimal lysozyme production. *Stanford Med Bull* 1960;18:34-39.
11. Crandall DC, Leopold IH. The influence of systemic drugs on tear constituents. *Ophthalmology* 1979;86:115-125.
12. Miller D. Role of the tear film in contact lens wear. *Int Ophthalmol Clin* 1973;13:247-262.
13. Koeffler BH, Lemp MA. The effect of an antihistamine (chlorpheniramine maleate) on tear production in humans. *Am J Ophthalmol* 1980;12:217-219.
14. Leopold IH, Comroe JH. Effect of intramuscular administration of morphine, atropine, scopolamine and neostigmine on the human eye. *Arch Ophthalmol* 1948;40:285-290.
15. Ahmad S. Disopyramide: pulmonary complications and glaucoma. *Mayo Clin Proc* 1990;65:1030-1031.
16. Lieberman E, Stoudemiere A. Use of tricyclic antidepressants in patients with glaucoma. Assessment and appropriate precautions. *Psychosomatics* 1987;28:145-148.
17. Frucht J, Freimann I, Merin S. Ocular side effects of disopyramide. *Br J Ophthalmol* 1984;68:890-891.
18. Hiatt RL, Fuller IB, Smith L, et al. Systemically administered anticholinergic drugs and intraocular pressure. *Arch Ophthalmol* 1970;84:735-740.
19. Mackie IA, Seal DV, Pescod JM. Beta-adrenergic receptor blocking drugs: tear lysozyme and immunological screening for adverse reactions. *Br J Ophthalmol* 1977;61:354-359.
20. Almog Y, Monselise M, Almog CH, et al. The effect of oral treatment with beta blockers on tear secretion. *Metab Pediatr Syst Ophthalmol* 1983;6:343-345.

21. Yablonski ME, Zimmerman TJ, Waltman SR, Becker B. A fluorophotometric study of the effect of topical timolol on aqueous humor dynamics. *Exp Eye Res* 1978;27:135-142.
22. Coakes RL, Brubaker RF. The mechanism of timolol in lowering intraocular pressure in the normal eye. *Arch Ophthalmol* 1978;96:2045-2048.
23. Zimmerman TJ, Harbin R, Pett M, Kaufman HE. Timolol and facility of outflow. *Invest Ophthalmol Vis Sci* 1977;16:623-624.
24. Sonntag JR, Brindley GO, Shields MB, et al. Timolol and epinephrine. Comparison of efficacy and side effects. *Arch Ophthalmol* 1979;97:273-277.
25. Schenker HI, Yablonski ME, Podos SM, Linder L. Fluorophotometric study of epinephrine and timolol in human subjects. *Arch Ophthalmol* 1981;99:1212-1216.
26. Vareilles P, Lotti VJ. Effect of timolol on aqueous humor dynamics in the rabbit. *Ophthalmic Res* 1981;13:72-79.
27. Reiss GR, Brubaker RF. The mechanism of betaxolol, a new ocular hypotensive agent. *Ophthalmology* 1983;90:1369-1372.
28. Neufeld AH. Experimental studies on the mechanism of action of timolol. *Surv Ophthalmol* 1979;23:363-370.
29. Felix FH, Ive FA, Dahl MGC. Cutaneous and ocular reactions with practolol administration. Oculomucocutaneous syndrome. *Br Med J* 1975;1:595-598.
30. Scott D. Another beta blocker causing eye problems. *Br Med J* 1977;2:1221.
31. Smith SE, Smith SA, Reynolds F, et al. Ocular and cardiovascular effects of local and systemic pindolol. *Br J Ophthalmol* 1979;63:63-66.
32. Borthne A. The treatment of glaucoma with propranolol (Inderal). A clinical trial. *Acta Ophthalmol* 1976;54:291-300.
33. Rennie IG, Smerdon DL. The effect of a once-daily oral dose of nadolol on intraocular pressure in normal volunteers. *Am J Ophthalmol* 1985;100:445-447.
34. Macdonald MJ, Cullen PM, Phillips CI. Atenolol vs. propranolol. *Br J Ophthalmol* 1976;60:789-791.
35. Heel RC, Brogden RN, Speight TM, Avery GS. Atenolol: a review of its pharmacological properties and therapeutic efficacy in angina pectoris and hypertension. *Drugs* 1979;17:425-460.
36. Duff GR. The effect of twice daily nadolol on intraocular pressure. *Am J Ophthalmol* 1987;104:343-345.
37. Wettrell K, Pandolfi M. Effect of oral administration of various beta-blocking agents on the intraocular pressure in healthy volunteers. *Exp Eye Res* 1975;21:451-456.
38. Ohrstrom A. Dose response of oral timolol combined with adrenaline. *Br J Ophthalmol* 1982;66:242-246.
39. Chew E, Ghosh M, McCulloch C. Amiodarone-induced corneal verticillata. *Can J Ophthalmol* 1982;17:96-99.
40. Gittinger JW, Asdourian GK. Papillopathy caused by amiodarone. *Arch Ophthalmol* 1987;105;349-351.
41. Ghosh M, McCulloch C. Amiodarone-induced ultrastructural changes in human eyes. *Can J Ophthalmol* 1984;19:178-186.
42. D'Amico DJ, Kenyon KR, Ruskin JN. Amiodarone keratopathy. Drug-induced lipid storage disease. *Arch Ophthalmol* 1981;99:257-261.
43. Haug SJ, Friedman AH. Identification of amiodarone in corneal deposits. *Am J Ophthalmol* 1991;111:518-520.
44. Bron AJ. Vortex patterns of the corneal epithelium. *Trans Ophthalmol Soc UK* 1973;43:455-472.
45. Flach AJ, Dolan BJ. Amiodarone-induced lens opacities: an eight-year follow-up study. *Arch Ophthalmol* 1990;108:1668-1669
46. Gibson HC, Smith DM, Alpern M. II5 specificity in digitoxin toxicity. A case report. *Arch Ophthalmol* 1965;74:154-158.
47. Binnin PF, Frazer G. ^{3}H digoxin in the optic tract in digoxin intoxication. *J Cardiovasc Pharmacol* 1980;2:699-706.
48. Weleber RG, Shults WT. Digoxin retinal toxicity. Clinical and electrophysiologic evaluation of a cone dysfunction syndrome. *Arch Ophthalmol* 1981;99:1568-1572.
49. Orlando RG, Dangel ME, Schaal SF. Clinical experience and grading of amiodarone keratopathy. *Ophthalmology* 1984;91:1184-1187.
50. Dolan BJ, Flach AJ, Peterson JS. Amiodarone keratopathy and lens opacities. *J Am Optom Assoc* 1985;56:468-470.

51. Ingram DV, Jaggarao NSV, Chamberlain DA. Ocular changes resulting from therapy with amiodarone. *Br J Ophthalmol* 1982;66:676-679.
52. Kaplan LJ, Cappaert WE. Amiodarone keratopathy. Correlation to dosage and duration. *Arch Ophthalmol* 1982;100:601-602.
53. Nielsen CE, Andreasen F, Bjerregaard P. Amiodarone-induced corneal verticillata. *Acta Ophthalmol* 1983;61:474-480.
54. Flach AJ, Dolan BJ, Sudduth B, et al. Amiodarone-induced lens opacities. *Arch Ophthalmol* 1983;101:1554-1556.
55. D'Amico DS, Kenyon RR. Drug-induced lipidoses in the cornea and conjunctiva. *Int Ophthalmol* 1981;4:67-76.
56. Reifler DM, Verdier DD, Davy CL, et al. Multiple chalazia and rosacea in a patient treated with amiodarone. *Am J Ophthalmol* 1987;103:594-595.
57. Sykowski P. Digitoxin intoxication resulting in retrobulbar optic neuritis. *Am J Ophthalmol* 1949;32:572-574.
58. Robertson DM, Hollenhorst RW, Callahan JA. Ocular manifestations of digitalis toxicity. Discussion and report of three cases of central scotomas. *Arch Ophthalmol* 1966;76:640-645.
59. Robertson DM, Hollenhorst RW, Callahan JA. Receptor function and digitalis therapy. *Arch Ophthalmol* 1966;76:852-857.
60. Rietbrock N, Alken RG. Color vision deficiencies: a common sign of intoxication in chronically digoxin-treated patients. *J Cardiovasc Pharmacol* 1980;2:93-99.
61. Haustein K-O, Oltmanns G, Rietbrock N, et al. Differences in color vision impairment caused by digoxin, digitoxin, or pengitoxin. *J Cardiovasc Pharmacol* 1982;4:536-541.
62. Deluise VP, Flynn JT. Asymmetric anterior segment changes induced by chlorpromazine. *Ann Ophthalmol* 1981;13:953-955.
63. Davidorf FH. Thioridazine pigmentary retinopathy. *Arch Ophthalmol* 1973;90:251-255.
64. Potts AM. The concentration of phenothiazines in the eye of experimental animals. *Invest Ophthalmol* 1962;1:522-530.
65. Kimbrough BO, Campbell RJ. Thioridazine levels in the human eye. *Arch Ophthalmol* 1981;99:2188-2189.
66. Miller FS, Bunt-Milam AH, Kalina RE. Clinical ultrastructural study of thioridazine retinopathy. *Ophthalmology* 1982;89:1478-1488.
67. Krupin T, Kolker AE, Becker B. Alcohol and intraocular pressure. *Invest Ophthalmol* 1967;6:559-560.
68. Houle RE, Grant WM. Alcohol, vasopressin and intraocular pressure. *Invest Ophthalmol* 1967;6:145-154.
69. Thaler JS, Curinga R, Kiracofe G. Relation of graded ocular anterior chamber pigmentation to phenothiazine intake in schizophrenics. Quantification procedures. *Am J Optom Physiol Opt* 1985;62:600-604.
70. Mathalone MBR. Ocular effects of phenothiazine derivatives and reversibility. *Dis Nerv Syst* 1968;29:29-35.
71. Siddall JR. Ocular complications related to phenothiazines. *Dis Nerv Syst* 1968;29:10-13.
72. Prin RF, DeLong SL, Cole JO, et al. Ocular changes occurring with prolonged high dose chlorpromazine therapy. *Arch Gen Psychiatry* 1970;23:464-468.
73. Rasmussen K, Kirk L, Faurbye A. Deposits in the lens and cornea of the eye during long-term chlorpromazine medication. *Acta Psychiatr Scand* 1976;53:1-6.
74. Alexander LJ, Bowerman L, Thompson LR. The prevalence of the ocular side effects of chlorpromazine in the Tuscaloosa Veterans Administration patient population. *J Am Optom Assoc* 1985;56:872-876.
75. Kjaer GCD. Retinopathy associated with phenothiazine administration. *Dis Nerv Syst* 1968;29:316-319.
76. Meredith TA, Aaberg TM, Willerson D. Progressive chorioretinopathy after receiving thioridazine. *Arch Ophthalmol* 1978;96:1172-1176.
77. Miyata M, Imai H, Ishikawa S, et al. Change in human electroretinography associated with thioridazine administration. *Ophthalmologica* 1980;181:175-180.
78. Godel V, Loewenstein A, Lazar M. Spectral electroretinography in thioridazine toxicity. *Ann Ophthalmol* 1990;22:293-296.
79. Neves MS, Jordan K, Dragt H. Extensive chorioretinopathy associated with very low dose thioridazine. *Eye* 1990;4:767-770.

80. Cameron ME, Lawrence JM, Olrich JG. Thioridazine (Mellaril) retinopathy. *Br J Ophthalmol* 1972;56:131-134.
81. Marmor MF. Is thioridazine retinopathy progressive? Relationship of pigmentary changes to visual function. *Br J Ophthalmol* 1990;74:739-742.
82. Hays GB, Lyle CB, Wheeler CE. Slate grey color in patients receiving chlorpromazine. *Arch Dermatol* 1964;90:471-476.
83. Cairns RH, Capoore HS, Gregory JDR. Oculocutaneous changes after years of high doses of chlorpromazine. *Lancet* 1965;1:239-241.
84. Siddall JR. The ocular toxic findings with prolonged and high dosage chlorpromazine intake. *Arch Ophthalmol* 1965;74:460-464.
85. McClanahan WS, Harris JE, Knobloch WH, et al. Ocular manifestations of chronic phenothiazine derivative administration. *Arch Ophthalmol* 1966;75:319-125.
86. Editorial. Iatrogenic symptoms in ophthalmology. *Br Med J* 1969;2:199-200.
87. Durkee DP, Bryant BG. Drug therapy reviews: drug therapy of glaucoma. *Am J Hosp Pharm* 1978;35:682-690.
88. Alkemade PPH. Phenothiazine retinopathy. *Ophthalmologica* 1968;155:70-76.
89. Thaler JS. The effect of multiple psychotropic drugs on the accommodation of prepresbyopes. *Am J Optom Physiol Opt* 1979;56:259-261.
90. Thaler JS. Effects of benztropine mesylate (Cogentin) on accommodation in normal volunteers. *Am J Optom Physiol Opt* 1982;59:918-919.
91. Peczon JD, Grant WM. Glaucoma, alcohol, and intraocular pressure. *Arch Ophthalmol* 1965;73:495-501.
92. Jaanus SD. Hyperosmotic drugs. In: Bartlett JD, Jaanus SD, eds. *Clinical ocular pharmacology*. Boston: Butterworth, 1989;275-283.
93. Wilkinson IMS, Kime R, Purnell M. Alcohol and human eye movement. *Brain* 1974;97:785-792.
94. Bittencourt P, Wade P, Richens A, et al. Blood alcohol and eye movements. *Lancet* 1980;16:981.
95. Wilson G, Mitchell R. The effect of alcohol on the visual and ocular motor systems. *Aust J Ophthalmol* 1983;11:315-319.
96. Rosenberg ML. Reversible downbeat nystagmus secondary to excessive alcohol intake. *J Clin Neuro Ophthalmol* 1987;7:23-25.
97. Henkes HE. Electro-oculography as a diagnostic aide in phenothiazine retinopathy. *Trans Ophthalmol Soc UK* 1967;87:285-287.
98. Halperin E, Yolton RL. Is the driver drunk? Oculomotor sobriety testing. *J Am Optom Assoc* 1986;57:654-657.
99. Tiffany DV. Optometric expert testimony. Foundation for the horizontal gaze nystagmus test. *J Am Optom Assoc* 1986;57:705-708.
100. Melon J, Register M. Passage into normal salivary, lacrimal and nasal secretions of ampicillin and erythromycin administered intramuscularly. *Acta Otorhinolaryngol Belg* 1976;30:643-651.
101. Fraunfelder FT. Orange tears. *Am J Ophthalmol* 1980;89:752.
102. Lyons RW. Orange contact lenses from rifampin. *N Engl J Med* 1979;300:372.
103. Alvaro ME. Effects other than antiinfections of sulfonamide compounds on eye. *Arch Ophthalmol* 1943;29:615-632.
104. Tilden ME, Rosenbaum JT, Fraunfelder FT. Systemic sulfonamides as a cause of bilateral, anterior uveitis. *Arch Ophthalmol* 1990;109:67-69.
105. Mattsson R. Transient myopia following the use of sulphonamides. *Acta Ophthalmol* 1952;30:385-398.
106. Chirls IA, Norris JW. Transient myopia associated with vaginal sulfanilamide suppositories. *Am J Ophthalmol* 1984;98:120-121
107. Maddallena MA. Transient myopia associated with acute glaucoma and retinal edema. *Arch Ophthalmol* 1968;80:186-188.
108. Brothers DM, Hidayat AA. Conjunctival pigmentation associated with tetracycline medication. *Ophthalmology* 1981;88:1212-1215.
109. Messmer E, Font RL, Sheldon G, et al. Pigmented conjunctival cysts following tetracycline/minocycline therapy. *Ophthalmology* 1983;90:1462-1468.
110. Huang NN, Harley RD, Promadhattavedi V, et al. Visual disturbances in cystic fibrosis following chloramphenicol administration. *J Pediatr* 1966;68:32-44.
111. Harley RD, Huang NN, Macri CH, et al. Optic neuritis and optic atrophy following chloramphenicol in cystic fibrosis patients. *Trans Am Acad Ophthalmol Otolaryngol* 1970;74:1011-1031.

112. Godel V, Nemet P, Lazar M. Chloramphenicol optic neuropathy. *Arch Ophthalmol* 1980;98:1417-1421.
113. Lieberman TW. Ocular effects of prolonged systemic drug administration (corticosteroids, chloramphenicol, and anovulatory agents). *Dis Nerv Syst* 1968;29:44-50.
114. Walker GF. Blindness during streptomycin and chloramphenicol therapy. *Br J Ophthalmol* 1961;45:555-559.
115. Hook SR, Holladay JT, Prager, TC, et al. Transient myopia induced by sulfonamides. *Am J Ophthalmol* 1986;101:495-496.
116. Bovino JA, Marcus DF. The mechanism of transient myopia induced by sulfonamide therapy. *Am J Ophthalmol* 1982;94:999.
117. Spaide RF, Diamond G, D'Amico RA, et al. Ocular findings in cystic fibrosis. *Am J Ophthalmol* 1987;103:204-210.
118. Keith CG. Optic atrophy induced by chloramphenicol. *Br J Ophthalmol* 1964;48:567-570.
119. Roberts SM. A review of the papers on the ocular toxicity of ethambutol hydrochloride (Myambutol), an anti-tuberculosis drug. *Am J Optom Physiol Opt* 1974;51:987-992.
120. Van Dijk BW, Spekreijse H. Ethambutol changes the color coding of carp retinal ganglion cells reversibly. *Invest Ophthalmol Vis Sci* 1983;24:128-133.
121. Kakisu Y, Adachi-Usami E, Mizota A. Pattern electroretinogram and visual evoked cortical potential in ethambutol optic neuropathy. *Doc Ophthalmol* 1988;67:327-334.
122. Carr RE, Henkind P. Ocular manifestations of ethambutol. Toxic amblyopia after administration of an experimental anti-tuberculosis drug. *Arch Ophthalmol* 1962;67:50-55.
123. Addington WW. The side effects and interactions of anti-tuberculosis drugs. *Chest* 1979;76(suppl):782-784.
124. Karamon G, Savir H, Zevin D, et al. Bilateral optic neuropathy due to combined ethambutol and isoniazid treatment. *Ann Ophthalmol* 1979;11:1013-1017.
125. Trusiewicz D. Farnsworth 100-Hue test in the diagnosis of ethambutol-induced damage to optic nerve. *Ophthalmologica* 1975;171:425-431.
126. Kuming BS, Braude L. Anterior optic neuritis caused by ethambutol toxicity. *S Afr Med J* 1979;55:4.
127. Bronté-Stewart J, Pettigrew AR, Foulds WS. Toxic optic neuropathy and its experimental production. *Trans Ophthalmol Soc UK* 1976;96:355-358.
128. Polak BCP, Leys M, van Lith GHM. Blue-yellow colour vision changes as early symptoms of ethambutol oculotoxicity. *Ophthalmologica* 1985;191:223-226.
129. Salmon JF, Carmichael TR, Welsh NH. Use of contrast sensitivity measurement in the detection of subclinical ethambutol toxic optic neuropathy. *Br J Ophthalmol* 1987;71:192-196.
130. Yiannikas C, Walsh JC, McLeod JG. Visual evoked potentials in the detection of subclinical optic toxic effects secondary to ethambutol. *Arch Neurol* 1983;40:645-648.
131. Barron GJ, Tepper L, Iovine G. Ocular toxicity from ethambutol. *Am J Ophthalmol* 1974;77:256-260.
132. DeVita EG, Miao M, Sadun AA. Optic neuropathy in ethambutol-treated renal tuberculosis. *J Clin Neuro Ophthalmol* 1987;7:77-83.
133. DePalma P, Franco F, Bragliani G, et al. The incidence of optic neuropathy in 84 patients treated with ethambutol. *Metab Pediatr Syst Ophthalmol* 1989;12:80-82.
134. Garrett CR. Optic neuritis in a patient on ethambutol and isoniazid evaluated by visual evoked potentials: case report. *Milit Med* 1985;150:43-46.
135. Citron KM, Thomas GO. Ocular toxicity from ethambutol. *Thorax* 1986;41:737-739.
136. Guerra R, Casu L. Hydroxycobalamin for ethambutol-induced optic neuropathy. *Lancet* 1981;2:1176.
137. Bernstein HN. Chloroquine ocular toxicity. *Surv Ophthalmol* 1967;12:415-447.
138. Beebe WE, Abbott RL, Fung WE. Hydroxychloroquine crystals in the tear film of a patient with rheumatoid arthritis. *Am J Ophthalmol* 1986;101:377-378.
139. Cullen AP, Chou BR. Keratopathy with low dose chloroquine therapy. *J Am Optom Assoc* 1986;57:368-372.
140. Calkins LL. Corneal epithelial changes occurring during chloroquine (Aralen) therapy. *Arch Ophthalmol* 1958;60:981-988.
141. Shearer RV, Dubois EL. Ocular changes induced by long-term hydroxychloroquine (Plaquenil) therapy. *Am J Ophthalmol* 1967;64:245-252.
142. Rosenthal AR, Kolb H, Bergsma D, et al. Chloroquine retinopathy in the rhesus monkey. *Invest Ophthalmol Vis Sci* 1978;17:1158-1175.

143. Bernstein HN, Ginsberg J. The pathology of chloroquine retinopathy. *Arch Opthalmol* 1964;71:238-245.
144. Ramsey MS, Fine BS. Chloroquine toxicity in the human eye. Histopathologic observations by electron microscopy. *Am J Ophthalmol* 1972;73:229-235.
145. Wetterholm DH, Winter FC. Histopathology of chloroquine retinal toxicity. *Arch Ophthalmol* 1964;71:116-121.
146. Rubin ML, Thomas WC. Diplopia and loss of accommodation due to chloroquine. *Arthritis Rheum* 1970;13:75-82.
147. Yospaiboon Y, Lawtiantong T, Chotibutr S. Clinical observations of ocular quinine intoxication. *Jpn J Ophthalmol* 1984;28:409-415.
148. Brinton GS, Norton EWD, Zahn JR, et al. Ocular quinine toxicity. *Am J Ophthalmol* 1980;90:403-410.
149. Dyson EH, Proudfoot AT, Bateman DN. Quinine amblyopia: is current management appropriate? *Clin Toxicol* 1985-86;23:571-578.
150. Gangitano JL, Keltner JL. Abnormalities of the pupil and visual-evoked potential in quinine amblyopia. *Am J Ophthalmol* 1980;89:425-430.
151. Hobbs HE, Eadie SP, Somerville F. Ocular lesions after treatment with chloroquine. *Br J Ophthalmol* 1961;45:284-298.
152. Bernstein NH. Some iatrogenic ocular diseases from systemically administered drugs. *Int Ophthalmol Clin* 1970;10:553-619.
153. Goldhammer Y, Smith JL. Bitemporal hemianopia in chloroquine retinopathy. *Neurology* 1974;24:1135-1138.
154. Petrohelos MA. Chloroquine-induced ocular toxicity. *Ann Ophthalmol* 1974;6:615-618.
155. Mantyjarvi M. Hydroxychloroquine treatment in the eye. *Scand J Rheumatol* 1985;14:171-174.
156. Abel A, Leopold III. Ocular diseases. In: Avery JS, ed. *Drug treatment*. New York: Adis Press, 1980;Chap. 12.
157. Lozier JR, Friedlaender MH. Complications of antimalarial therapy. *Int Ophthalmol Clin* 1989;29:172-178.
158. Marks JS, Power BJ. Is chloroquine obsolete in treatment of rheumatic disease? *Lancet* 1979;1:171-173.
159. Tobin DR, Krohel GB, Rymes RI. Hydroxychloroquine. Seven-year experience. *Arch Ophthalmol* 1982;100:81-83.
160. Cruess AF, Schachat AP, Nicholl J, et al. Chloroquine retinopathy. Is fluorescein angiography necessary? *Ophthalmology* 1985;92:1127-1129.
161. Henkind P, Parr RE, Siegel IM. Early chloroquine retinopathy: clinical and functional findings. *Arch Ophthalmol* 1964;71:157-165.
162. Percival SPB, Behrman P. Ophthalmological safety of chloroquine. *Br J Ophthalmol* 1969;53:101-109.
163. Percival SPB, Meanock I. Chloroquine: ophthalmological safety and clinical assessment in rheumatoid arthritis. *Br Med J* 1968;3:579-584.
164. Carberg O. Three cases of chloroquine retinopathy. A follow-up investigation. *Acta Ophthalmol* 1966;44:367-374.
165. Martin LJ, Bergen RL, Dobrow HR. Delayed onset chloroquine retinopathy: case report. *Ann Ophthalmol* 1978;10:723-726.
166. Brinkley JR, Dubois EL, Ryan SJ. Long-term course of chloroquine retinopathy after cessation of medication. *Am J Ophthalmol* 1979;88:1-11.
167. Lowes M. Peripheral visual field restriction in chloroquine retinopathy. Report of a case. *Acta Ophthalmol* 1976;54:819-826.
168. Nylander U. Ocular damage in chloroquine therapy. *Acta Ophthalmol* 1966;44:335-348.
169. Krill AE, Potts AM, Johanson CE. Chloroquine retinopathy. Investigation of discrepancy between dark adaptation and electroretinographic findings in advanced stages. *Am J Ophthalmol* 1971;71:530-543.
170. Banks CN. Melanin: blackguard or red herring? Another look at chloroquine retinopathy. *Aust NZ J Ophthalmol* 1987;15:365-370.
171. Kolb H. Electro-oculogram findings in patients treated with antimalarial drugs. *Br J Ophthalmol* 1965;49:573-589.
172. Finbloom DS, Silver K, Newsome DA, et al. Comparison of hydroxychloroquine and chloroquine use and the development of retinal toxicity. *J Rheumatol* 1985;12:692-694.

173. Ehrenfeld M, Mesher R, Merin S. Delayed-onset chloroquine retinopathy. *Br J Ophthalmol* 1986;70:281-283.
174. Easterbrook M. Dose relationships in patients with early chloroquine retinopathy. *J Rheumatol* 1987;14:472-475.
175. Easterbrook M. Ocular effects and safety of antimalarial agents. *Am J Med* 1988;85:23-29.
176. Ogawa S, Kurumatani N, Shibaike N, et al. Progression of retinopathy long after cessation of chloroquine therapy. *Lancet* 1979;1:1408.
177. Terrell WL, Haik KG, Haik GM. Hydroxychloroquine sulfate and retinopathy. *South Med J* 1988;81:1327-1328.
178. Rynes RI, Krohel G, Falbo A, et al. Ophthalmologic safety of long-term hydroxychloroquine treatment. *Arthritis Rheum* 1979;22:832-836.
179. Mills PV, Beck M, Tower BJ. Assessment of the retinal toxicity of hydroxychloroquine. *Trans Ophthalmol Soc UK* 1981;101:109-113.
180. Johnson MW, Vine AK. Hydroxychloroquine therapy in massive total doses without retinal toxicity. *Am J Ophthalmol* 1987;104:139-144.
181. Howell R. Treatment of discoid lupus erythematosus. *St John's Hosp Dermat Soc* 1957;39:48.
182. Fleck BW, Bell AL, Mitchell JD, et al. Screening for antimalarial maculopathy in rheumatology clinics. *Br Med J* 1985;291:782-784.
183. Bishara SA, Matamoros N. Evaluation of several tests in screening for chloroquine maculopathy. *Eye* 1989;3:777-782.
184. Hart WM, Burde RM, Johnston GP, et al. Static perimetry in chloroquine retinopathy. Perifoveal patterns of visual field depression. *Arch Ophthalmol* 1984;102:377-380.
185. Easterbrook M. Is corneal deposition of antimalarial any indication of retinal toxicity? *Can J Ophthalmol* 1990;25:249-251.
186. Burns RP. Delayed onset of chloroquine retinopathy. *N Engl J Med* 1966;275:693-696.
187. Kaiser-Kupfer MI, Kupfer C, Rodriques MM. Tamoxifen retinopathy. A clinicopathologic report. *Ophthalmology* 1981;88:89-93.
188. Shingleton BJ, Bienfang DC, Albert DM, et al. Ocular toxicity associated with high-dose carmustine. *Arch Ophthalmol* 1982;100:1766-1772.
189. Miller DF, Bay JW, Lederman RJ, et al. Ocular and orbital toxicity following intracarotid injection of BCNU (carmustine) and cisplatinum for malignant gliomas. *Ophthalmology* 1985;92:402-406.
190. Kaiser-Kupfer MI, Lippman ME. Tamoxifen retinopathy. *Cancer Treat Rep* 1978;62:315-320.
191. McKeown CA, Swartz M, Blom J, et al. Tamoxifen retinopathy. *Br J Ophthalmol* 1981;65:177-179.
192. Beck M, Mills PV. Ocular assessment of patients treated with tamoxifen. *Cancer Treat Rep* 1979;63:1833-1834.
193. Longstaff S, Sigurdsson H, O'Keeffe M, et al. A controlled study of the ocular effects of tamoxifen in conventional dosage in the treatment of breast carcinoma. *Eur J Cancer Clin Oncol* 1989;25:1805-1808.
194. Griffiths MFP. Tamoxifen retinopathy at low dosage. *Am J Ophthalmol* 1987;104:185-186.
195. Pickrell L, Purvin V. Ischemic optic neuropathy secondary to intracarotid infusion of BCNU. *J Clin Neuro Ophthalmol* 1987;7:87-91.
196. Chrousos GA, Oldfield EH, Doppman JL, et al. Prevention of ocular toxicity of carmustine (BCNU) with supraophthalmic intracarotid infusion. *Ophthalmology* 1986;93:1471-1475.
197. Kupersmith MJ, Frohman LP, Choi IS, et al. Visual system toxicity following intra-arterial chemotherapy. *Neurology* 1988;38:284-289.
198. Bigby M, Stern RS. Adverse reactions to isotretinoin. A report from the adverse drug reaction reporting system. *J Am Acad Dermatol* 1988;18:543-552.
199. Lerman S. Photosensitizing drugs and their possible role in enhancing ocular toxicity. *Ophthalmology* 1986;93:304-313.
200. Weleber RG, Denman ST, Hanifin JM, et al. Abnormal retinal function associated with isotretinoin therapy for acne. *Arch Ophthalmol* 1986;104:831-837.
201. Milson J, Jones DH, King K. Ophthalmological effects of 13-cis-retinoic acid therapy for acne vulgaris. *Br J Dermatol* 1982;107:491-495.
202. Fraunfelder FT, Baico JM, Meyer SM. Adverse ocular reactions possibly associated with isotretinoin. *Am J Ophthalmol* 1985;100:534-537.
203. Ensink BW, VanVoorst Vader PC. Ophthalmological side effects of 13-cis-retinoic therapy. *Br J Dermatol* 1983;108:637-641.

204. Ubels JL, MacRae SM. Vitamin A is present as retinol in tears of humans and rabbits. *Curr Eye Res* 1984;3:815-817.
205. Gold JA, Shupack JL, Nemec MA. Ocular side effects of the retinoids. *Int J Dermatol* 1989;28:218-225.
206. Black RL, Oglesby RB, vonSallmann L, et al. Posterior subcapsular cataracts induced by corticosteroids in patients with rheumatoid arthritis. *JAMA* 1960;174:166-171.
207. Fraunfelder FT, Meyer SM. Posterior subcapsular cataracts associated with nasal or inhalation corticosteroids. *Am J Ophthalmol* 1990;109:489-490.
208. Urban RC, Cotlier E. Corticosteroid-induced cataracts. *Surv Ophthalmol* 1986;31:102-110.
209. Harris JE, Gruber L. The electrolyte and water balance of the lens. *Exp Eye Res* 1962;1:372-384.
210. Mayman CI, Miller D, Tigerina ML. In vitro production of steroid cataract in bovine lens: II. Measurement of sodium-potassium adenosine triphosphatase activity. *Acta Ophthalmol* 1979;57:1107-1116.
211. Bucala R, Fishman J, Cerami A. Formation of covalent adducts between cortisol and 16 α-hydroxyesterone and protein: possible role in the pathogenesis of cortisol toxicity and systemic lupus erythematosus. *Proc Natl Acad Sci USA* 1982;79:3320-3324.
212. Feiler-Ofry V, Godel V, Stein R. Systemic steroids and ocular fluid dynamics. III. The genetic nature of the ocular response and its different levels. *Acta Ophthalmol* 1972;50:699-706.
213. Lindholm B, Linner E, Tengroth B. Effects of long-term systemic steroids on cataract formation and on aqueous humour dynamics. *Acta Ophthalmol* 1965;43:120-127.
214. Godel V, Feiler-Ofry V, Stein R. Systemic steroids and ocular fluid dynamics. I. Analysis of the sample as a whole. Influence of dosage and duration of therapy. *Acta Ophthalmol* 1972;50:655-663.
215. Godel V, Feiler-Ofry V, Stein R. Systemic steroids and ocular fluid dynamics. II. Systemic vs. topical steroids. *Acta Ophthalmol* 1972;50:664-676.
216. Diotallevi M, Bocci N. Effect of systemically administered corticosteroids on intraocular pressure and fluid dynamics. *Acta Ophthalmol* 1965;43:524-527.
217. Spaeth GL, Rodrigues MM, Weinreb S. Steroid-induced glaucoma. A. Persistent elevation of intraocular pressure. B. Histopathological aspects. *Trans Am Ophthalmol Soc* 1977;75:353-381.
218. Kobayashi Y, Akaishi K, Nishio T, et al. Posterior subcapsular cataract in nephrotic children receiving steroid therapy. *Am J Dis Child* 1974;128:671-673.
219. Furst C, Smiley WK, Ansell BM. Steroid cataract. *Ann Rheum Dis* 1966;25:364-368.
220. Oglesby RB, Black RL, vonSallmann L, et al. Cataracts in patients with rheumatic diseases treated with corticosteroids. Further observations. *Arch Ophthalmol* 1961;66:625-630.
221. Giles CL, Mason GL, Duff IF, et al. The association of cataract formation and systemic corticosteroid therapy. *JAMA* 1962;182:719-722.
222. Crews SJ. Posterior subcapsular lens opacities in patients on long-term corticosteroid therapy. *Br Med J* 193;1:1644-1647.
223. Kristensen P. Posterior subcapsular cataract (PSC) and systemic steroid therapy. *Acta Ophthalmol* 1968;46:1025-1032.
224. Skalka HW, Prchal JT. Effect of corticosteriods on cataract formation. *Arch Ophthalmol* 1980;98:1773-1777.
225. Limaye SR, Pillai S, Tina LU. Relationship of steroid dose to degree of posterior subcapsular cataracts in nephrotic syndrome. *Ann Ophthalmol* 1988;20:225-227.
226. Loredo A, Rodriguez RS, Murillo L. Cataracts after short-term corticosteroid treatment. *N Engl J Med* 1972;286:160.
227. Rooklin AR, Lampert SI, Jaeger EA, et al. Posterior subcapsular cataracts in steroid-requiring asthmatic children. *J Allergy Clin Immunol* 1979;63:383-386.
228. Astle JN, Ellis PP. Ocular complications in renal transplant patients. *Ann Ophthalmol* 1974;6:1269-1274.
229. Covell LL. Glaucoma induced by systemic steroid therapy. *Am J Ophthalmol* 1958;45:108-109.
230. Bluming AZ, Zeegen P. Cataracts induced by intermittent Decadron used as an antiemetic. *J Clin Oncol* 1986;4:221-223.
231. Pavlin CR, deVeber GA, Cook GT, et al. Ocular complications in renal transplant recipients. *Can Med Assoc J* 1977;117:360-362.
232. Wilson DM, Martin JHS, Niall JF. Raised intraocular tension in renal transplant recipients. *Med J Aust* 1973;482-484.
233. Henkes HE, vanLith GHM, Canta LR. Indomethacin retinopathy. *Am J Ophthalmol* 1972;73:846-856.

234. Palimeris G, Kolipoulis J, Velissaropoulos P. Ocular side effects of indomethacin. *Ophthalmologica* 1972;164:339-353.
235. Burns CA. Indomethacin, reduced retinal sensitivity, and corneal deposits. *Am J Ophthalmol* 1968;66:825-835.
236. Mortada A, Abboud I. Retinal hemorrhages after prolonged use of salicylates. *Br J Ophthalmol* 1973;57:199-200.
237. Werblin TP, Peiffer RL. Persistent hemorrhage after extracapsular surgery associated with excessive aspirin ingestion. *Am J Ophthalmol* 1987;105:426.
238. Kingham JD, Chen MC, Levy MH. Macular hemorrhage in the aging eye: the effects of anticoagulants. *N Engl J Med* 1988;318:1126-1127.
239. Graham CM, Blach RK. Indomethacin retinopathy: case report and review. *Br J Ophthalmol* 1988;72:434-438.
240. Koliopoulos J, Palimeris G. On acquired colour vision disturbances during treatment with ethambutol and indomethacin. *Mod Probl Ophthalmol* 1972;11:178-184.
241. McCormick SA, DiBartolomeo G, Raju VK, et al. Ocular chrysiasis. *Ophthalmology* 1985;92:1432-1435.
242. Gottlieb NL, Major JC. Ocular chrysiasis correlated with gold concentrations in the crystalline lens during chrysotherapy. *Arthritis Rheum* 1978;21:704-708.
243. Tierney DW. Ocular chrysiasis. *J Am Optom Assoc* 1988;59:960-962.
244. Roberts WH, Wolter JR. Ocular chrysiasis. *Arch Ophthamol* 1956;56:48-52.
245. Weidle EG. Lenticular chrysiasis in oral chrysotherapy. *Am J Ophthalmol* 1987;103:240-241.
246. Wood JR. Ocular complications of oral contraceptives. *Ophthalmol Sem* 1977;2:371-402.
247. Koetting RA. The influence of oral contraceptives on contact lens wear. *Am J Optom Arch Am Acad Optom* 1966;43:268-274.
248. Ruben M. Contact lenses and oral contraceptives. *Br Med J* 1966;1:1110.
249. Varga M. Recent experiences on the ophthalmologic complications of oral contraceptives. *Ann Ophthalmol* 1976;8:925-934.
250. Connell EB, Kelman CD. Ophthalmologic findings with oral contraceptives. *Obstet Gynecol* 1968;31:456-460.
251. Drill VA, Rao KS, McConnell RG, et al. Ocular effects of oral contraceptives. I. Studies in the dog. *Fertil Steril* 1975;26:908-913.
252. Faust JM, Tyler ET. Ophthalmologic findings in patients using oral contraception. *Fertil Steril* 1966;17:1-6.
253. Andelman MB, Zackler J, Slutsky HL, et al. Family planning and public health. *Int J Fertil* 1968;13:405-414.
254. Smith MS, Kreiger A. Visual loss associated with oral contraceptives. *Am J Ophthalmol* 1970;69:874-876.
255. Goren SB. Retinal edema secondary to oral contraceptives. *Am J Ophthalmol* 1967;64:447-449.
256. Schenker JG, Ivry M, Oliver M. The effect of oral contraceptives on microcirculation. *Obstet Gynecol* 1972;39:909-916.
257. Stowe GC, Zakov ZN, Albert DM. Central retinal vascular occlusion associated with oral contraceptives. *Am J Ophthalmol* 1978;86:798-801.
258. Ruskiewicz JP. Birth control linked to vein occlusion. *Rev Optom* 1983;120:58-60.
259. McGrand JC, Cory CC. Ophthalmic disease and the pill. *Br Med J* 1969;2:187.
260. Gombos GM, Moreno DA, Bedrossian PB. Retinal vascular occlusion induced by oral contraceptives. *Ann Ophthalmol* 1975;7:215-217.
261. Marre M, Neubauer O, Nemetz U. Colour vision and the "pill." *Mod Probl Ophthalmol* 1974;13:345-348.
262. Radnot M, Follmann P. Ocular side effects of oral contraceptives. *Ann Clin Res* 1973;5:197-204.
263. Lerman S, Megaw J, Gardner K. Psoralens. Long-wave ultraviolet therapy and human cataractogenesis. *Invest Ophthalmol Vis Sci* 1982;23:801.
264. Lerman S, Megaw J, Willis I. The photoreactions of 8-methoxypsoralen with tryptophan and lens proteins. *Photochem Photobiol* 1980;31:235.
265. Stern RS, Parrish JA, Fitzpatrick TB. Ocular findings in patients treated with PUVA. *J Invest Dermatol* 1985;85:269.
266. Cox NH, Jones SK, Downey DJ, et al. Cutaneous and ocular side effects of oral photochemotherapy: results of an 8-year follow-up study. *Br J Dermatol* 1987;116:145-152.

267. Michelson JB, Whitcher JP, Wilson S, et al. Possible foreign body granuloma of the retina associated with intravenous cocaine addiction. *Am J Ophthalmol* 1979;87:278-280.
268. Tse DT, Ober RR. Talc retinopathy. *Am J Ophthalmol* 1980;90:624-640.
269. AtLee WE. Talc and cornstarch emboli in eyes of drug abusers. *JAMA* 1972;219:49-51.
270. Kaga N, Tso MOM, Jampol LM. Talc retinopathy in primates: a model of ischemic retinopathy. III. An electron microscopic study. *Arch Ophthalmol* 1982;100:1649-1657.
271. Bluth LL, Hanscom TA. Retinal detachment and vitreous hemorrhage due to talc emboli. *JAMA* 1981;246:980-981.
272. Paré JAP, Fraser RG, Hogg JC, et al. Pulmonary "mainline" granulomatosis: talcosis of intravenous methadone abuse. *Medicine* 1979;58:229-239.
273. Kingele TG, Alves LE, Rose EP. Amiodarone keratopathy. *Ann Ophthalmol* 1984;16:1172-1176.
274. Jaanus SD. Anti-inflammatory drugs. In: Bartlett JD, Jaanus SD, eds. *Clinical ocular pharmacology*. Boston: Butterworth, 1989;163-203.
275. McCormick SA, diBartolomeo AG, Raju VK, et al. Ocular chrysiasis. *Ophthalmology* 1985;92:1432-1435.

Ophthalmic Toxicology, edited by
George C. Y. Chiou. Raven Press, Ltd.,
New York © 1992.

7

Ophthalmic Toxicity by Local Agents

George C. Y. Chiou

Institute of Ocular Pharmacology and Department of Medical Pharmacology and Toxicology, Texas A & M University College of Medicine, College Station, Texas 77843

Ever since the methods of chemical synthesis were invented, tens of thousands of new chemicals have been introduced into the world every year. A large portion of these compounds are reported to be irritating to the eyes. Obviously, it is not possible to cover all these agents in this chapter. Only a very small portion of these agents will be mentioned here by giving some representative chemicals in each class of agents, based on their uses.

ADRENERGIC STIMULANTS AND BLOCKERS

Adrenergic drugs may be either direct-acting or indirect-acting. Direct-acting adrenergics break down into alpha-adrenergics, such as **phenylephrine** (which is discussed more in mydriatics), and beta-adrenergics, such as **isoprenaline**. Direct-acting adrenergics have the side effects of decreased intraocular pressure (IOP) and allergy and irritation of the eye of sensitized individuals. There are also adrenergics that are not specific for either alpha- or beta-adrenergic sites: **bamethan** (discussed under glaucoma tests) and **epinephrine** (discussed under antiglaucoma drugs). Other direct-acting adrenergics are **methoxamine** and **norepinephrine** (1–4).

Indirect acting adrenergics produce a variety of side effects that tend to vary with the drug. **Amphetamine** falls within this class; it has the side effects of mydriasis and retraction of the upper lid. **Ephedrine** has many side effects, including conjunctival vasoconstriction, decreased vision, allergic reactions of the eyelids or conjunctiva of sensitized individuals, conjunctivitis, irritation (with the further symptoms of lacrimation, rebound hyperemia, and photophobia), mydriasis, and aqueous "floaters" (bits of pigment debris). Another indirect adrenergic is **naphazoline**. These drugs have the side effects of mydriasis and punctate epithelial keratitis. **Norepinephrine** may cause a decrease in the IOP, and **methoxamine** may cause widening of the palpebral fissure (1,5–9).

There are many dopaminergic drugs that act on the central nervous system, but the only one used on the eyes is **dopamine**. Ten percent eyedrops of **dopamine** produced mydriasis; however, they do not affect accommodation (10).

Adrenergic blockers may be either direct-acting or indirect-acting. The direct-acting blockers also are divided in alpha-adrenergic blocking agents, beta-adrenergic blocking agents, and nonspecific agents. The most prominent alpha-adrenergic blocking agent is **moxisylyte**. This drug has side effects that depend on the dosage. A 0.1% solution causes brief miosis. A 5% solution produces transient ptosis, hyperemia of the conjunctiva, and reduced IOP in glaucoma (side effects are not always objectionable). The primary beta-adrenergic blocking agent is **betadine**. This agent has the side effects of ptosis, miosis, and hyperemia of the conjunctiva, and it decreases IOP. Nonspecific adrenergic blockers include **practolol, propranolol**, and **oxprenolol**. These drugs have the side effect of decreased IOP. **Oxprenolol** causes punctate keratitis and miosis. **Propranolol** also causes miosis; it also can cause decreased corneal reflect, conjunctival hyperemia, and irritation (1,11-16).

Indirect-acting adrenergic blockers include **guanethidine** and **bretylium**, which are discussed under antiglaucoma agents (17).

ANTIGLAUCOMA AGENTS

One test for open-angle glaucoma is the use of **tolazoline**, an alpha-adrenergic blocking agent. This drug has the side effect of increasing IOP when injected subconjunctivally. Another test for open-angle glaucoma uses the alpha- plus beta-adrenergic agent **bamethan**. This agent has the side effects of increased IOP and of redness and swelling of the eye (1,18-20).

A large number of drugs of several classes are used to control glaucoma. Some of the most common are adrenergic drugs. **Epinephrine** (adrenaline) is an adrenergic agonist that has an extensive list of reported side effects: decreased vision, mydriasis, allergic reactions of the eyelids or conjunctiva of sensitized persons, blepharoconjunctivitis (follicular), vasoconstriction of the conjunctiva, poliosis, and pemphigoid lesions of the eyelids and conjunctiva. It may produce hyperplasia of the sebaceous glands of the eyelids, or symptoms of irritation (lacrimation, rebound hyperemia, photophobia, ocular pain, and ocular burning sensations). There may be adrenochrome deposits in the conjunctiva, in the cornea, or in the nasolacrimal system, cystoid macular edema, punctate keratitis, corneal edema, narrowing or occlusion of lacrimal canaliculi, subconjunctival or retinal hemorrhages, loss of eyelashes or eyebrows, paradoxical pressure elevation in open-angle glaucoma, scotomas, aqueous floaters (pigment debris), periorbital edema, iritis, cysts, and, in infected individuals, reactivation of corneal herpes simplex. Some of these symptoms may be secondary to changes in blood circulation in the eye and surrounding tissues produced by the continuously elevated levels of epinephrine used to treat glaucoma. The prodrug of epinephrine, **dipivefrin** (**DPE**) has much fewer side effects, including irritation, erythema of the eyelids, conjunctivitis, decreased vision, and mydriasis (1,6,21-24).

The most common beta-adrenergic blocker for treatment of glaucoma is **L-timolol**. This drug has the reported side effects of irritation (with hyperemia, ocular pain, and burning sensations), allergic reactions and erythema of the eyelids or conjunctiva, blepharoconjunctivitis, urticaria, purpura of the conjunctiva, decreased vision, myopia, visual hallucinations, decreased corneal reflex, keratoconjunctivitis, and myasthenic neuromuscular blocking effect (paralysis of the extraocular muscles and ptosis) (1,25–27).

Guanethidine and **bretylium** are antiadrenergic norepinephrine-releasing blockers. They act by blocking the release of endogenous norepinephrine. **Guanethidine** has the side effects of irritation (with hyperemia, photophobia, ocular pain, edema, and burning sensations), Horner's syndrome (with miosis, ptosis, and enophthalmos), mydriasis, decreased IOP, and punctate keratitis. **Bretylium** (10% to 25%) causes some reduction of ocular pressure in glaucoma and slight ptosis, but no irritation or injury (1,28–29).

Glycerin is an osmotic agent given for acute glaucoma. Its side effects include irritation (with lacrimation, hyperemia, ocular pain, and burning sensations) and subconjunctival hemorrhages (1,30–32).

Direct-acting cholinomimetics include **carbachol** and **methacholine**. These agents have the side effects of allergic reactions and hyperemia of the eyelids or conjunctiva of sensitized individuals, blepharoclonus, and myopia. **Carbachol** can produce miosis, decreased vision, accommodative spasms, follicular conjunctivitis, ocular pain, retinal detachment, and, after intracameral injection, corneal edema. **Methacholine** can produce Adie's pupil (myosis), lacrimation, and even blood tears. Another drug in this family is **bethanechol**. It has the side effects of severe itching, burning, and tearing of the eyes (1,8,10,33–36).

MIOTICS AND MYDRIATICS

There are two main classes of miotics in general use: (a) cholinergic agents (cholinergic agonists), such as **aceclidine**, **carbachol**, **acetylcholine**, **methacholine**, and **pilocarpine**; and (b) anticholinesterases, such as **demecarium**, **echothiophate**, **isoflurophate (DFP)**, **neostigmine**, **physostigmine**, **paraoxon**, and **nibufin**. General side effects of miotics include miosis, accommodative spasm, decreased vision, irritation of the eyes, decreased IOP, decreased anterior chamber depth, cataract, and even retinal detachment (of diseased retinas) (10,37–42).

One example of a cholinergic miotic is **pilocarpine**. Its side effects include an initial increase in IOP after administration, allergic reactions, and hyperemia of the eyelids or conjunctiva of certain sensitive individuals, follicular conjunctivitis (after long-term use), transient myopia, and punctate keratitis. Other side effects can include blepharoclonus, increased axial lens diameter, decreased scleral rigidity, and, sometimes, retinal detachment or problems with color vision (dyschromatopsia) (1,10,37,40,41).

An example of an anticholinesterase miotic is **isoflurophate (DFP)**. This miotic may produce allergic reactions of the eyelids or conjunctiva in sensitive individuals, follicular conjunctivitis, edema of the eyelids or conjunctiva, pemphigoid lesion and depigmentation of the eyelids or conjunctiva, blepharoclonus, and iris or ciliary body cysts. Other side effects can include iritis, myopia, an initial increase in IOP, decreased scleral rigidity, occlusion of lacrimal canaliculi, or vitreous hemorrhages. Individuals who have had a surgical implant of a filtering bleb to control IOP may find the filtration decreased. **Nibufin** is another common anticholinesterase. Its side effects include increased tear production and changes in the b-wave of the electroretinogram (ERG) (1,10,42).

Mydriatics fall into two classes: anticholinergic drugs and adrenergic drugs. Examples of the anticholinergic mydriatics include **amprotropine, atropine, cyclopentolate, tropicamide, hemicholinium, eucatropine, homatropine**, and **scopolamine**. Adrenergic mydriatics include **hydroxyamphetamine, phenylephrine, pholedrine**, and **epinephrine**. **Epinephrine** and its side effects are presented under antiglaucoma drugs. Anticholinergic mydriatics have the general side effects of cycloplegia and decreased vision. They produce mydriasis, which may precipitate narrow-angle glaucoma, and they may increase intraocular pressure (with the exception of hemicholinium). Some drugs have more specific side effects. An example is **cyclopentolate**, which may produce irritation (with hyperemia, photophobia, ocular pain, and burning sensations), decrease or paralysis of accommodation, allergic reactions of the eyelids or conjunctiva in sensitized individuals, blepharoconjunctivitis, visual hallucinations, synechiae, keratitis, and shallow anterior chamber (1,8,33,43-46).

CHOLINESTERASE INHIBITORS AND REACTIVATORS AND CHEMICAL WARFARE AGENTS

Edrophonium is a drug used to diagnose myasthenia gravis that has a number of ocular side effects. These include photophobia, allergic reactions of the eyelids or conjunctiva, conjunctivitis, iritis, iris cysts, a decreased depth of the anterior chamber, vitreous hemorrhages, and cataracts (1,8,42).

Diphenylchloroarsine, diphenylcyanoarsine, and **hexachloroethane** are three chemical warfare agents that have the side effects of ocular irritation and lacrimation. **Hexachloroethane** can cause blepharospasm, photophobia, and reddening of the conjunctiva. **Diphenylcyanoarsine** may cause necrosis of the corneal epithelium (47-50). **Sarin** is a nerve gas with ocular side effects. This toxic agent can produce miosis and spasm of accommodation for viewing near objects (48,50).

Pralidoxime is the cholinesterase reactivator most associated with ocular toxicity. This drug has the side effects of irritation (with hyperemia and burning sensations), subconjunctival hemorrhages, and iritis. It reverses miosis and accommodative spasms (1,51-52).

AUTACOIDS AND ANTIHISTAMINES

Autacoids are mediators of inflammatory responses; most can occur endogenously. Autocoids of interest in ocular toxicity include **bradykinin, prostaglandins, prot-**

amine, and **serotonin**. When **bradykinin** was injected into the vitreous of rabbits, it produced hyalitis and subcapsular changes in the lens (10,53,54).

There are many kinds of endogenous and exogenous **prostaglandins**. In the eye, a **prostaglandin** from the iris, known as **irin,** is a local mediator of a specific reaction to irritation in the eyes (10). This reaction is characterized by vasodilation in the iris, leakage of protein from the blood to the aqueous humor (breakdown of the blood-aqueous barrier), miosis, and a rise in IOP lasting 1 to 2 hr (53,55,56).

When **protamine** was injected into the cornea of rabbits, it produced an immediate chalk-white opacity, apparently caused by the precipitation of acid mucopolysaccharides (53). **Serotonin** produced less severe side effects, including slight miosis and a slight reduction in IOP (10).

Antihistamines of interest for their ocular side effects include **antazoline, diphenhydramine, mepyramine**, and **prophenpyridamine**. Side effects of antihistamines include an atropine-like action characterized by slight dilation of the pupils and impairment of accommodation for far vision. **Mepyramine** and **antazoline** may cause rapid clouding of the corneal epithelium, local anesthesia, and transitory swelling of the cornea. High concentrations of **antazoline** can cause temporary keratitis epithelialis (1,8,10,57,58).

CARDIOVASCULAR DRUGS

Cardiovascular drugs with ocular side effects include **digoxin**, **erythrophleum alkaloids**, **gitalin**, **ouabain**, and **squill**. All these drugs decrease IOP and all except **ouabain** produce corneal edema. **Digoxin** may produce wrinkling of Descemet's membrane, **erythrophleum alkaloids** may produce chemosis, and intravitreal injection of **ouabain** may cause loss of vision (1,10,30,42,59,60). A 9.7% solution of **potassium thiocyanate** can cause loosening of the corneal epithelium (10).

Amyl nitrite is an agent for treatment of angina pectoris. Ocular side effects include stinging and transient lacrimation. There may be slight superficial injury of the eye or severe corneal damage (1,10,61,62).

Several classes of drugs are used as vasodilators; the side effects depend on the individual drug. **Acetylcholine** has the side effects of lacrimation, miosis, and clouding of the aqueous humor. **Isoxsuprine** has the side effects of increased IOP, edema, and hyperemia of episcleral tissues. **Nicodan-percutan** has the side effects of loss of corneal epithelium, clouding of the corneal stroma, corneal opacity, and vascularization and wrinkling of Descemet's membrane (1,10).

BLOOD-RELATED AGENTS

The usual plasma expanders are **dextran** and **dextran sulfate**. These agents may cause clouding of the vitreous. **Dextran sulfate** has severe side effects of severe irritation, intraocular hemorrhage, and distention of the globe. **Dextran** may produce phthisis bulbi (1,63,64).

The ocular side effects of anticoagulants depend on the agent given. **Citric acid** has the side effects in some patients of a severe conjunctival reaction, with corneal ulceration or severe, dense opacification of the cornea. **Heparin** has different side effects. Subconjunctival injection of **heparin** may cause subconjunctival or periocular hemorrhages, subconjunctival scarring, chemosis, and decreased IOP. Intracameral injection of **heparin** may cause corneal edema and opacification, conjunctival chemosis, hyperemia of the iris, and a transient increase in IOP. Three percent eyedrops of **heparin** may affect the corneal epithelium (1,8,10,42,65).

Phenylhydrazine is a hemolytic that was injected intravitreally in one study. It caused inflammation of the eye, chorioretinitis, and degeneration of the retina (10). **Saponins** are hemolytic agents also. Topical contact of **saponins** with the eye causes irritation, tearing, pain, photophobia, chemosis, and hyperemia. There may be conjunctivitis, damage to the corneal epithelium, keratitis, corneal ulceration, and corneal leukoma (66,67).

Choline is an agent in this class. Its ocular side effects include inflammation and hemorrhages in the conjunctiva and superficial corneal opacities with edema (42,68).

VITAMINS

Some vitamins (**menadione [vitamin K]** and **vitamin A**) have ocular side effects. **Vitamin K** may have the effects of discomfort of the eye, conjunctival congestion, and moderate injury to the eye. **Vitamin A** may produce blepharoconjunctivitis and loss of hair from the lids (1,10,69,70).

AGENTS FOR DEFICIENCY ANEMIAS

A number of agents are used to treat deficiency anemias. Many of the agents with ocular side effects are iron compounds: **ferrocholinate, ferrous fumarate, ferrous gluconate, ferrous succinate, ferrous sulfate, iron dextran, iron sorbitex**, and **polysaccharide-iron complex**. These agents have the side effects of irritation (with hyperemia and photophobia), yellow-brown discoloration or deposits in the eyelids, conjunctiva, cornea, and sclera. There may be hypopyon and ulceration of the eyelids, conjunctiva, and cornea (1,10,58,71).

SEDATIVES, HYPNOTICS, AND TRANQUILIZERS

Some agents classified as sedative or hypnotic have ocular side effects. **Chlorobutanol** has the side effects of irritation (foreign body sensation) and keratitis epithelialis (72,73). **Alcohol (ethanol)** has the side effects of irritation (with ocular pain, hyperemia, edema, lacrimation, and burning sensation), keratitis, paralysis of the extraocular muscles, nystagmus, ptosis, corneal ulceration or necrosis, corneal opacities, and decreased vision (1,74–76).

Reserpine is a tranquilizer with the side effects of decreased IOP and hyperemia of the conjunctiva (1,77,78).

ANTIDEPRESSANTS AND ANTIPARKINSONISM AGENTS

Protriptyline is an antidepressant with a mydriatic side effect. It also may cause corneal opacities of unknown composition (1,79).

Antiparkinsonism agents include **L-dopa (levodopa)** and **trihexyphenidyl**. These drugs may produce mydriasis and irritation; **trihexyphenidyl** may have an anesthetic action. **Amantadine** may cause decreased vision (1,10,80).

LOCAL ANESTHETICS

Local anesthetics may be used for local ophthalmic use, or the eyes may be exposed unintentionally. Local anesthetics include **benoxinate, bulacaine, bupivacaine, cocaine, cornecaine, dibucaine, dyslonine, lidocaine, phenacaine, piperocaine, proparacaine, procaine**, and **tetracaine**. These drugs produce a variety of ocular side effects. All can produce irritation, with lacrimation, hyperemia, ocular pain, or burning sensations. There may be allergic reactions of the eyelids or conjunctiva in sensitized individuals, or blepharoconjunctivitis. There may be punctate keratitis, a gray, ground glass appearance of the cornea, corneal edema, corneal softening, erosions, sloughing, filaments, ulceration, vascularization, or scarring. Corneal wound healing may be delayed. **Bupivacaine, lidocaine**, and **procaine** may produce decreased vision, paresis or paralysis of the extraocular muscles, or a decrease in IOP. Other reported side effects include a decrease in the blink reflex, subconjunctival hemorrhages, hypopyon, or iritis. **Cocaine** can cause conjunctival vasoconstriction; it also may induce mydriasis, paralysis of accommodation, or even visual hallucinations (1,10,81–84).

ANALGESICS

Analgesics fall into two main classes: narcotic analgesics and antipyretic analgesics. Narcotic analgesics include **meperidine** and **morphine**. **Meperidine** has the side effects of blepharitis and nonspecific conjunctivitis. **Morphine** has the side effects of miosis and, possibly, increased IOP (1,10).

Antipyretic analgesics include **aspirin, sodium salicylate, ethylmorphine, ethylmorpholine**, and **trichloroethylene**. **Aspirin** and **sodium salicylate** have the side effects of conjunctival edema or scarring and of keratitis, with or without ulceration. **Ethylmorphine** has the side effects of conjunctival vasodilation and edema, and may either increase or decrease IOP. **Ethylmorpholine** may produce corneal epithelium injury, hazy cornea, blurring of vision, and colored halos around lights. **Trichloroethylene** may cause chemical burns of the lids, conjunctiva, and cornea. There may be smarting pain and injuries to the corneal epithelium or disturbances of vision (1,10,58,85–88).

ANTIRHEUMATIC AND ANTIGOUT AGENTS

Antirheumatic agents include **aurothioglucose, aurothioglycanide, gold (Au), gold sodium thiomalate (sodium aurothiomalate)**, and **gold thiosulfate (sodium aurothiosulfate)**. These agents have the ocular side effects of irritation, corneal clouding, and iritis (1,20,30,89,90).

Colchicine is an antigout agent with the ocular side effects of decreased vision, conjunctival hyperemia, corneal clouding, vascularization of the cornea, and opacification of the cornea (1,20,91).

AGENTS FOR RESPIRATORY DISEASES

Polyoxyethylene dodecanol (Laurithyl) is an agent for the treatment of respiratory diseases. Reported ocular side effects include irritation and corneal damage (10,92).

ANTISPASMODICS

Antispasmodics include a large number of agents of differing classes of drugs: **adiphenine, ambutonium, anisotropine, belladonna clidinium, dicyclomine, dephemanil, glycopyrrolate, hexocylium, isopropamide, mepenzolate, methantheline, methixene, methylatropine, oxyphencyclamine, oxyphenonium, pipenzolate, piperidolate, poldine, propantheline**, and **tridihexethyl**. **Atropine** and **homatropine** (94) are also used as antispasmodics; they are discussed with the mydriatics.

Side effects vary with the drug in question. Many antispasmodics produce mydriasis (which may, in turn, precipitate narrow-angle glaucoma), a decrease or paralysis of accommodation or irritation (with hyperemia, edema, and photophobia). **Belladonna** may produce decreased vision or follicular blepharoconjunctivitis. **Oxyphenonium** may produce nonspecific conjunctivitis. Both **belladonna** and **oxyphenonium** may induce allergic reactions of the eyelids or conjunctiva; they also may increase IOP, decrease lacrimation, or cause micropsia and brawny scleritis (1,8,10,30,33,58,93,94).

GASTROINTESTINAL AGENTS

The ocular effects of cathartics depend on the specific agent. **Gamboge** that comes in contact with the eye can produce purulent keratitis (10). **Mercurous chloride** will cause slight transient redness and swelling of the eye, and inflammation or scarring of the conjunctiva. When soluble iodides or soluble bromides were given systemically at the same time that mercurous chloride was applied to the eye of experimental animals, they produced edema of the lids, hyperemia of the eye, tearing and mucoid or purulent discharge, erosions of the corneal epithelium, and clouding of the cornea (10,53,95). **Croton oil** is very toxic to the eyes, causing severe keratoconjunctivitis with pain, swelling, and purulent discharge. When croton oil is injected intracamerally, it causes violent iritis and necrosis of the cornea. When injected into the vitreous, it causes devastating endophthalmitis (96–98).

Bile and **bilirubin** are toxic when they come into contact with the eyes. **Bile** causes corneal epithelial injury, corneal opacity, cataract, degeneration of the retina, and choroid and hypertrophy of the iris and ciliary process. **Bilirubin** causes severe loss of vision, intraocular hemorrhages, loss of the electroretinogram (ERG), and yellow staining of the retina (10).

CHEMOTHERAPEUTIC AGENTS

Copper sulfate is an antitrachoma agent. Its side effects include temporary inflammation and purulent reaction, discoloration of the cornea, local necrosis, and corneal opacity symblepharon (99).

Antibacterials include several classes of agents of diverse chemical structure. Antibiotics are drugs derived from natural sources. Penicillin antibiotics include **amoxicillin, ampicillin, carbenicillin, cloxacillin, dicloxacillin, hetacillin, methicillin, nafcillin, oxacillin, benzathine penicillin G, hydrabamine penicillin V, potassium penicillin G, potassium penicillin V, potassium phenethicillin**, and **procaine penicillin G**. Polypeptide antibiotics include **bacitracin, colistimethate, colistin, polymyxin B**, and **capreomycin**. Cephalosporins include **cefazolin, cephalexin, cephaloglycin, cephaloridine, cephalothin**, and **cephradine**. **Chloramphenicol** is a bacteriostatic antibiotic. Bacteriostatic derivatives of polycyclic naphthalene carboxamide include **chlortetracycline, demeclocycline, doxycline, methacycline, minocycline, oxytetracycline**, and **tetracycline**. Aminoglycosidic antibiotics include **framycetin, neomycin, gentamicin, kanamycin**, and **streptomycin**. Other antibiotics include **clindamycin, erythromycin, lincomycin**, and **vancomycin** (1,8,10,20,30,34,42,58,100–106).

Sulfa drugs are synthetic compounds (in contrast to antibiotics, which are natural compounds) with antibacterial action. Sulfonamides include **sulfacetamide, sulfachlorpyridazine, sulfacytine, sulfadiazine, sulfadimethoxine, sulfamerazine, sulfameter, sulfamethazine, sulfamethizole, sulfamethoxazole, sulfamethoxypyridazine, sulfanilamide, sulfaphenazole, sulfapyridine, sulfasalazine, sulfathiazole**, and **sulfisoxazole**.

Side effects depend somewhat on the class of antibacterial agents (107,108). All of the antibiotics may produce irritation, allergic reactions, and/or edema of the eyelids or conjunctiva in sensitized individuals and overgrowth of nonsusceptible organisms. After intracameral injection, they produce uveitis, corneal edema, and lens damage (with the exceptions of the cephalosporins).

Other side effects depend on the specific antibiotic. **Cloxacillin** may produce corneal opacities. **Nafcillin** may produce conjunctival necrosis. Polypeptides can produce blepharoconjunctivitis, urticaria, and keratitis. **Cephalosporins** can produce urticaria. **Chloramphenicol** can produce depigmentation and optic neuritis. **Lincomycin** can produce subconjunctival hemorrhages, and **erythromycin** may produce mydriasis. Retrobulbar injection of **clindamycin** can cause optic neuritis and optic atrophy. **Framycetin** and **neomycin** may cause urticaria, erythema, and follicular conjunctivitis. **Gentamycin** may also cause follicular conjunctivitis. **Synermycin**, after intracameral injection, may cause intense inflammation involving, principally, the uveal tissues. **Sparsomycin** may cause the retinal pigment to gather together in coarse clumps and produce disturbance of vision and ring scotomas. **Pleomycin** after topical application of a 0.1% solution causes corneal opacity (10,109). Sulfonamides cause follicular conjunctivitis, deposits, and delayed corneal wound healing. Some of the sulfonamides, particularly **sulfadiazine, sulfanilamide, sulfapyridine**, and **sulfathiazole**, cause acute myopia and shallowing of the anterior chamber (1,107,108).

Silver-containing antibacterial agents include **colloidal silver, silver nitrate**, and **silver protein**. These agents have the side effects of silver deposits in the cornea, conjunctiva, eyelids, lens, and lacrimal sac. They produce irritation with hyperemia, photophobia, ocular pain, and edema. There may be allergic reactions and edema of the eyelids or conjunctiva in sensitized individuals, or conjunctivitis and symblepharon. **Silver nitrate**, at caustic concentrations, can cause scarring or opacities of any ocular structure. There may be decreased vision and problems with color vision: objects will appear to have a yellow tinge (1,110–112).

Other antibacterial agents may have ocular side effects. **Ethylhydrocupreine** may cause corneal anesthesia and clouding of the corneal epithelium. **Hydragaphene** may cause irritation, and **1-(5-nitro-2-furfunylideneamino) guanidine** may cause depigmentation of the eyelashes and the skin of the eyelids (10,107).

There are a variety of fungicide agents: **amphotericin B, chloranil, Nemagon, dodine, drazoxolon, ferban, 2-heptadecyl-2-imidazoline, methyl mercury compounds, mylone, nystatin, propionic acid, sulfur dust, tetrachlorophenol, tomatine, trichlorophenol, triphenyltin hydroxide, undecylenic acid**, and **zinc dimethyldithiocarbamate**. The side effects depend on the agent. **Methyl mercury compounds, sulfur dust**, and **undecylenic acid** can cause irritation and keratitis. **Mylone** can cause loss of the corneal epithelium. **Chloranil** can cause corneal necrosis. **Methyl mercury compounds** can cause opacity of the cornea. **Amphotericin B** and **nystatin** can cause allergic reactions of the eyelids or conjunctiva, and treatment may lead to overgrowth of nonsusceptible organisms; **amphotericin B** and **undecylenic acid** can cause conjunctivitis. **Amphotericin B** also may cause edema of the conjunctiva (as may **tomatine**), corneal ulceration, necrosis, and nodules or yellow discoloration, or may produce uveitis (1,8,10,30,33,34,42,58).

Some antiviral agents have ocular side effects; the effects depend on the agent. ***p*-Fluorophenylalanie** may cause delayed regeneration of the corneal epithelium. **Cytarabine** may cause ocular pain, iritis, and corneal opacities and ulceration. **Idoxuridine (IDU), trifluridine (F3T)**, and **vidarabine** have similar side effects.

They produce irritation, with lacrimation, hyperemia, photophobia, and ocular pain. There may be superficial punctate keratitis, corneal filaments, delayed wound healing, erosions or indolent ulceration, stromal opacities and superficial vascularization. There may be allergic reactions and hyperemia of the eyelids or conjunctiva in sensitized individuals. There may be follicular conjunctivitis, conjunctival punctate staining, and conjunctival scarring. There may be narrowing or occlusion of the lacrimal punctum and ptosis (1,10,33,113,114).

Neoarsphenamine is an antisyphilis drug with the side effects of corneal edema and opacity. **Oxophenarsine**, injected into the corneal stoma, causes moderate to moderately severe injury to the cornea (115).

DISINFECTANTS

Disinfectants with ocular toxicity include **cresols, propiolactone**, **propylene oxide**, **savlon**, **triethylene glycol**, and **xylenol**. All produce ocular irritation. **Cresols, propiolactone**, **savlon**, and **triethylene glycol** produce corneal haziness or opacity. **Cresols** also may produce conjunctival and lid reactions. **Savlon** also may produce corneal edema, hyphemia, and wrinkling of Descemet's membrane. **Xylenol** causes severe and, presumably, permanent injury to the eye. **Propylene oxide** is moderately injurious to the eye. **Propiolactone** may cause miosis (116–122).

SCABICIDES AND PEDICULICIDES

Lindane is the most common drug used to kill mites and lice. It has the side effects of irritation, conjunctivitis, and hyperemia (10,53).

ANTINEOPLASTIC AGENTS

There are several classes of antineoplastic agents, and the side effects vary somewhat from group to group. **Cyclophosphamide** and **thiotepa** are alkylating agents. **Cyclophosphamide** may cause damage to the cornea. **Thiotepa** causes irritation, allergic reactions in sensitized individuals, poliosis, and depigmentation of the eyelids or conjunctiva. There may be delayed corneal wound healing, keratitis, corneal edema, occlusion of the lacrimal punctum, or corneal ulceration (1,10,123,124).

Fluorouracil is an antimetabolite. It may cause irritation, allergic reactions, hyperpigmentation, photosensitivity, and subconjunctival hemorrhages of the eyelids or conjunctiva. After intradermal eyelid injection, there may be periorbital edema and cicatricial ectropion (42,125).

Chromomycin A3-Adriamycin and **mitomycin C** are antibiotics with antineoplastic effects. **Chromomycin A3** destroys the retina when injected into the vitreous. **Mitomycin C** may cause blepharoconjunctivitis, uveitis, scleral degeneration, increased IOP, prolapse of the iris, and destruction of the retina (10,126).

Vinblastine and **vincristine sulfate** are Vinca alkaloids. **Vinblastine** causes irritation, with lacrimation, hyperemia, and photophobia. It may cause keratitis, superficial gray opacities of the cornea, blepharospasm, decreased vision, and astigmatism. **Vincristine sulfate** causes degeneration of the retina after injection into the vitreous (127-130).

Other antineoplastic agents have different specific ocular side effects. **Actinomycin D** may cause a severe intraocular reaction of both the anterior and posterior segments of the eye, with opacification of the lens and cornea. **Alloxan** can cause severe injury to the eye. There may be corneal edema, opacity, and vascularization or glaucoma may develop. **Methotrexate** can cause irritation, such as foreign body sensation, tearing, and blurring of vision. There may be defects of the epithelium, wrinkling of Descemet's membrane, and hyperemia of the conjunctiva. **Triaziquone** may produce local pain or a violent local reaction, with extensive necrosis of the conjunctiva and glaucoma (10,42,131,132).

ANTIWART AGENTS

Chelidonium majus and **podophyllin** are antiwart agents with toxic effects to the eyes. They cause irritation, with burning, epiphora, and blepharospasm. There can be keratoconjunctivitis and iritis. **Chelidonium majus** can cause hypopyon. **Podophyllin** causes conjunctival hyperemia, loss of corneal epithelium, and deposits in the back of the cornea (10,42,133-135).

ANTIMALARIAL AGENTS

Modern antimalarial agents include **amodiaquine chloroquine, hydroxychloroquine, mepacrine,** and **quinoline**. All except **quinoline** can cause corneal deposits. **Mepacrine** may cause conjunctival deposits or corneal haziness and edema. **Quinoline** can cause moderately severe injury to the eyes (1,10,146-138).

ANTHELMINTICS AND AMEBICIDES

Quinacrine is used in the treatment of tapeworm infestations. Also, it is used in prophylaxis against worm infections and for the treatment of malaria. It has the side effects of producing blue haloes around lights, edema of the eyelids, conjunctiva, or cornea, and yellow discoloration of the eyes. There may be irritation, with lacrimation and ocular pain (1,139-140).

Piperazine is used in the treatment of oxyuriasis and ascariasis. It is very toxic when applied topically to the eyes; a drop of 10% solution causes very severe injury to rabbit eyes within 24 hr (10,20,30).

Emetine and **Ipecac** are used in the treatment of acute amebic dysentery, amebic hepatitis, and amebic abscesses. They have the side effects of irritation, with lacrimation, hyperemia, and photophobia. There may be allergic reactions of the eyelids or conjunctiva in sensitized individuals, conjunctivitis, or keratitis. **Emetine** causes conjunctival edema, blepharospasm, corneal ulceration, corneal opacities, and iritis. **Ipecac** causes miosis (1,10,141,142).

ADRENAL CORTICOSTERIODS

There are a variety of adrenal corticosteriods and preparations: **adrenal cortex injection, aldosterone, betamethasone, cortisone, desoxycorticosterone, dexamethasone, fludrocortisone, fluorometholone, fluprednisolone, hydrocortisone, midrysone, meprednisone, methylprednisolone, paramethasone, prednisolone, prednisone,** and **triamcinolone**. These agents produce a great variety of ocular side effects. There may be increased IOP, decreased resistance to infection, delayed healing of corneal or scleral wounds, mydriasis, or glaucoma. There may be ptosis, posterior subcapsular cataracts, or decreased vision. The drugs may enhance the lytic action of collagenase. There may be a changing of visual fields, with scotomas, constriction, an enlarged blind spot, or glaucoma field defect. There may be problems with color vision, such as dyschromatopsia or colored halos around lights. Sensitized people may have allergic reactions to these drugs. There may be persistent erythema, telangiectasis of the eyelids or conjunctiva, or eyelid or conjunctiva depigmentation, poliosis, or scarring. There may be fat atrophy and skin atrophy of the eyelids. Some patients develop paralysis of accommodation, punctate keratitis, irritation (with lacrimation, photophobia, ocular pain, or burning sensations) or anterior uveitis. The corneal or scleral thickness may change, initially increasing and then decreasing. There may be development of toxic amblyopia, optic atrophy, granulomas, or retinal embolic phenomenon. Adrenal corticosteroids may enhance facultative intraocular pathogens or cause development of retinal hemorrhages, retinal degeneration, and detachment or ascending optic atrophy. Adrenal corticosteroids may aggravate certain diseases, including scleromalacia perforans, corneal "melting" diseases, Behcet's disease, Eales' disease, or presumptive ocular toxoplasmosis (1,10,143–146).

DERMATOLOGIC AGENTS

Dematologic agents with ocular side effects include **benzoyl peroxide, chrysarobin, dithranol, exolan, hexachlorophene, resorcinol,** and **salicylic acid**. All these agents may produce irritation with lacrimation, hyperemia, photophobia and burning sensations; all except **dithranol** and **exolan** can produce conjunctivitis. **Chrysarobin** can cause allergic reactions of the eyelids or conjunctiva in sensitized persons, edema or brown-violet discolorations. **Chrysarobin** and **hexachlorophene** can produce keratitis, **hexachlorophene** and **exolan** can produce corneal edema. **Resorcinol** can produce corneal vascularization, necrosis, and perforation. Treatment with **benzoyl**

peroxide can lead to corneal opacity, and **exolan** can increase the IOP (1,8,10,18,58,147–149).

ANTISEPTICS

A variety of chemicals and compounds are used as antiseptics; their ocular side effects depend on the specific agent.

Local antiseptics include **brilliant green, chlorhexidine** (see **Savlon** in Disinfectants section), **gentian violet, hexylresorcinol, oxychlorosene, picric acid, silver proteinates,** and **mercuric chloride.**

All local antiseptics can produce ocular irritation (with the exception of **silver proteinates**). **Silver proteinates** can cause discoloration of the conjunctiva (110–112,150). **Gentian violet** can produce dark purple staining of the cornea and conjunctiva, loss of corneal epithelium and corneal stroma cloudiness. **Hexylresorcinol** can cause corneal edema or hyperemia of the iris. **Brilliant green** can produce keratitis and corneal opacity and, sometimes, hypopyon. **Mercuric chloride** can produce moderate to moderately severe corneal damage (graded from 22 to 75 on a scale of 0 to 100) (1,10,150–154).

Camphor is an antiseptic that can produce superficial keratitis with temporary loss of corneal epithelium (155,156).

Cetrimonium bromide has the same side effects as **Savlon** (157).

Creosote has the side effects of irritation (with burning sensations, itching, hyperemia, photophobia, and ocular discharge). It also is reported to be a carcinogen (53,158,159).

***n*-Hexanol** has the potential to cause severe eye injury (graded at 9 on a scale of 0 to 10) (10,160).

Mercuric oxycyanide can produce the side effects of corneal edema, wrinkling of Descemet's membrane, hyperemia of the iris, cataract and posterior synechiae, disturbance of vision, and secondary glaucoma (53,161).

Methylene blue can produce irritation, with stinging and epiphora (10,171).

Phenol can produce corneal ulceration and opacity, chemotic, entropion, and scarring of the conjunctiva. Edema of the lids may develop, along with iritis and disturbance of vision (162,163).

Zinc phenosulfonate may cause corneal necrosis and opacity (164).

Mercuric oxide (yellow) may cause deposits of the pigment in the lids, conjunctiva, cornea, and lens. There may be blepharitis or conjunctivitis. Injection of **mercuric oxide** into the anterior chamber cause inflammation and purulent exudate (53,165,166).

PRESERVATIVES

Ophthalmic preservatives may belong to several categories; many are either quaternary ammonium agents or organomercurial agents. **Benzalkonium** is the most important quaternary ammonium agent. It has the side effects of irritation (with lacrimation, hyperemia, photophobia, and edema), punctate keratitis, gray corneal epithelia haze, pseudomembrane formation, decreased corneal epithelial microvilli, and cytotoxicity to the corneal epithelial cells. It also is suggested that it may cause delayed corneal wound healing (1,167).

Organomercurials include **mercuric oxide, nitromersol, phenylmercuric acetate, phenylmercuric nitrate**, and **thimerosal**. These compounds have the side effects of allergic reactions in sensitized individuals, erythema, edema, and hyperemia of the eyelids or conjunctivitis. They may produce blepharoconjunctivitis. **Mercuric oxide** may produce bluish-gray mercury deposits on the eyelids, conjunctiva, and cornea; **mercuric oxide** and **phenylmercuric acetate** or **nitrate** also may leave deposits on the lens. **Thimerosal** can produce cytotoxicity of the corneal epithelial cells (1,10,147,168–170).

Chlorobutanol is another preservative. It has the side effect of cytotoxicity to corneal epithelial cells. Phenylmercuric salts include **dinaphylmethane disulfonate** and the **phenylmercuric** salts of acetate, chloride, nitrate, and oleate. These compounds have the side effect of mercurialentis (10,170).

DYES

Ophthalmic dyes frequently are used for ocular diagnostic tests. Commonly used dyes are **alcian blue, fluorescein, rose bengal**, and **trypan blue**. These dyes have the side effects of staining mucus, connective tissue, ocular fluids, and degenerated epithelial cells. They will produce irritation (with ocular pain and burning sensations) and blue, yellow-orange, or red discolorations of the eyelids or conjunctiva. **Fluorescein** may produce problems with color vision (objects will have a yellow tinge) (1,10).

Normally, the ocular side effects due to these ophthalmic dyes are rare and transient. However, if the corneal epithelium is not intact, the topical application of alcian blue may cause long-term, or even permanent, stromal deposits of the dye (1,10).

Methylene blue is a dye used during ocular surgery as a tissue marker. It has the side effects of producing a burning sensation, and it stains corneal nerves (10,33,171).

Nonophthalmic dyes normally are not placed deliberately in the eye, though some ophthalmic dyes also have nonophthalmic uses. They are a class of potentially toxic compounds that may accidentally contaminate the eye. The list of nonophthalmic dyes is fairly long: **acridine red, acridine yellow, acriflavine, alkali violet, amethyst violet, alisolin concentrate, auramine, Bindschedler's green, Bismarck green, brilliant cresyl blue, brilliant firnblau, brilliant green, brilliant phoaphin 5G, brilliant victoria blue RB, chrysoidine, clematin, coriphosphine, crystal violet, diamond fuchsin, 2,3-dichlorophenolindophenol, echtblau 2B, ethyl violet, basic fuchsin, gentian violet, homacridine yellow, indelible pencils, indigo, indoin, Janus black, Janus green B, malachite green, Mendola blue, mepacrine,**

methyl green, methyl rosaniline, methyl violet, methylene blue, methylene green, new blue R, new fuchsin, night blue, pararosaniline, patent phosphin G, phenosafranin, *p*-phenylenediamine, phloxine B, phosphine, prune pure, rhodamine B, rhodamine 6G, rhodamine S, safranin O, setocyanin, setoglaucin, spirit blue, thiazin blue, thionin, toluidine blue, Victoria blue R, Victoria pure blue BO, Dupont FDL 316, Victoria R.B., and **violet 4RN**.

All of these dyes have the potential to produce injury to the eye. **Bindschedler's green** and **phloxine B** may produce opacification and vascularization of the cornea. **Brilliant green** may produce destructive keratitis with hypopyon. **Janus green B** may produce corneal edema and damage to the epithelium, and **2,3-dichlorophenolindophenol** may produce histologic and metabolic disturbances of the retina (1,10,53,172–174).

OPHTHALMIC IMPLANTS

Flaxseeds sometimes have been placed in the conjunctival sac as a form of home remedy. **Flaxseeds** may produce erythema, edema, and a local gray mucoid discharge. Corneal edema and abrasions inferior to the conjunctival sac also have been observed (10).

Ivalov is used as an implant in orbits after enucleation of the eyes they contain. This procedure may produce a foreign body type of cellular reaction, like rejection of a foreign substance (10).

Silicone has been used for implants; **silicone** implants increase postoperative infections and glaucomatous reactions. Liquid **silicone** applied topically causes a burning sensation. Liquid **silicone** used intraocularly can produce cataracts and endothelial damage with corneal edema or vascularization (1,175–177).

Polygenline is used as a substitute for the vitreous humor in patients being treated for retinal detachment. Signs of inflammation with clouding of the vitreous have been noted in rabbits who received intravitreal injection of **polygenline** at concentrations of 7% or greater (10).

ANTIPERSPIRANTS

Antiperspirants contain compounds such as **aluminum chloride**, employed in the form of liquids, powders, sprays, and sticks. Contamination of the eyes with antiperspirants can cause transient irritation, ocular pain, blepharospasm, transient epithelial damage, and persistent faint nebula in the corneal stroma (10,53,178).

COUNTERIRRITANTS

Drugs used as counterirritants include **allylisothiocyanate**, **arnica**, **veratrine**, and **2-naphthol**. All of these agents can produce irritation and lacrimation. **Veratrine** can induce irritation of the conjunctiva; **arnica** can produce edema of the lids or hyperemia of the conjunctiva. **Allylisothiocyanate** can cause keratitis, and **2-naphthol** causes cataracts, white, yellow-white, or pigmented spots, edema in the retina, and disturbance of vision (10,179–181).

CHELATING AGENTS

A number of chelating agents are used clinically. **Deferoxamine** is used in the treatment of ocular siderosis and hematogenous pigment of the cornea. It has the side effects of causing allergic reactions in sensitized individuals and hyperemia of the eyelids or the conjunctiva. When a 5-μg sample of **deferoxamine** was injected intravitreally, it caused widespread hemorrhagic necrosis, particularly affecting the rods and cones of the retina and extinguishing the ERG. When 200 μ of **deferoxamine** was injected intravitreally, there was congestion of the uvea and exudative detachment of the choroid and retina (1,8,10,42).

Dimercaprol is used in the treatment of arsenic, gold, or mercury poisonings. It has the side effects of causing irritation, with lacrimation, photophobia, burning sensations, and blepharospasm. There may be severe iritis, corneal infiltration, corneal vascularization, and permanent scarring (1,10,182,183).

Edetate (BEDTA) has the side effects of a mild stinging sensation, localized faint opacity of the cornea, and hyperemia of the iris and the conjunctiva (183).

DECONGESTANTS

Decongestants with ocular side effects include **naphazoline** and **tetrahydrozoline**. These agents can cause conjunctival vasoconstriction, irritation, lacrimation, reactive hyperemia, and burning sensations. There may be punctate keratitis, decreased vision or mydriasis which, in turn, may precipitate narrow-angle glaucoma. There may be allergic reactions of the eyelid or conjunctiva in sensitized individuals or increases in pigment granules in the anterior chamber. **Naphazoline** may produce conjunctivitis; **tetrahydrozoline** may cause blepharoconjunctivitis or a decrease in IOP pressure (1,8,10,30,42).

ASTRINGENTS

Alum has been employed topically as an astringent and styptic and in the treatment of trachoma. It can cause corneal incrustation and turbidity (10).

Potassium permanganate can cause a hardened, eroded lesion of the eye, swelling of the lids, and conjunctiva, subconjunctival hemorrhages, turbidity, and brown discoloration of the cornea (10).

Tannic acid has been employed topically as an astringent and hemostatic. It has the side effects of a slight or mild reaction, discoloration, and, sometimes, corneal injury (10).

Lead acetate can cause irritation, opacity, and lead incrustation of the cornea and conjunctiva (10,184-186).

SURFACTANTS

Surfactants fall into three classes: cationic surfactants, anionic surfactants, and nonionic surfactants. Cationic surfactants include **benzalkonium, benzethonium, cetrimonium (CTAB), cetylpyridinium, decyltrimethylammonium, dodecyltrimethylammonium, Emcol E607, Emulsol 607, 607M, G271, hexadecyltrimethylammonium, Isothan Q15**, and **tetradecyltrimethylammonium**. These agents all can cause irritation and injury to the eyes; **benzalkonium** can cause degeneration of the iris or chorioretinitis (10,73,187-189).

Anionic surfactants include **Aerosol OS, Aerosol OT, alkyl sodium sulfate series** from **octyl** to **octadecyl, Armour #600 KOP soap, dodecyl sodium sulfate, Duponol ME, Duponol WAT, Eutsufon, Igepon AP, Ivory soap, Lissapol N, Naconol NRSF, Santomerse D, sodium lauryl sulfate, Duponol C, Tergitol-4, Tergitol-07, Tergitol-08, triethanolamine lauryl sulfate (Drene), Triton W30, Triton X30, Ultrawet 30DS**, and **Ultrawet 60L**.

All anionic surfactants cause irritation, discomfort, and potential injury to the eyes. There may be hyperemia of the conjunctiva, edema of the corneal epithelium, and temporary clouding of the cornea (10,53,190-194).

Nonionic surfactants include **Brij-30, G1690, G2132, G3721, Laurithyl**, and **Triton X155**. Side effects include irritation, with ocular pain and photophobia, loss of the corneal epithelium, and corneal opacity (10,53,190-191,195).

COSMETICS

Cosmetics usually are not single substances but are mixtures of substances, both natural and synthetic. **Eye cosmetics** contain numerous inert oily or waxy substances and coloring materials, such as **lecithin, cholesterin, cocoa butter, paraffin, diethylene glycol stearate, triethanolamine, stearic acid, carbon black, iron oxide**, and other inorganic pigments. Contamination of the eye with **eye cosmetics** can produce pigmentation of the palpebral conjunctiva, slight irregularities of the surface of the conjunctiva, mild burning or foreign-body sensations, and tearing (10,53,196-204).

Hair cosmetics include a variety of preparations for a variety of purposes, none of which should bring them in contact with the eyes (204). Hair dyes may be either ***p*-phenylenediamine-type hair dyes** or **henna** or **2,4-diaminophenol**. ***p*-Phenylenediamine** derived dyes can cause irritation, with burning sensations, ocular pain, tearing, redness, swelling, and edema of the lids. There also may be edema and hyperemia of the conjunctiva. There may be loss of the corneal epithelium and corneal ulceration. Dyes also may produce iritis, iridocyclitis, exophthalmos, lost vision, or retrobulbar neuritis with central scotoma (53,205–208).

Henna is a natural compound. It may have the side effects of swelling of the lids, tearing, discharge, and severe pain (53,207–211).

2,4-Diaminophenol may cause dark brown staining of the corneal stroma or permanent corneal opacification and vascularization (10).

Hair sprays and **lacquers** may produce ocular irritation, a transient stinging sensation, or a temporary fine keratitis epithelialis (204,210,211).

Hair tonics that contact the eye may cause stinging and burning sensations, ocular pain, swelling, and redness of the lids (10).

Hair-waving preparations, such as **thioglycolates**, generally produce keratitis. They also may produce irritation, burning sensations, conjunctival inflammation, corneal epithelial erosion, turbidity of the cornea, mydriasis, cycloplegia, loss of convergence, and disturbance of vision (10).

Skin lotions, such as **Parabens** and **Triacetin**, can cause eye irritation. **Parabens** causes redness and swelling of the eyelids. **Triacetin** causes ocular pain and much redness of the conjunctiva (10,212).

Nail hardener may cause allergic reactions of the eye and conjunctiva in sensitized individuals. **Nail polish** and **nail polish remover** can cause temporary solvent burns, swelling, and vesiculization of the lids and itching (10,53).

Lip Magik is a cosmetic preparation that should be mentioned, because it can cause discomfort and blurred vision, hyperemia, and chemosis of the conjunctiva (212).

Some common cosmetic ingredients can cause ocular side effects. **Isopropyl alcohol** and **hexylene glycol** both can cause irritation and mild transitory injury (graded 4 on a scale of 1 to 10), and **2-cyanoacrylic acid methyl ester**, an ingredient in glue, can cause irritation, haze of the cornea, inflammation of the eye, and blurred vision (213–223).

INSECTICIDES

A variety of compounds used as insecticides have unpleasant or dangerous effects on accidental topical contact with the eyes. These insecticides include **bis(tri-*n*-butyltin)oxide**, **mixtures of carbaryl** and **dimethoate**, **copper acetoardenite**, **Delna**, **Derris**, **1,1-dichloro-1-nitroethane**, **Deet**, **HETP**, **hexachlorocyclopentadiene**, **irsbornyl thiocyanoacetate**, **lead arsenate**, **malathione**, **methyl isothiocyanate**, **naphthalene**, **nicotine**, **parathion**, **Paris green**, **phenothiazine**, **pyrethrum**, **trichloroacetonitrile**, **tetraethylpyrophosphate (TEPP)**, and **trichlorobenzene**. All of these compounds can produce irritation and ocular pain (**nicotine, parathion, trichlorobenzene**), photophobia (**phenothiazine**), or lacrimation (**1,1-dichloro-1-nitroethane, Deet, trichloroacetonitrile**.). The eyelids or conjunctiva often are affected by topical contamination; there may be edema (**Deet, malathione,** or **pyrethrum**), hyperemia (**malathione** or **pyrethrum**), conjunctivitis (after **Delna** or **Deet**), injury (after **lead arsenate**), reaction (**nicotine**), or swelling of the lids (after a mixture of **carbaryl** and **dimethoate**). **Phenothiazine** and **pyrethrum** may cause corneal edema; corneal clouding or opacity may be induced by **bis(tri-*n*-butyltin)oxide, Deet, methyl isothiocyanate**, or **nicotine**. There may be corneal ulceration, vascularization and scarring, hemorrhages of the iris, or hypopyon after exposure to **bis(tri-*n*-butyltin)oxide**. There may be corneal epithelium injury after **Deet** or **methyl isothiocyanate**, a corneal haze or serious injury to the eye after **pyrethrum** exposure, corneal infiltration after **nicotine**, or keratitis epithelialis after a mixture of **carbaryl** and **dimethoate**. Miosis may be induced by **HETP, parathion, tetraethylpyrophosphate**, or **trichlorfon**. **Parathion** and **tetraethylpyrophosphate** may cause disturbed vision (8,10,53,224–241).

FISH AND JELLYFISH

Some kinds of **fish** are actually toxic; most of them can produce gases when decomposing that are toxic to the eyes. **Trimethylamine** is a gas released during the putrefaction of fish. **Trimethylamine** can cause hemorrhagic conjunctivitis, loss of corneal epithelium, corneal edema, opacity, and vascularization. Decomposing **fish** evolve gases that have induced bilateral keratitis epithelialis in fishermen. **Eel blood** is especially irritating. **Eel blood** can produce a burning sensation and purulent discharge of the eyes, photophobia, inflammation and chemosis of the conjunctiva, keratitis, and swelling of the lids. **Jellyfish** and other coelenterates possess stinging cells that can inject anything they contact with toxins. **Jellyfish** can produce irritation, ocular pain and blepharospasm, photophobia, swelling of the lids, and injury to the corneal epithelium (10,53,242–244).

TOXINS AND VENOMS

Moths flying into the eyes may cause irritation (245). **Caterpillar hairs** of many species are really spines containing a toxin. If spines enter the eye, they can cause irritation, conjunctivitis, keratitis, uveitis, and necrosis (246–248). **Cantharides** can cause conjunctivitis, keratitis, iritis, edema of the skin, a fibrinous exudate, hyperemia, and necrosis of the eyes (249). **Bee stings** cause ocular pain, photophobia, clouding and swelling of the cornea, corneal infiltration and vascularization, keratitis, conjunctivitis, iritis, hypopyon, cataract, abscess of the lens, and, more rarely, cause glaucoma. There may be optic atrophy or optic neuritis (250,251). **Tarantula hairs** also can irritate the eye (252).

Skunks spray anything that threatens them with a powerful irritant and may aim for the eyes. Spray from a **skunk** causes irritation, conjunctivitis, and, sometimes, corneal opacity and vascularization (10,53).

Diphtheria toxin is topically toxic to the eyes, causing hyperemia and edema of the conjunctiva and opacification of the cornea (10).

Spider venoms can cause ocular irritation, with swelling of the lids, conjunctival edema, and subconjunctival hemorrhages (253).

Toad poisons are produced in the toad's skin and may contact the eyes if a toad is handled and then the eyes touched. **Toad poisons** can cause irritation, swelling of the lids, hyperemia of the conjunctiva, conjunctivitis, corneal and conjunctival anesthesia, paresis of the eye muscles, ptosis and corneal clouding, keratitis, iritis, mydriasis, decreased IOP, and central retinal edema (10,254).

Wasp stings can cause swelling of the lids, ocular pain and bullous keratitis (255; see Bee Stings also).

Tetanus toxin is a neurotoxin. The effect of **tetanus toxin** on the iris has been shown to resemble postganglionic parasympathectomy (10).

PLANTS

A great variety of **plants** and **plant products** can cause irritation or changes in the eyelids, conjunctiva, or cornea. Some of the species are ***Acacia***, ***Actaea rubra***, ***Agrostemma*** **seed**, ***Araroba***, **burdock burs, cactus, capsaicin, carrageenan, cashew nut shell oil, castor beans, chamomile, chestnut shell, crownflower,** ***Datura***, ***Dieffenbachia*** **plants,** ***Ecballium elaterium***, ***Euphorbia***, **wild fig,** ***Hura crepitans***, ***Hyacinth*** **bulbs, jequirity bean, manchineel, mesquite thorn, morel,** ***Mucuna pruriens***, **mustard oil, onion, pepper, peppermint oil, pigweed, poison ivy** and related species of ***Rhus***, **primula,** ***Psyllium***, ***Pyracanthus*** **extract, ricin, snuff, tea, teakwood,** and **tobacco** and **wood dust** (256–278).

All of these plants and plant-derived substances can cause irritation, ocular pain, lacrimation, burning, photophobia, tearing, blurring of vision, blepharospasm, and itching (10). Other effects depend somewhat on the agent. **Capsaicin** causes abnormal permeability of the blood vessels of the conjunctiva (256–258). Edema or swelling of the eyelids or conjunctiva can be produced by **burdock burs** (10,259), **cashew nut shell oil** (260,261), **crownflower** (279), ***Ecballium elaterium*** (262), ***Euphorbia*** (10), **manchineel** (10,280), **pepper** (10), **poison ivy** (263), **primula** (10), **tobacco smoking** (264–265), or **wood dust** (266–268). Conjunctivitis can be induced by **cashew nut shell oil, castor beans** (269), ***Ecballium elaterium***, ***Euphorbia***, **wild fig** (10), ***Hura crepitans*** (10,280), ***Mucuna pruriens*** (270), **mustard oil** (10), ***Pyracanthus*** **extract** (271), **ricin** (269), **snuff,** or **tea** (10). Hyperemia of the conjunctiva can be produced by contact with ***Euphorbia***, **manchineel** (280), **primula** (273), or **wood dust** (266–268,275). Chemosis can be induced by ***Euphorbia*** (10), **mustard oil** (10), or **manchineel** (280). Conjunctival necrosis or ulcer can be produced by **chestnut shell** or **jequirity bean** (10). **Teakwood** can cause dermatitis in the lids (275). Damage of the corneal epithelium can be produced by **crownflower** (10), **morel,** or **peppermint oil** (10). **Wild fig** and **burdock burs** can cause corneal ulcers, **burdock burs** also cause scarring and erosion of the cornea and corneal edema, as does **crownflower**. Corneal clouding or opacity may be produced by **burdock burs, carrageenan** (272), ***Ecballium elaterium*** (262), **wild fig, jequirity**

beans, or **mustard oil** (10). **Burdock burs** and **carrageenan** (272) can cause corneal vascularization. Keratitis can be produced by ***Euphorbia***, **peppermint oil**, or ***Rhizoma galanga*** (10). Corneal infiltration can be induced by **jequirity beans** or **peppermint oil**. Keratitis epithelialis can be induced by **mustard oil, primula** (273), or **wood dust**. **Peppermint oil** can cause deposits on the cornea or release of pigment into the anterior chamber (10). Keratoconjunctivitis can be induced by ***Agrostemma* seed** (10), **manchineel** (280), or **morel** (10). **Castor beans** can produce symblepharon (269), whereas **jequirity bean** and **burdock burs** can produce inflammation of the anterior chamber (10). **Carrageenan** (272) can cause an acute rise in IOP, and **crownflower** (10) can cause a wrinkling of Descemet's membrane. Iritis may be produced by ***Euphorbia***, **jequirity bean, mustard oil, primula, *Pyracanthus* extract**, or ***Rhizoma galanga*** (268,271,273-277,281-283).

Some other plants also are known to cause ocular problems. ***Aloe*** barbs cause uveitis. ***Acacia* extract** (267) can cause nonnecrotizing inflammation, and ***Acacia* thorn** (278) can cause iridocyclitis. **Belladonna** causes blurring of the vision and impairment of accommodation for near objects, with pupil dilation, shallow anterior chamber, and increased IOP (1,283).

Datura cornigera can cause mydriasis and cycloplegia (277). ***Laminaria digitata*** can induce glaucoma (283).

GASES

Many substances are used in tear gases: **bromoacetone, bromomethyl ethyl ketone, bromoxylene, chloroacetone, chloroacetophenone, *o*-chlorobenzylidene malononitrile, dichloroformoxime, ethyl bromoacetate, alpha-iodotoluene, pelargonic acid morpholide, trichloroethane, trichloromethane sulfonyl chloride**, and **trichloromethanediol**. All tear gases can produce irritation, lacrimation, and smarting of the eyes (10,284-291).

Chloroacetophenone can produce blepharospasm, and ***o*-chlorobenzylidene malononitrile** can produce burning and pain. Corneal opacity can be induced by **bromoacetone, chloroacetone, chloroacetophenone**, or **ethyl bromoacetate**. Corneal necrosis or ulceration can be induced by **bromoacetone, bromomethyl ethyl ketone**, or **chloroacetophenone**. Corneal edema can be produced by **ethyl bromoacetate**; this substance and **bromomethyl ethyl ketone** can produce corneal scarring. **Dichloroformoxime** may even produce blindness (284-291).

War gases include **allyl alcohol alpha-bromobenzylcyanide, chlorine, chloropicrin, cyanogen chloride, ethylarsine dichloride, lewisite, methyl arisine dichloride, mustard gas, nitrogen mustard, nitrosamines, phenarsazine chloride, phenylcarbylamine, phosgene, sulfuryl chloride, tetrachlorosilane, thiodiglycol**, and **xylyl bromides** (10,292,293). All of these agents can produce irritation. Many are lacriminatory: **allyl alcohol, chlorine, chloropicrin, cyanogen chloride, ethylarsine dichloride, lewisite, methyl arisine dichloride, mustard gas, nitrogen mustard, phenarsazine chloride, phenylcarbylamine, sulfuryl chloride**, and **xylyl bromides**.

Many produce ocular pain (**allyl alcohol, chloropicrin, lewisite, thiodiglycol**), blepharospasm (**chlorine, cyanogen chloride, lewisite, mustard gas, nitrogen mustard, phenylcarbylamine**, and **phosgene**) or photophobia and burning sensations (**allyl alcohol, chlorine, cyanogen chloride, mustard gas, nitrogen mustard**, and **phenylcarbylamine**). There may be edema and hyperemia of the eyelids and conjunctiva (**allyl alcohol, cyanogen chloride, mustard gas, phosgene**, or **thiodiglycol**) or conjunctivitis (**cyanogen chloride**). Many cause corneal clouding or opacity (**allyl alcohol, mustard gas, nitrogen mustard, phenylcarbylamine**, or **phosgene**), corneal edema (**allyl alcohol, alpha-bromobenzylcyanide, mustard gas**, and **nitrogen mustard**), or corneal necrosis or ulceration (**ethylarsine dichloride, lewisite, methyl arisine dichloride, mustard gas, nitrogen mustard, phenarsazine chloride, phenylcarbylamine, phosgene**, or **sulfuryl chloride**). There may be keratitis (**allyl alcohol, ethyl isothiocyanate, mustard gas, or nitrogen mustard**). Other symptoms of exposure may be uveitis from **nitrosamines**, injury of the iris from **nitrogen mustard** or **nitrosamines**, or lens damage from **nitrogen mustard**.

Nerve gas has been dealt with elsewhere; **savin** can produce miosis and spasm of accommodation for near objects.

Other gases of interest in ocular toxicology include **arsine, carbon dioxide, carboxide, chlorine dioxide, chlorine monofluoride, chlorine oxide, chlorine trifluoride, cyanogen, dichlorodifluoromethane (F12, Freon F-12), dimethyl ethylamine, ethylamine, fluorine, formaldehyde, germanium tetrafluoride, hydrogen chloride gas, hydrogen selenide, nitrosyl chloride**, and **triethylamine** (294–307). All these gases can cause irritation. **Formaldehyde** can cause lacrimation and photophobia, corneal vascularization, chemosis, and iritis. There may be swelling of the lids after exposure to **formaldehyde** and **arsine**. Corneal edema may follow exposure to **chlorine dioxide, chlorine monofluoride, F-12**, or **formaldehyde**. Some gases cause corneal ulcer or erosion: **chlorine trifluoride, ethylamine, formaldehyde**, and **hydrogen chloride gas**; the latter two gases also may cause corneal clouding or opacity. **Chlorine dioxide** and **formaldehyde** can cause cataract; **chlorine dioxide** also may cause pupil dilation and paralysis of obduction (308–310).

Sodium chloroacetate is a chemical defoliant. Contact with the eyes causes temporary corneal clouding and ulceration (311).

IODIDES

Iodides have the effects on topical contact of lacrimation, edema of the eyelids, conjunctival hyperemia, keratoconjunctivitis, hypopyon, hemorrhagic iritis, and vitreous opacities (10,312,313).

SOLVENTS

A great variety of substances and preparations are used as solvents. The effects of topical exposure of the eyes to solvents depend on the nature of the solvent

(314–404). Some solvents only produce irritation of the eyes; these include **benzyl acetate, *n*-butyl formate, *n*-butyl methyl ketone, ethyl benzene, isoamyl alcohol, isopropyl acetate, methyl cyclohexanol, methyl cyclohexanone, methyl formate, methyl isobutyl ketone, 2,5-tetrahydrofurandimethanol,** and **tetrahydronaphthalene.**

Other solvents produce irritation and slight to severe injuries to the eyes. Slight injury is produced by contact with **dichloroethyl ether, *N,N*-dimethylacetamide, dimethyl phthalate, dioxane, epichlorophydrin, 2-ethoxyethanol,** or **isophorone** (314). Moderate injury follows contact with ***n*-butanol, cyclohexanol, cyclohexanone, diacetone alcohol, dimethylaniline, ethyl formate, isobutyl alcohol, methyl acetate, methyl propyl ketone, *n*-propyl alcohol,** or **pyridine**. Severe injury follows exposure to **ethylenediamine, ethyl chloroacetate,** or **bisphenol A**. Other solvents with toxic properties on the eyes include **acetone, amyl acetate, amyl alcohol, benzyl alcohol, 2-butoxyethanol, butyl acetate, *p*-tertiary-butyltoluene, diacetin, 1,2-dichloroethane** (323), **diethyleneglycol monoethyl ether, *N,N*-dimethylformamide, dimethyl sulfoxide (DMSO), ethyl alcohol, ethyl acetate, ethyl ethyl ketone, glycerol, methanol, methyl cellosolve, morpholine, nitroparaffins, phosphorus oxychloride, alpha-picoline, sulfolane, tetrachloroethylene, toluene, turpentine,** and **xylene** (319).

All these solvents, except **benzyl alcohol**, cause irritation. Burning, stinging sensations, lacrimation, ocular pain, blurring of vision, blepharospasm, and conjunctival injury follow exposure to **acetone** or **sulfolane**. Many solvents cause hyperemia of the conjunctiva: **amyl acetate, amyl alcohol, butyl acetate, 2-butoxyethanol, diacetin, 1,2-dichloroethane, ethyl alcohol, methyl cellosolve, methanol, methyl ethyl ketone, toluene, turpentine,** and **xylene**. Chemosis or swelling follow exposure to **2-butoxyethanol, *p*-tertiary-butyltoluene,** or **methyl cellosolve**. **DMSO** and **glycerol** cause dilation of blood vessels in the eye. **Ethyl alcohol** and **morpholine** can cause necrosis or ulceration. **Diethyleneglycol monoethyl ether** cause conjunctivitis. **Amyl alcohol** and **phosphorus oxychloride** cause corneal injury; many agents cause corneal epithelial injury and edema: **acetone, amyl acetate, 1,2-dichloroethane, DMSO, ethyl acetate, ethyl alcohol, tetrachloroethylene, toluene, turpentine,** and **xylene**. Several agents cause corneal edema (**acetone, benzyl alcohol, ethyl alcohol, glycerol,** and **methyl ethyl ketone**) or corneal opacity (**acetone, 2-butoxyethanol, diethyleneglycol monoethyl ether, ethyl alcohol, methyl ethyl ketone, morpholine,** or **turpentine**). **Benzyl alcohol** and **xylene** cause corneal keratopathy. **Toluene, isobutyl alcohol,** and ***n*-butanol** can cause vacuolar keratitis. **Benzyl alcohol, 1,2-dichloroethane, ethyl alcohol,** and **glycerol** can cause endothelial injury; **ethyl alcohol** also produces corneal infiltration and vascularization. **Acetone** can cause cataract, and **diethyleneglycol monoethyl ether** can cause iritis. **Nitroparaffins** can cause mydriasis, and **alpha-picoline** can cause diplopia. **Toluene** causes dilation of the pupil and impairment of pupillary reaction to light. **Glycerol** may cause retinal edema, and **amyl acetate** can cause retrobulbar neuritis. **Turpentine**, injected intracamerally, causes fibrinopurulent inflammation, and, injected subconjunctivally, causes phthisis bulbi (314–404).

FOREIGN BODIES

The ocular side effects of foreign bodies in the eye depend on the nature of the foreign body; some substances produce specific reactions of the eye. **Glass, lead metal foreign bodies, peat dust**, and **plastics** cause irritation and can cause injury mechanically (405,406).

Copper metal foreign bodies and **alloys of brass, bronze**, or **aluminum containing copper** also can cause purulent inflammation, fibrinous iritis, changes of the vitreous and retina, widespread inflammatory and degenerative changes, pigment migration, or macular injury. There may be development of cataract, chalcosis, and glaucoma (407,408).

Iron and **iron compounds** cause siderosis on various ocular tissues. There may be discolorations of ocular tissues. The pupil may become larger or smaller (mydriasis or miosis), and there may be poor reaction to light. Cataract, retinal degeneration, disturbance of vision, or glaucoma may develop (408–410).

The materials packed in a golf ball may include **sodium hydroxide, barium sulfate**, and **zinc sulfide**. These materials may be corrosive; they may produce deposits in conjunctival and palpebral tissues and macrophage reaction (10).

Common dusting powders are **starch powder** and **talc. Talc** can cause conjunctival inflammation and symblepharon. Injected into the anterior chamber, it produces pseudohypopyon (10). **Starch powder** has been associated with petechial hemorrhages in the retina; injected into the anterior chamber, **starch powder** produces granulomatous reactions and transitory leukocytic and fibrinous exudate (411–413).

GUN POWDER

Gun powder can produce corneal injury, with coagulation of the epithelium and stippling of the epithelium with black particles (10).

Mercury fulminate is a detonator, a powerful explosive. Exposure to **mercury fulminate** may produce conjunctival irritation and itching erythema, and swelling of the eyelids (10,53).

SMOG

Smog (see also chapter by Way, Baxter, and Cannon) contains **nitro-olefins, peroxyacetyl nitrate, peroxybenzoyl nitrate, ozone, aldehydes**, and **organic peroxides**. These compounds cause irritation, lacrimation, conjunctival hyperemia, and whitening of the corneal epithelium. **Nitro-olefins** can cause inflammation of the conjunctiva and lids, and dilation of superficial blood vessels (10).

PENCILS AND INK

Indelible pencils and **colored pencils** cause injury that depends on the location of the foreign material and its content of cationic dye. Injury from a pencil may cause permanent corneal opacification, ulceration of the conjunctiva, panophthalmis, or necrosis (10). **Hectograph ink** can cause burning sensations if it contacts the eyes (10).

TAR

Tar and carbon come in several forms. **Charcoal** has the side effects of irritation, discoloration, and inflammation of the anterior segment of the eye, and can cause fine particles to become embedded in the cornea and conjunctiva. **Coal tar** can cause reddening and squamous eczema of the lid margins, erosions of the corneal epithelium, superficial changes in the corneal stroma, conjunctivitis, discoloration of the cornea, and epithelioma of the lid margin. **Pitch** can cause irritation, chemosis, ulceration and infiltration of the cornea, hypopyon, staining of the cornea, conjunctival discoloration, and deformities of the lids (159,414–418).

ACIDS AND BASES

Some acids produce specific ocular injury. **Acetic acid** causes irritation, lacrimation, photophobia, swelling of the lids, corneal edema, anesthesia, epithelial injury, and opacity. There may be conjunctival hyperemia, iritis, or a small pupil fixed by posterior synechiae (419,420). **Chrysophanic acid** can cause ocular inflammation (10).

Chromic acid can cause corneal infiltration, vascularization, opacification, and ulceration. There may be brown staining of the eye and keratitis. It may also cause occlusion of the central retinal vein (421).

Citroconic acid can cause slight transient injury of the eye (10).

Diphenylarsenic acid can cause tearing, swelling of the lids, and conjunctival hyperemia (10).

Formic acid causes corneal opacity, loss of the endothelium, and infiltration, vascularization, and swelling of the epithelium and stroma. There may be hypopyon, iritis, and opacity (10). **Mesaconic acid** causes moderate acid-type injury (10).

Pimelic acid causes moderate irritation, swelling of the lids, and corneal opacity (422).

Alkalies include **ammonium hydroxide (ammonia), calcium hydroxide (lime), diethylethanolamine, diethylenetriamine, diisopropylamine, 3-dimethylaminopropylamine, sodium hydroxide (lye), tetraethylammonium hydroxide**, and **tetramethylammonium hydroxide**. All alkalies are highly toxic to the eyes, causing irritation, corneal opacification, sloughing of the epithelium, edema, necrosis, infiltration, ulceration perforation, vascularization, scarring, regeneration of the epithelium and endothelium, and loss of corneal mucoid. There may be iritis, followed by disappearance of iritis, cataract, glaucoma, ischemic necrosis, edema of the conjunctiva and limbal region of the sclera, symblepharon, or staphyloma (165,423–436).

Other substances classified as alkalies are **neurine** and **putrescine**. **Neurine** causes hemorrhagic conjunctivitis and corneal edema with opacities. **Putrescine** causes mucoid discharge and a slight reaction of the eyes (10).

Ethanolmaine and **ethanolamine oleate** are sclerosing agents. **Ethanolamine** causes injury similar to that caused by ammonia. Subconjunctival injection of **ethanolamine oleate** causes a severe local reaction (10,436).

Substances classified as amines include **aliphatic amines, 2-chloroethylamines, cyclic amines, 2-aminoethoxyethanol,** and ***N*-aminoethylmorpholine**. These amines cause severe injury to the eyes. Contact with the eyes causes irritation, burning sensations, photophobia, destruction of the corneal epithelium, edema of the corneal epithelium, and keratitis (10,437–441).

ENZYMES

Hyaluronidase is an enzyme used as a spreading agent. It can cause redness and irritation of the eyes, myopia, astigmatism, iritis, and glaucoma; it causes changes in the trabecular meshwork (10).

A number of proteolytic enzymes can have toxic effects on the eyes. **Chymotrypsin** can cause corneal edema, uveitis, scleritis, or an increase in the IOP; it lyses zonular fibers causing forward displacement of the lens. **Fibrinolysin** can cause disturbance of the endothelium. **Ficin** can be injurious to the eye. **Protease** can cause corneal edema and severe exudative and fibrinous reactions. **Streptokinase** can cause iritis or retinitis. **Trypsin** can cause burning sensations of the eyes, loss of epithelium, destruction of the burning cornea, chorioretinitis, retinal degeneration, or cataract. **Urokinase** can cause irritation, clouding of the cornea, uveitis, increased or decreased IOP, hypopyon, or chemosis (10,442–444).

RARE-EARTH SALTS

Commonly encountered rare-earth salts include **dysprosium chloride, erbium chloride, gadolinium chloride, gadolinium nitrate, praseodymium chloride, samarium chloride, scandium chloride,** and **terbium chloride**. These salts all can cause irritation and redness and edema of the conjunctiva. Many produce conjunctival ulcers (**erbium chloride, dysprosium chloride, scandium chloride,** and **terbium chloride**) or corneal opacity and vascularization (**praseodymium chloride, samarium chloride, scandium chloride,** and **terbium chloride**). **Praseodymium chloride** also produces conjunctival hyperemia and corneal leukoma, and **terbium chloride** causes hyperemia of the iris (10,445–447).

Other rare-earth salts that cause irritation and conjunctival ulceration are **holmium chloride, thulium chloride, ytterbium chloride,** and **neodymium chloride** (446).

AGENTS FOR AGRICULTURAL USE

Blasticidin s is an antimicrobial agent used in agriculture. Accidental topical contamination can produce conjunctivitis, keratitis, or hyperemia of the iris (10,448).

Herbicides (weed killers) include **isocil, 4(2-methyl-4-chlorophenoxy) butryic acid, Natrin, monochloroacetic acid**, and **pentachlorophenol**. Herbicides can cause ocular irritation. **Monochloroacetic acid** can cause corneal epithelial injury. **Natrin** can cause severe damage to the eyes, and **pentachlorophenol** is suspected of causing retrobulbar neuritis (10,53,449–450).

Other herbicides include: **barban, *N-N*-diallyl-2-chloroacetamide (CDAA), 2,6-ditert-butyl-*p*-tolylmethylcarbamate (Azak), butofen, dinitro-*o*-cresol (DNOC), diquat, endothal, paraquat**, and ***s*-propyl butylethylthiocarbamate** (10,451–453). All of these chemicals can cause irritation. **Diquat** can cause hyperemia of the conjunctiva. **Paraquat** can cause loss of the conjunctival epithelium or loss of the corneal epithelium and corneal scarring (449,453). **Butofen** can cause damage to the cornea, and **CDAA** can cause serious damage to the whole eye.

Fertilizers include **ammonia, cyanamide, basic slag, superphosphate, sodium nitrate**, and **urea**. All can cause irritation and are caustic to the eyes. **Urea** may cause loosening of the epithelium from the stroma or a slow decrease in electrical resistance of the cornea. **Ammonia** (426–430) has many topical effects, including irritation, stinging and pain, tearing, and blepharospasm. Rarely, there is keratitis epithelialis. There may be fine, band-shaped cornea clouding, corneal endothelial damage, or corneal stroma edema. There may be iritis or lens damage; severe **ammonia** burns develop all the serious complications caused by strong alkalies in general (1,10,33,53,454–463).

Sodium nitrate may cause irritation, with tearing, blepharitis, conjunctival hyperemia, and conjunctivitis. There may be corneal infiltration, superficial corneal clouding, or clouding of the lens (53,445,464). **Calcium superphosphate** may cause irritation and corneal burns or even superficial necrosis of the cornea (10).

Soil fumigants include **sodium *N*-methyl-dithiocarbamate** and the so-called **DD mixture**. They can cause ocular irritation (465,466).

Arsenic trioxide is used in agriculture. It can cause the effects of irritation, itching, burning, lacrimation, and photophobia. There may be conjunctivitis, hyperemia, chemosis, or edema of the lids after topical contamination. Corneal injury and opacity may develop. When placed in the anterior chamber, **arsenic trioxide** produces a local necrotizing action (467–470).

SUBSTANCES FOR COMMERCIAL USE

A number of substances are used as bleaches: **chlorinated lime, hypochlorites, hypochlorite** and **ammonia mixtures, potassium persulfate**, and **sulfur dioxide**.

All bleaches could cause irritation, with a smarting, burning, or stinging sensation, pain and lacrimation. All but **potassium persulfate** cause hyperemia of the conjunctiva. **Hypochlorite** and **ammonia mixtures, sodium hypochlorite**, and **sulfur dioxide** can cause keratitis; **sulfur dioxide** also can cause conjunctivitis, corneal opacity, and vascularization and disturbance of vision. **Chlorinated lime** can cause caustic lime burns to the eye (10,53,471,472).

Cleaning agents include **nitrogen trichloride** and mixtures of compounds used as **oven cleaners**. These preparations can cause irritation and damage to the corneal epithelium and conjunctiva. **Drano** is a drain cleaner; in granular, solid form, it consists mainly of sodium hydroxide and can cause devastating damage to the eye (10,423–425,473–474).

Ozone, sodium hydroxide, and **sulfamic acid** are industrial cleaners. All three are irritating (475–477); **sulfamic acid** may cause swelling of the lids and blepharospasm and also may cause moderate conjunctivitis, edema, and keratitis (478,479). **Sodium hydroxide** causes erosion of the conjunctiva, devastating injuries of the eye, and increased IOP (10,53,423–425,475,480–484).

Shampoos may contain **pyrinate, cherimoya** or **cherimoya seeds, "Duponol WAT,"** or **selenium sulfide**. Topical side effects of shampoos can include ocular pain (after **pyrinate** or **cherimoya** or **cherimoya seeds),** irritation or superficial keratitis (**selenium sulfide**). There may be mild injury to the cornea (**"Duponol WAT"**), erosion of the epithelium (from **cherimoya** or **cherimoya seeds**), or loss of the corneal epithelium (**pyrinate**) (10,53,485–490).

Glues for gluing wood contain a urea-formaldehyde resin. This resin can cause photophobia, blepharospasm, and corneal disturbance (10,53,222,491–494).

Gold is sometimes toxic in industrial settings. Metallic **gold dust** can cause atrophic changes in the retina when introduced into the corneal stroma. **Gold chloride** can cause slight irritation, brown stains of the eye, iritis, nebula, or leukoma with vascularization. **Gold cyanide** induces corneal clouding and severe iritis. **Gold sodium thiosulfate** has been injected into the anterior chamber and has been found to cause injury to the endothelium, corneal edema, and vascularization (10,53,495–499).

Ethylene oxide is used as a fumigant for foodstuffs and medical devices. It can produce irritation, with soreness and a foreign-body sensation in the eye, tearing, conjunctivitis, or keratitis (500).

Matches ignite with a release of irritating oxides. They may cause allergic blepharitis and conjunctivitis (10).

Chemicals used in photography include **hydroquinone, lithium hydroxide,** and **trisodium phosphate**. These chemicals can produce irritation, photophobia, lacrimation, corneal injury, ulceration, or corneal opacification and vascularization. Chronic injury from **hydroquinone** can arise with discoloration, hypesthesia, distortion of the cornea, brownish staining in the cornea and conjunctiva, scarring of the corneal epithelium, corneal flattening, and stigmatism or disturbance of vision (10,501,502).

Depilatories are intended to remove hair and cause breakdown of beta-keratin. They are thus corrosive and cause injuries to the cornea resembling severe calcium hydroxide burns (10,53).

Ethylene glycol is used in antifreeze. Exposure to the vapor or spray causes ocular irritation, edema of the lids, and corneal opacity. When it is splashed into the eyes, there is discomfort with a temporary conjunctival reaction. After intracameral injection, iritis and corneal opacity develop (53,503–505).

***p*-Dichlorobenzene** is used to protect clothing against moths. This agent can cause irritation, ocular pain, or cataracts (53,506,507).

Sodium hexametaphosphate is the principal ingredient in water softeners. Side effects of topical contact with this compound include chemosis and hemorrhages in the conjunctiva and nictitating membrane (of species with a nictitating membrane), corneal edema, and hyperemia of the iris (10).

Many kinds of detergents are used in industry; many of them have been dealt with in the section on Surfactants. Other detergent agents are **carbon tetrachloride, polyethyleneglycol ethers, soaps, enzyme-detergent combinations,** and **pHisoHex. Soap** can cause stinging pain, conjunctival hyperemia, and damage of the corneal epithelium. **Polyetheyleneglycol ethers** can produce inflammation, corneal hypesthesia, corneal edema, ulceration, vascularization, and keratitis epithelialis. **pHisoHex** also can cause corneal edema, and **enzyme-detergent** combinations can cause transient conjunctivitis. **Carbon tetrachloride** can cause reduction of central visual acuity and visual field abnormalities (10,53,485,487,508,509).

Fire-extinguisher fluids may contain **carbon tetrachloride, methyl bromide, chlorobromomethane,** or **tetrachloroethylene.** These compounds may cause superficial injury to the eye. **Chlorobromomethane,** in particular, causes severe burning sensations, photophobia, hyperemia, and edema of the conjunctiva and lids; there may be transient corneal epithelial injury (53,510–516).

Acriflavine is a germicide with the side effects of irritation and of corneal injury, opacity, and vascularization (517).

Sodium chloride is used in many industrial situations and is also used as a topical agent to reduce corneal edema. Side effects include hyperemia and a transitory rise in the IOP (1,10,20,518,519). Solutions of **sodium chloride** that are used as topical osmotic agents may produce irritation, hyperemia, ocular pain and burning sensations, corneal dehydration, subconjunctival hemorrhages, or increases in IOP (520).

Antimony trichloride is highly corrosive. Topical effects include strong irritation and destruction of the cornea and conjunctiva (10,53).

SUBSTANCES FOR MEDICINAL USE

Ammonium chloride can cause hyperemia of the iris or hemorrhages of the iris. It may induce a salt cataract, or increase in the IOP or fibrin in the anterior chamber with corneal edema (521,522).

Ointments that contact the eye may cause interference with corneal wound healing. There may be intraocular penetration of ointment bases and oils. Water-soluble or greaseless ointment bases may cause keratitis (523).

Paraffin may cause considerable tissue reaction. There may be loss of vision following an embolic of **paraffin** reaching the retinal arteries. When paraffin is put into the anterior chamber, it causes slight inflammatory reactions and clouding of the cornea (10,524).

Radiopaque x-ray media are used in orbitography. One procedure involved retrobulbar injection of a mixture of 25% sodium diatrizoate and 1% lidocaine. This procedure caused rapidly reduced vision, dilation of the pupil, weakness of abduction, and nystagmus (525). In another case, an unidentified **radiopaque medium** caused pain, edema, diplopia, and severe granulomatous reaction when injected along the floor of the orbit (10).

Orbital injection of **diodone** causes edema of the lids and transient loss of vision (10). **Amylopectin sulfate** and **polyethylene sulfonic acid** were injected into the eye in a study of experimental retinal detachment. **Amylopectin** caused iritis and contraction of vitreous strands and retinal adhesions. **Polyethylene sulfonic acid** caused uveitis, vitreous opacities, partial liquefaction and formation of strands, detachment of the retina, cataract, dislocation of the lens, band keratopathy, and superficial calcification of the cornea (10,526).

Tattooing of the cornea may cause uveitis (10).

Gastric juice contaminating the eyes can cause corneal ulceration (10).

Hemoglobin, injected in the vitreous, caused damage of the rods; the so-called AU visual cells disappeared (527).

Catechol, in solid form, causes burns of the eye (528).

AGENTS OF INDUSTRIAL USE

Workers with aircraft and missiles have the potential danger of ocular contamination with some unusual agents. **Dural** causes irritation, conjunctivitis, and blepharitis. Propellants may be ocular toxins. **Pentaborane** produces miosis. **Tetranitromethane** produces irritation, and **methylhydrazine** causes corneal edema, swelling, and injury of the corneal epithelium (10,529–531).

Workers in building and masonry can come into contact with **calcium hydroxide** (slacked lime) and **calcium oxide** (quicklime). These agents have caustic effects resembling lime burns (532–536).

The chemical industry brings workers into proximity with a number of toxic chemicals. Methylating agents include **dimethyl sulfate, methyl bromide, methyl chloride**, and **methyl iodide**. All these agents produce irritation, and all except **methyl chloride** produce lacrimation. **Dimethyl sulfate** produces pain and photophobia, corneal opacity, and necrosis and edema of the lids. Conjunctival hyperemia is reported after exposure to **dimethyl sulfate** and **methyl chloride**. **Methyl bromide** and **methyl chloride** can produce blurring of vision and diplopia. **Methyl bromide** can produce retinal hemorrhage; **methyl chloride** can produce ptosis (537–541).

Agents used in routine organic synthesis can be toxic. The nature of the injury depends on the agent. **Acetonitrile** causes damage like acetone. **Diketene** and **thionyl chloride** cause irritation. **Methylamine** causes irritation, hemorrhages in the conjunctiva, corneal opacity, and edema. **Red phosphorus** is sometimes used in organic synthesis; when injected into the anterior chamber, it produces hypopyon and dilation of blood vessels of the iris. **Potassium metal** produces severe ocular injuries (10,542–545).

Other agents commonly used in chemical manufacture are **acetic anhydride, acetyl chloride, allyl chloride, barium hydroxide, boron tribromide, chlorosulfonic acid, cyanic acid, cyclododecatriene, ethylenimine, mercuric iodide, phosphorus trichloride, piperidine,** and **triethylamine** (546). All cause irritation; many cause severe damage to the eyes (**acetyl chloride, barium hydroxide, chlorosulfonic acid,** and **triethylamine**). **Acetic anhydride** causes burning sensations and photophobia and edema of the eyelids or conjunctiva. **Acetic anhydride, cyanic acid,** and **ethylenimine** can produce lacrimation. **Chlorosulfonic acid** causes swelling of the lids. **Cyclododecatriene, ethylenimine,** and **phosphorus trichloride** can produce conjunctivitis; **cyclododecatriene** can also cause dermatitis of the lids. **Acetic anhydride** and **chlorosulfonic acid** can cause corneal edema; **ethylenimine** can cause keratitis. Many agents (**acetic anhydride, barium hydroxide, boron tribromide, phosphorus trichloride,** and **piperidine**) can cause clouding or opacity of the cornea; **boron tribromide** also causes corneal hypesthesia, scarring, and vascularization. **Acetic anhydride, boron tribromide,** and **triethylamine** all can cause erosions to the eye; when injected into the anterior chamber they produce damage to the eye, purulent exudate, and inflammation (10,547–551).

Many substances are used as catalysts in industrial synthesis. Common catalysts with ocular toxic properties include **aluminum alkyls, antimony pentachloride, *t*-butyl hydroperoxide, cyclohexanone peroxide, diacetyl peroxide, *N*-methyl morpholine, osmium tetroxide,** various **organic peroxides, phosphorus pentachloride, silver(II)oxide, tetramethylbutanediamine, triethylenediamine,** and **vanadium pentoxide** (10,546,552,553).

Antimony pentachloride can cause severe injury to the eyes. **Cyclohexanone peroxide** can cause moderately severe corneal injury with superficial opacity and associated conjunctival inflammation. ***t*-Butyl hydroperoxide** and ***N*-methyl morpholine** can cause moderate injury of the eyes; ***N*-methyl morpholine** can also cause sloughing of the epithelium, corneal haze or conjunctival hyperemia. **Osmium tetroxide** can cause keratitis epithelialis or blurring of vision by fixing corneal proteins. **Diacetyl peroxide** (546), **tetramethylbutanediamine,** and **triethylenediamine** can all cause corneal damage, irritation, lacrimation, burning sensations, ocular pain, and photophobia. Corneal epithelial edema can be produced by ***N*-methyl morpholine, osmium tetroxide, tetramethylbutanediamine,** or **triethylenediamine; tetramethylbutanediamine** also can cause mydriasis and cycloplegia. **Vanadium pentoxide** can cause conjunctivitis (10).

Calcium chloride and **phosphorus peroxide** are used as drying and dehydrating agents. They can cause irritation on topical exposure. **Calcium chloride** can produce superficial injuries to the eye and miosis (554–557); **phosphorus peroxide** is more dangerous, causing burns to the lids, conjunctiva, and cornea, and leaving blue-white opacities (10,546).

Many chemicals are used in the manufacture of dyes, including **acrylamide, anthraquinone, aniline, benzene, barium chloride, bis-(chloromethyl) anthra-**

cene, **benzoyl chloride, 2,4-dinitrophenol (DNP), lactic acid, manganese compounds, nitric acid, *m*-nitroaniline, nitronaphthalene, oxalic acid, *p*-phenylenediamine, phthalic anhydride, quinones, sodium hydrosulfite, titanium tetrachloride**, and ***o*-toluidine**. All these agents can produce ocular irritation; other side effects depend on the agent. **Anthraquinone** can produce inflammation, and injuries to the eyes can follow exposure to **benzoyl chloride, 2,4-dinitrophenol, *o*-toluidine**, or **titanium tetrachloride. Bis-(chloromethyl) anthracene** can induce blepharospasm and, like ***p*-phenylenediamine**, may produce conjunctival hyperemia. Conjunctival edema may follow exposure to ***p*-phenylenediamine** or **sodium hydrosulfite**. Conjunctivitis may be induced by ***p*-phenylenediamine** and **phthalic anhydride. Nitric acid** can produce necrosis of the eyelids or conjunctiva, and sometimes symblepharon. **Quinones** and ***m*-nitroaniline** can stain the conjunctiva. Superficial corneal injury can follow exposure to **acrylamide**; there also may be vitreous opacities. Corneal opacity and clouding can be produced by **bis-(chloromethyl) anthracene, *m*-nitroaniline, oxalic acid, *p*-phenylenediamine**, and **nitric acid. Lactic acid** can cause corneal epithelial coagulation and, sometimes, corneal necrosis, perforation, and vascularization or hypopyon; **nitronaphthalene** can cause keratitis. Corneal ulceration can be produced by ***p*-phenylenediamine**, and corneal opacification and vascularization can be produced by **manganese compounds. Acrylamide, barium chloride**, and ***p*-phenylenediamine** can produce iritis or iridocyclitis. **Phthalic anhydride** can produce exophthalmos or proptosis. Cataract can follow exposure to **acrylamide, lactic acid**, or **nitronaphthalene** (558–576).

Agents used in the explosives industry include **nitrogen dioxide, sulfuric acid, sulfur trioxide, tetryl, trinitrobenzene, fulfuric acid**, and **trinitrotoluene (TNT)**. All these substances except **trinitrobenzene** can cause irritation. **Sulfuric acid** and **sulfur trioxide** can cause devastating damage to the eye. **Tetryl** can cause dermatitis of the eyelids and conjunctivitis or keratitis and iridocyclitis. **Nitrogen dioxide** can cause damage of the corneal epithelium and corneal opacity. **Sulfuric acid** and **trinitrotoluene** can induce cataract, and **fulfuric acid** can induce glaucoma. **Trinitrobenzene** can cause yellowing of the conjunctiva or sclera or optic neuritis and amblyopia. **Trinitrotoluene** can cause disturbance of vision, pupil dilation, blurring, and hyperemia of the optic nerve heads (10,577–579).

Fuels are of many kinds; some of the fuels used in industry or in hobbies include **dimethylamineborane, dimethylhydrazine, fuel for model airplanes** (a mixture of methyl alcohol, nitromethane or nitropropane, and castor oil), **hydrazine, petroleum products** and, at some places, **uranium compounds**. All can cause irritation. **Dimethylamineborane** and **petroleum products** cause hyperemia of the conjunctiva; **dimethylamineborane** and **fuel for model airplanes** can cause conjunctival edema. **Uranium compounds** are capable of producing moderately severe injury to the eyes and necrosis of the eyelids and conjunctiva; they also may produce perforating ulceration of the cornea. **Fuel for model airplanes** and **petroleum products** can cause injury to the corneal epithelium. **Petroleum products** can cause cataract and, after subconjunctival injection, they may cause chemosis and exophthalmos and corneal clouding (10,580–583).

The manufacture of lubricants involves some special compounds: **barium oxide, decyl alcohol,** and **silicone oil. Decyl alcohol** is slightly injurious to the eyes, but **barium oxide** causes severe alkali burns of the eyes (584). **Silicone oil** causes corneal edema, vascularization and scarring, glaucoma, and cataract (585–588).

The manufacture of apparatus for laboratory use involves the use of some particular compounds: **platinum salts** and **polytetrafluoroethylene**. These substances cause irritation and lacrimation. **Platinum salts** cause burning sensations, photophobia, and conjunctival hyperemia. **Polytetrafluoroethylene** can cause etching of the cornea (588–591).

Some compounds encountered in the pharmaceutic industry include **bromal *n*-butyl amine, dichloroethyl acetate** (592), **halazone, methyl cellulose, *o*-nitrobenzylchloride, phenothiazine, phosphoric acid, polysorbate 80, tartaric acid**, and **triethanolamine**. All these substances, except **methylcellulose** and **polysorbate 80**, cause irritation. Severe injury to the eyes can be induced by ***n*-butyl amine. Phosphoric acid** and **triethanolamine** can cause hyperemia of the conjunctiva. **Dichloroethyl acetate** can cause conjunctivitis and corneal ulceration. Corneal edema can be induced by **phosphoric acid, polysorbate 80**, and **triethanolamine. Triethanolamine** also can produce hyperemia of the iris. **Methyl cellulose** can produce iridocyclitis and increases in the IOP, and **phenothiazine** can cause corneal keratitis (10,593–596).

Compounds used in the manufacture of plastics include **acrylic acid, acrylonitrile, dibutyl phthalate, dibutyl tin dichloride, ethyl acrylate, furfural, levulinic acid, methocryonitrile, methyl acrylate, polyvinyl chloride, toluene diisocyanates, tributyl phosphate**, and **vinyl acetate**. Side effects depend on the compound. **Vinyl acetate** can cause slight injury to the eyes; **methyl acetate** causes mild injury, whereas **acrylic acid** and **levulinic acid** cause severe injury to the eyes. **Methocryonitrile** and **toluene diisocyanates** cause irritation and blepharospasm; these compounds, as well as **methyl acrylate** and **dibutyl tin dichloride** can cause lacrimation. **Furfural** and **toluene diisocyanates** can cause swelling of the eyelids or corneal edema. **Toluene diisocyanates** can cause hyperemia of the conjunctiva, and **fufural** can cause hemorrhage of the conjunctiva. **Acrylonitrile** can cause transient disturbance of the cornea. **Ethyl acrylate** and **tributyl phosphate** can cause injury to the epithelium (10,597–608).

Gilsonite is a mineral hydrocarbon used in making roads and roofs and causes irritation (609).

Arsenic trichloride is used in the ceramic industry. It can produce irritation, blepharospasm, photophobia, or lacrimation. There may be redness of the conjunctiva after exposure, corneal ulceration, and corneal opacity (610).

Lead chloride is used in the manufacture of white lead. It causes moderate purulent reactions and general inflammation of the eye (10).

Agents used in the manufacture of perfumes include **acetophenone** (608), **allyl bromide, menthol, methylal, methyl salicylate, 1-naphthol, octanol, oil of citro-**

nella, phenethyl alcohol, and **propyl acetate. Oil of citronella** and **methyl salicylate** can cause slight eye injury; **acetophenone, menthol,** and **1-naphthol** can cause severe injury. **Octanol** can cause irritation and corneal epithelial injury, whereas **phenethyl alcohol** can cause clouding of the epithelium (10,611-615).

Industrial reducing agents include **calcium carbide** and **lithium hydride. Calcium carbide** causes injuries like lime burns. **Lithium hydride** causes irritation, inflammation, corneal opacity, and ulceration (10,616).

The manufacture of matches uses **white phosphorus** and **phosphorus sesquisulfide. White phosphorus** causes blepharospasm, photophobia, lacrimation, corneal opacity, interstitial vascularization, episcleritis, and inflammation of the eye. **Phosphorous sesquisulfide** causes irritation, blepharitis, and conjunctivitis (10,162).

Chemicals used in the manufacture of rubber include **chloroprene, cyclohexylamine, diethanolamine, dibenzathiazyl disulfide, diethylamine, 1,3-diethylthiourea, dimethylamine, diphenyl guanidine, 1-mercaptobenzothiazole, methyl vinyl ketone, styrene, sulfur monochloride,** and **thiram. Cyclohexylamine** and **dimethylamine** can cause severe injury to the eye; **diethanolamine** causes moderate injury. **Sulfur monochloride** causes irritation and corrosion. **Diphenyl guanidine** causes conjunctival edema, whereas **styrene** causes hyperemia of the conjunctiva. **Dimethylamine** can cause hemorrhage of the conjunctiva or corneal edema and infiltration, and **1,3-diethylthiourea** can cause keratitis or ocular pain with photophobia and blurred vision. **Chloroprene** and **methyl vinyl ketone** can cause conjunctivitis; these agents, as well as **diethylamine** and **styrene** can cause corneal epithelial injury. **Diphenyl guanidine** and **1,3-diethylthiourea** can cause punctate corneal epithelial defects, whereas **cyclohexylamine, diethylamine,** and **dimethylamine** can cause corneal opacity (10,617-632).

The manufacture of soaps involves the use of **oleic acid, potassium carbonate, potassium hydroxide, sodium aluminate, sodium carbonate,** and **sodium silicate. Potassium hydroxide** and **sodium aluminate** cause injuries like alkali burns. **Oleic acid** causes inflammation, scarring, necrosis, and vascularization of the eyes and corneal abscess. **Potassium carbonate** induces ocular pain and slight transient optical irregularities of the epithelium. **Sodium carbonate** and **sodium silicate** cause damage of the corneal epithelium (10,633-640).

Thioglycolic acid is a reagent that causes ocular pian, conjunctival edema, hyperemia, necrotic neovascularization, and corneal opacity (641).

Synthesis of resins involves the use of **diglycidylresorcinol, epon, maleic acid,** and **maleic anhydride.** These agents produce irritation. **Maleic anhydride** produces burning sensations in the eyes, whereas **maleic acid** causes conjunctival hyperemia and corneal edema, opacity, and vascularization (642-647).

Manufacture of textiles, woolens, and cloth involves some special reagents. Manufacture of textiles involves **carbon disulfide, divinyl sulfone, glycolic acid, naphthalenebutylsulfonate sodium,** and **thioformaldehyde. Divinyl sulfone** causes severe burns; **glycolic acid** causes irritation and moderately severe injury. **Carbon disulfide** causes keratitis epithelialis, retrobulbar neuritis, and disturbance of vision. Manufacture of woolens involves **ficin,** which induces injuries to the eyes. Manufacture of some kinds of cloth involves **urea-formaldehyde,** which causes irritation of the eye. Manufacture of nylon involves **1,6-hexanediamine,** which causes ocular irritation (648–652).

Nitrocellulose paint or **lacquer** can cause keratitis, cataract, and optic neuritis (10,653).

Manufacture of glass requires **silica,** which causes inflammation of the eye, corneal edema, opacity and vascularization, necrosis of the retina, and atrophy of the choroid. Removing color from glass involves **sodium selenite,** which causes severe injury to the eyes (654–656).

Compounds used in soldering are **fluorides, zinc chloride,** and **zinc sulfate. Zinc chloride** causes pain and redness of the eye, it can cause corneal ulcer, vascularization, and opacity. It also may cause iritis or acute angle-closure glaucoma. **Fluorides** are necrotic to the conjunctiva and cause inflammation of the eye or corneal edema. Both **fluorides** and **zinc chloride** can cause injury of the epithelium or hemorrhages of the iris. **Zinc chloride** and **zinc sulfate** can cause cataract (10,657–661).

Manufacture of batteries involves **lead sulfate** and **nickel metal.** When **lead sulfate** was placed in the anterior chamber, it produced a moderate purulent reaction and inflammation of the eye. **Nickel metal** can cause conjunctivitis and epiphora (20,662).

Allyl amines are used in the manufacture of mercurial diuretics. They cause severe ocular irritation (10).

Compounds used in the cotton industry include **aniline, pyridine, formaldehyde, nitrogen oxide, hydrochloric acid, sulfuric acid,** and **sodium hydroxide.** Some of these substances are discussed elsewhere in this chapter. All of them cause clouding of the corneal stroma, vitreous opacities, retinal arteriosclerosis, and myopia (637,663–668).

Fiberglass dust can cause irritation of the conjunctiva and cornea (669,670).

Strontium hydroxide is used in the refining of sugar. It causes serious burns to the eyes like other strong alkalies (10).

Hydrofluoric acid (HF) is used in the cleaning of cast iron, copper, and brass, and in etching glass. It causes irritation, ocular pain, conjunctival hyperemia, loss of the epithelium from the cornea and conjunctiva, and edema of the lid, conjunctiva, and cornea (671,672).

Yttrium chloride is a rare-earth metal salt used in preparation of pure metal. It can cause corneal opacity and corneal vascularization (673,674).

Indium trichloride is used in electroplating; it causes irritation (675).

Copper cyanide plating bath is used in the electroplating of copper and can cause alkali burns (162).

Some chemicals and substances used in the automotive industry are ocular toxins. **Brake fluid** is composed of alcohols, glycols, and a lubricant, such as castor oil. Topical contamination causes severe smarting and burning sensations and injury of the corneal epithelium (10).

Tetraethyl lead is a gasoline additive. It can cause slight mydriasis, photophobia, smarting sensations, blepharospasms, and contractions of the visual field (10).

Cobalt compounds are used to make metal alloys. These compounds can cause corneal injury, corneal opacification and vascularization, and uveitis (676,677).

The manufacture of mirrors involves the use of **mercury metal (liquid)** or of **silver metal, silver ammonium compounds,** or **silver nitrate. Liquid mercury metal** causes corneal opacity, band keratopathy, purulent reactions, local abscesses, detachment of the retina, and shrinkage and atrophy of the eye. **Silver nitrate** can cause argyria and edema of the conjunctiva and lids, symblepharon, or cataract. **Silver ammonium compounds** and **silver nitrate** can cause corneal opacity and scarring, whereas exposure to **silver metal** can cause retinal atrophy (678–680).

Makare is a wood used in cabinet making. Exposure to **makare** dust causes ocular irritation with lacrimation and swelling of the eyelids (10).

Pinha is a substance employed in the preparation of an alcoholic tincture used in repelling lice. It can induce the side effects of edema and erosions of the corneal epithelium, chemosis of the conjunctiva, and dermatitis of the lids (10).

The synthesis of polymers can involve the use of **methyl polymers** and **diepoxybutane. Methyl polymers** can cause ocular irritation. **Diepoxybutane** can cause severe injury, with loosening and sloughing of the epithelium, and opacification of the corneal stroma with scarring and vascularization (10,681,682).

Bicycloheptadiene dibromide is an alkylating agent. It can cause conjunctivitis and hemorrhage in the fundus (10).

Difluoro ia an intermediate in the chemical manufacture of **sarin. Difluoro** can cause irritation and opacity (see War Gases).

There are a number of miscellaneous compounds used in manufacturing that can be ocular toxins. **Nitrosomethyl urethane** is used in the synthesis of diazomethane (683). It can produce irritation, hyperemia, blepharospasm, chemosis, and loss of the corneal epithelium or edema of the corneal epithelium. There may be keratitis, epithelialis, and blurring of vision after exposure. **Sulfosalicylic acid** is used in the precipitation of proteins. It can cause hazing of the cornea and hyperemia of the iris. **Tetraethoxysilane** is used as a water-proofing agent. It can cause ocular irritation and opacities of the cornea; **1,3-butadiene** and **1,4-butynediol** can cause irritation. **Copper chloride** can cause severe injury to the cornea with permanent opacification. **Iodine monobromide** can cause corrosion of the eye. **Methyl *n*-butyl ketone** causes moderate irritation (683). **Tantalum fluoride** causes burns of the cornea (684). **Mortar, plaster,** and **Portland cement** cause injuries like a lime burn (10,162,681,685–689).

References

1. Fraunfelder FT. *Drug-induced ocular side effects and drug interactions*, 2nd ed. Philadelphia: Lea & Febiger, 1982;364–372.
2. Fraunfelder FT, Scafidi AF. Possible adverse effects from topical ocular 10% phenylephrine. *Am J Ophthalmol* 1978;85:447.
3. Haddad NJ, Moyer NJ, Riley FC. Mydriatic effect of phenylephrine hydrochloride. *Am J Ophthalmol* 1970;70:729.

4. McReynolds WU, Havener WH, Henderson JW. Hazards of the use of sympathomimetic drugs in ophthalmology. *Arch Ophthalmol* 1956;56:176.
5. Mitchell DWA. The effect of ephedrine instillations on intraocular pressure. *Br J Phyiol Opt* 1957;14:38.
6. Drance SM, Ross RA. The ocular effects of epinephrine. *Surv Ophthalmol* 1970;14:330.
7. Hull DS. Effect of norepinephrine on the corneal epithelium. *Am J Ophthalmol* 1975;79:245.
8. Gilman AG, Goodman LS, Gilman A, eds. *The pharmacological basis of therapeutics*, 6th ed. New York: Macmillan, 1980;151-153,164-166.
9. Pollack IP, Rossi, H. Norepinephrine in the treatment of ocular hypertension and glaucoma. *Arch Ophthalmol* 1975;93:173.
10. Grant, WM. *Toxicology of the eye*, 3rd ed. Springfield, IL: Charles C. Thomas, 1986.
11. Cote G, Drance SM. The effect of propranolol on human intraocular pressure. *Can J Ophthalmol* 1968;3:207.
12. Felix RH, Ive FA, Dahl MGC. Cutaneous and ocular reactions to practolol. *Br Med J* 1973;2:452.
13. Rahi AHS. Pathology of practolol-induced ocular toxicity. *Br J Ophthalmol* 1976;60:312.
14. Bucci MG. Topical administration of oxprenolol (beta blocking agent) in the therapy of glaucoma. Preliminary note. *Bull Oculist* 1975;54:235.
15. Holt PJA, Waddington E. Oculocutaneous reaction to oxprenolol. *Br Med J* 1975;2:539.
16. Lewis BS, Setzen M, Kokoris N. Ocular reaction to oxprenolol. A case report. *S Afr Med J* 1976;50:482.
17. Wills JH. Toxicity of anticholinesterases and treatment of poisoning. In: Karacaman AG, ed. *Anticholinesterase agents, international encyclopedia of pharmacology and therapeutics*. Oxford: Pergamon Press, 1970;355.
18. Duke-Elder S. *System of ophthalmology*, vol 14, pt. 2. St. Louis: C.V. Mosby, 1972;1046.
19. Sugar S, Santos R. The priscoline provocation test. *Am J Ophthalmol* 1955;40:510.
20. Walsh FB, Hoyt WF. *Clinical neuro-ophthalmology*, vol 1, 3rd ed. Baltimore: Williams and Wilkins, 1969;447.
21. Kaback MB. The effects of dipivalyl epinephrine on the eye. *Am J Ophthalmol* 1976;81:768.
22. Theodore J, Leibowitz HM. External ocular toxicity of dipivalyl epinephrine. *Am J Ophthalmol* 1979;88:1013.
23. Becker B, Morton WR. Topical epinephrine in glaucoma suspects. *Am J Ophthalmol* 1966;62:272.
24. Waltman SR. Corneal endothelial changes with long-term topical epinephrine therapy. *Arch Ophthalmol* 1977;95:1357.
25. Fraunfelder FT. Interim report: National Registry of Possible Drug-Induced Ocular Side Effects. *Ophthalmology* 1980;87:87.
26. Van Buskirk EM. Adverse reactions from timolol administration. *Ophthalmology* 1980;87:447.
27. Wilson RP, Spaeth GL, Poryzees E. The place of timolol in the practice of ophthalmology. *Ophthalmology* 1980;87:451.
28. Bonomi L, Di Comite P. Outflow facility after guanethidine sulfate administration. *Arch Ophthalmol* 1967;78:337.
29. Davidson SI. Reports of ocular adverse reactions. *Trans Ophthalmol Soc UK* 1973;93:495.
30. *AMA drug evaluations*, 4th ed. New York: John Wiley, 1980;365-366, 403.
31. Hovland KR. Effects of drugs on aqueous humor dynamics. *Int Ophthalmol Clin* 1971;11:99.
32. Virno M. Oral glycerol in ophthalmology. *Am J Ophthalmol* 1963;55:1133.
33. Havener WH. *Ocular pharmacology*, 4th ed. St. Louis: C.V. Mosby, 1978;263-264.
34. Ellis PP. *Ocular therapeutics and pharmacology*, 5th ed. St. Louis: C.V. Mosby, 1977;16,47,50,187.
35. Fraunfelder FT. Corneal edema after use of carbachol. *Arch Ophthalmol* 1979;97:975.
36. Vaughn ED, Hull DS, Green K. Effect of intraocular miotics on corneal endothelium. *Arch Ophthalmol* 1978;96:1897.
37. Hockwin O, Swanson A. Comments on the influence of miotics on the lens. *Ann Ophthalmol* 1976;8:895-896.
38. Axelsohn U, Holmberg A. The frequency of cataract after miotic therapy. *Acta Ophthalmol* 1973;44:421-429.
39. Axelsohn U. Glaucoma, miotic therapy and cataract. *Acta Ophthalmol* 1986;46:83-105.
40. Muller HK, Kleifeld O, Hockwin O, Dardenne U. Der Einfluss von Pilocarpin und Mintacol auf den Stoffwechsel der Linse. *Ber dt Ophthal Ges* 1956;60:115-118.
41. Lebensohn JE. Spectacular adverse reactions from pilocarpine. *Am J Ophthalmol* 1977;83:281.
42. *Physician's desk reference*, 42nd ed. Oradell, NJ: Edward R. Barnhart, 1988;1334.

43. Awan KJ. Adverse systemic reactions of topical cyclopentolate hydrochloride. *Ann Ophthalmol* 1976;8:695.
44. Ostler HB. Cycloplegics and mydriatics. Tolerance, habituation and addiction after topical administration. *Arch Ophthalmol* 1975;93:432.
45. Simcoe CW. Cyclopentolate (Cyclogyl) toxicity. *Arch Ophthalmol* 1962;67:406.
46. German E, Siddiqui N. Atropine toxicity from eyedrops. *N Engl J Med* 1970;282:689.
47. Mann I, Pirie A, Pullinger BD. An experimental and clinical study of the reaction of the anterior segment of the eye to chemical injury, with special reference to chemical warfare agents. *Br J Ophthalmol (Suppl)* 1948;13:1.
48. Maumenee AE, Scholz RO. The histopathology of the ocular lesions produced by the sulfur and nitrogen mustards. *Bull Johns Hopkins Hosp* 1948;82:121.
49. NTP Working Group. Toxicology and carcinogenesis studies of hexachloroethane in F344/N rats (gavage study). *National Toxicology Program Technical Report Series* 1989;361:120.
50. Hochmeister M, Vycudilik W. Morpho-toxicological findings following war gas effect (S-Last). *Beitr Gerichtl Med* 1989;47:533–538.
51. Jager BV, Stagg GN. Toxicity of diacetyl monoxime and of pyridine-2-aldoxime methiodide in man. *Bull Johns Hopkins Hosp* 1958;102:203.
52. Byron HM, Posner H. Clinical evaluation of Protopam. *Am J Ophthalmol* 1964;57:409.
53. Haddad LM, Winchester JF. *Clinical management of poisoning and drug overdose*. Philadelphia: W.B. Saunders, 1990;130:315–316.
54. Spada CS, Woodward DF, Hawley SB, Nieves AL, Williams LS, Feldman BJ. Synergistic effects of LTB4 and LTD4 on leucocyte emigration into the guinea pig conjunctiva. *Am J Pathol* 1988;130:354–368.
55. Fleisher LN. Effects of inhibitors of arachidonic acid metabolism on endotoxin-induced ocular inflammation. *Curr Eye Res* 1988;7:321–327.
56. Campochiaro PA, Sen HA. Adenosine and its agonists cause retinal vasodilation and hemorrhages. Implication for ischemic retinopathies. *Arch Ophthalmol* 1989;107:412–416.
57. Wyngaarden VB, Seevers MH. Toxic effects of antihistamine drugs. *JAMA* 1951;145:277.
58. Dukes MNG, ed. *Meyler's side effects of drugs*, vol 9. Amsterdam: Excerpta Medica, 1980;265–268.
59. Robertson DM, Hollenhorst RW, Callahan JA. Ocular manifestations of digitalis toxicity. *Arch Ophthalmol* 1966;76:640.
60. Weleber RB, Shults WT. Digoxin retinal toxicity. Clinical and electrophysiologic evaluation of a cone dysfunction syndrome. *Arch Ophthalmol* 1981;99:1568.
61. Cristini G, Pagliarani N. Amyl nitrate test in primary glaucoma. *Br J Ophthalmol* 1953;37:741.
62. Robertson D, Steves RM. Nitrates and glaucoma. *JAMA* 1977;237:117.
63. Blake J, Cassidy H. Ocular hypersensitivity to dextran. *Ir J Med Sci* 1979;148:249.
64. Fothergill R, Heaney GA. Reactions to dextran. *Br J Med* 1976;2:11502.
65. Aronson SB, Elliott JH. *Ocular inflammation*. St. Louis: C.V. Mosby, 1972;91–92.
66. Chiou GCY, Chuang CY. Improvement of systemic absorption of insulin through eyes with absorption enhancers. *J Pharm Sci* 1989;78:815–818.
67. Chiou GCY, Chuang CY, Chang MS. Systemic delivery of insulin through eyes to lower the glucose concentration. *J Ocular Pharmacol* 1989;5:81–91.
68. Merchant JA. Epidemiological assessment of laboratory animal allergy. In: *Crisp data base*. Washington, DC: National Institutes of Health, 1988.
69. Oliver KT, Havener WH. Eye manifestations of chronic vitamin A intoxication. *Arch Ophthalmol* 1958;60:19.
70. Turtz CA, Turtz AL. Vitamin-A intoxication. *Am J Ophthalmol* 1960;50:165.
71. Chisholm JF. Iron pigmentation of the palpebral conjunctiva. *Am J Ophthalmol* 1930;3:1108.
72. BIBRA Working Group. Chlorobutanol. In: *Toxicity profile*. Brit Ind Biol Res Assoc, 1989;5.
73. Tripathi BJ, Tripathi RC. Cytotoxic effects of benzalconium chloride and chlorbutanol on human corneal epithelial cells *in vitro*. *Lens Eye Tox Res* 1989;6:395–403.
74. Adams AJ, Brown B. Alcohol prolongs time course of glare recovery. *Nature* 1975;257:481
75. Gramberg-Danielsen B. Ophthalmological findings after the use of alcohol. *Zentralbl Verkehrs-Med* 1965;11:129.
76. Olurin O, Osuntokun O. Complications of retrobulbar alcohol injections. *Ann Ophthalmol* 1978;10:474.
77. Kaplan MR, Pilger IS. The effect of rauwolfia serpentina derivatives on intraocular pressure. *Am J Ophthalmol* 1957;43:550.

78. Raymond LF. Ocular pathology in reserpine sensitivity. Report of two cases. *J Med Soc NJ* 1963;60:417.
79. Davidson SI. Reports of ocular adverse reactions. *Trans Ophthalmol Soc UK* 1973;93:495.
80. Spiers ASD. Mydriatic response to sympathomimetic amines in patients treated with L-dopa. *Lancet* 1969;2:1301.
81. *American hospital formulary service*, vol 2. Washington, DC: American Society of Hospital Pharmacists, 1974;72-100.
82. Burns RP, Gipson I. Toxic effects of local anesthetics. *JAMA* 1978;240:347.
83. Fraunfelder FT, Sharp JD, Silver BE. Possible adverse effects from topical anesthetics. *Doc Ophthalmol* 1979;18:341.
84. Siegel RK. Cocaine hallucinations. *Am J Psychiatry* 1978;135:309.
85. Ros AM, Juhlin L, Michaelsson G. A follow-up study of patient with recurrent urticaria and hypersensitivity to aspirin, benzoates, and azo dyes. *Br J Dermatol* 1976;95:19.
86. Gorn RA. The detrimental effect of aspirin on hyphema rebleed. *Ann Ophthalmol* 1979;11:351.
87. Smith GF. Trichloroethylene: a review. *Br J Ind Med* 1966;23:249.
88. Vernon RJ, Ferguson RK. Effects of trichloroethylene on visual motor performance. *Arch Environ Health* 1969;18:894.
89. Gibbons RB. Complications of chrysotherapy. A review of recent studies. *Arch Intern Med* 1979;139:343.
90. Roberts WH, Wolter JR. Ocular chrysiasis. *Arch Ophthalmol* 1956;56:48.
91. Estable JJ. The ocular effect of several irritant drugs applied directly to the conjunctiva. *Am J Ophthalmol* 1948;31:837.
92. Anon. Final report on the safety assessment of stearate-2, -4, -6, -7, -10, -11, -13, -15 and -20. *Am J Coll Toxicol* 1988;7:881-910.
93. Lazenby GW, Reed JW, Grant WM. Anticholinergic medication in open-angle glaucoma. Long term tests. *Arch Ophthalmol* 1970;84:719.
94. German E, Siddqui N. Atropine toxicity from eyedrops. *N Engl J Med* 1970;282:689.
95. EPA Working Group. Mercury health effects update. In: *Health Issue Reassessment*. Document EPA-600/8-84-019F, Washington, DC: EPA, 1984.
96. Mazzanti G, Bolle P, Martinoli L, Piccinelli D, Gagurina E, Animati F, Mugne Y. Croton acrostachys, a plant used in traditional medicine: purgative and inflammatory activity. *J Ethnopharmacol* 1987;19:213-219.
97. Hull DS. Drugs, pathological conditions and corneal epithelium (rabbits). In: *Crisp data base*. Washington, DC: National Institutes of Health, 1988.
98. Willis SM, Stephens CJM, Wilkinson J. Experimentally-induced irritant contact dermatitis. Determination of optimum initial concentrations. *Contact Dermatitis* 1988;18:20-24.
99. Thirumalaikolundusubramanian P, Chandramohen M, Johnson ES. Copper sulphate poisoning. *J Indian Med Assoc* 1984;82:6.
100. Crews SJ. Ocular adverse reaction to drugs. *Practitioner* 1977;219:72.
101. Cole JG, Cole HG, Janoff LA. A toxic ocular manifestation of chloramphenicol therapy. *Am J Ophthalmol* 1957;44:18.
102. Lamda PA, Sood NN, Moorthy SS. Retinopathy due to chloramphenicol. *Scott Med J* 1968;13:166.
103. Krejci L, Brettschneider I. Yellow-brown cornea: a complication of topical use of tetracycline. *Ophthalmic Res* 1978;10:131.
104. Lund MH. Colistin sulfate ophthalmic in the treatment of ocular infections. *Arch Ophthalmol* 1968;81:4.
105. Edwards TS. Transcient myopia due to tetracycline. *JAMA* 1963;186:69.
106. Francois J, Mortiers P. The injurious effects of locally and generally applied antibiotics on the eye. *T Geneestd* 1976;32:139.
107. Boettner EA, Fralick FB, Wolter JR. Conjunctival concretions of sulfadiazine. *Arch Ophthalmol* 1974;92:446.
108. Haviland JW, Long PH. Skin and ocular reactions to sulfathiazole therapy. *Bull Johns Hopkins Hosp* 1940;66:263.
109. Zylic Z, De Grip WJ, Wagener DJ, Van Rennes H, Van der Kleijn E, Van den Brock LA, Ottenheijm HD. Studies on retinotoxic potential of a novel antitumor antibiotic—sparsomycin—in rats. *Anticancer Res* 1989;9:923-927.
110. Goldstein JH. Effects of drugs on cornea, conjunctiva and lids. *Int Ophthalmol Clin* 1971;11:13.
111. Grayson M, Pieroni D. Severe silver nitrate injury to the eye. *Am J Ophthalmol* 1970;70:227.

112. Rosen E. Argyrolentis. *Am J Ophthalmol* 1950;33:797.
113. Elliott GA, Schut AL. Studies with cytarabine HCI (CA) in normal eyes of man, monkey and rabbit. *Am J Ophthalmol* 1965;60:1074.
114. Itoi M. Teratogenicities of ophthalmic drugs. I. Antiviral ophthalmic drugs. *Arch Ophthalmol* 1975;93:46.
115. Doukan G. Venerologie d'antefois. *Rev Prat* 1990;40:1689-1690.
116. Jones RD. Xylene/amitraz: a pharmacological review and profile. *Vet Hum Toxicol* 1990;32:446-448.
117. Meylan W, Papa L, De Rose CT, Stura JF. Chemical of current interest: propylene oxide: health and environmental effects profile. *Toxicol Ind Health* 1986;2:219-260.
118. Hayka BJ, Zhu L, Sens D, Tapert MJ, Crouch RK. Cytolysis of corneal epithelial cells by hydrogen peroxide. *Exp Eye Res* 1990;50:11-16.
119. Von Berg R. Toxicology update. *J Appl Toxicol* 1988;8:145-148.
120. Khurana AK, Ahluwalic BK, Scod S. Savlon keratopathy a clinical profile. *Acta Ophthalmol (Copenh)* 1989;67:465-466.
121. Anon. *Cresols, all isomers.* U.S. Department of Health and Human Services. Cincinnati: Public Health Service, Center for Disease Control, 1988.
122. Kanerva L, Estlander T, Jolanki R. Allergic contact dermatitis from dental composite resins due to aromatic epoxy acrylates and aliphatic acrylates. *Contact Dermatitis* 1989;20:201-211.
123. Berkow JW, Gills JP, Wise JB. Depigmentation of eyelids after topically administered thiotepa. *Arch Ophthalmol* 1969;82:415.
124. Olander K, Haik KG, Haik GM. Management of ptrygia. Should thiotepa be used? *Ann Ophthalmol* 1978;10:853.
125. Christoophidis N. Ocular side effects with 5-fluorouracil. *Aust NZ J Med*1979;9:143.
126. Van Dyk JJ. Adriamycin in the treatment of cancer. *S Afr Med J* 1976;50:61.
127. Albert DM, Wong VG, Henderson ES. Ocular complications of vincristin therapy. *Arch Ophthalmol* 1967;78:709.
128. Green WR. Retinal and optic nerve atrophy induced by intravitreous vincristine in the primate. *Trans Am Ophthalmol Soc* 1975;73:389.
129. McLendon BF, Bron AJ. Corneal toxicity from vinblastin solution. *Br J Ophthalmol* 1978;62:97.
130. Sanderson PA, Kuwabara T, Cogan DG. Optic neuropathy presumably caused by vincristin therapy. *Am J Ophthalmol* 1976;81:146.
131. Herse PR. Diurnal and long-term variations in corneal thickness in the normal and alloxan-induced diabetic rabbit. *Curr Eye Res* 1990;9:451-457.
132. Loprinzi CL, Love RR, Garrity JA, Ames MM. Cyclophosphamide, methotrexate and 5-fluorouracil (CMF) induced ocular toxicity. *Cancer Invest* 1990;8:459-465.
133. Holdright DR, Jahanqiri M. Accidental poisoning with podophyllin. *Hum Exp Toxicol* 1990;9:51-56.
134. Miller RA. Podophyllin. *Int J Dermatol* 1985;24:491-498.
135. Beutner KR, van Krogh G. Current status of podophyllotoxin for the treatment of genital warts. *Semin Dermatol* 1990;9:148-151.
136. Bernstein HN. Chloroquine ocular toxicity. *Surv Ophthalmol* 1967;12:415.
137. Burns RP. Delayed onset of chloroquine retinopathy. *N Engl J Med* 1966;275;693.
138. Lal S, Gupta AK. Lenticular deposits associated with chloroquine keratopathy. *Indian J Ophthalmol* 1974;22:34.
139. Chamberlain WP, Boles DJ. Edema of the cornea precipitated by quinacrine (Atabrine). *Arch Ophthalmol* 1946;35:120.
140. Ferrara A. Optic neuritis from high doses of Atebrin. *Rass Ital Ottalmol* 1943;12:123.
141. Duke-Elder S. *Systems of ophthalmology*, vol 14, part 2. St Louis: C.V. Mosby, 1972;1187.
142. Lasky MA. Corneal response to emetine hydrochloride. *Arch Ophthalmol* 1950,44.47.
143. Armaly MF. Effect of corticosteroids on intraocular pressure and fluid dynamics. I. Effect of dexamethasone in the normal eye. *Arch Ophthalmol* 1963;70:482.
144. Becker B. The side effects of corticosteroids. *Invest Ophthalmol* 1964;3:492.
145. David DS, Berkowitz JS. Ocular effects of topical and systemic corticosteroids. *Lancet* 1969;2:149.
146. O'Connor GR. Periocular corticosteroid injections: uses and abuses. *Eye Ear Nose Throat Mouth* 1976;55:83.
147. Willetts GS. Ocular side-effects of drugs. *Br J Ophthalmol* 1969;53:252.
148. Andersen KE, Maibach HI. Allergic reaction to drugs used topically. *Clin Toxicol* 1980;16:415.
149. Lerman S, Megaw J, Willis I. Potential ocular complications from PUVA therapy and their prevention. *J Invest Dermatol* 1980;74:197.

150. Hanna C, Fraunfelder FT, Sanchez J. Ultrastructural study of argyrosis of the cornea and conjunctiva. *Arch Ophthalmol* 1974;92:18.
151. Anon. Final report on the safety assessment of sodium borate and boric acid. *J Am Coll Toxicol* 1983;2:87-125.
152. Groden LR, Rodnite J, Brinser JH, Genvert GI. Acridine orange and gram stains in infectious keratitis. *Cornea* 1990;9:122-124.
153. Gomez JT, Robinson NM, Osato MS, Wilhelmus KR. Comparison of acridine orange and gram stains in bacterial keratitis. *Am J Ophthalmol* 1988;106:735-737.
154. Stevens E, Ectors M, Cornil A. Case of acute poisoning by mercuric oxycyanide. *Acta Clin Belg* 1989;44:116-122.
155. Anon. Camphor, synthetic. In: *Documentation of the threshold limit values of biological exposure indices*, 5th ed. Amer Conf Govt Ind Hygienists, 1986;94.
156. Committee on drugs. Camphor—who needs it? *Pediatrics* 1978;62:404.
157. Khurana AK, Ahluwalie BK, Scod S. Savlon keratopathy, a clinical profile. *Acta Ophthalmol (Copenh)* 1989;67:465-466.
158. Anon. Consensus report for creosote. *Arbete Och Halsa* 1989;32:18-25.
159. Liire J. Creosote. Nordiske-expertgruppen for gransvardesdocumentation. *Arbet Och Halsa* 1988;33:7-51.
160. Kennah HE, Albulesen D, Hignet S, Barrow CS. A critical evaluation of predicting ocular irritancy potential from an *in vitro* cytotoxicity assay. *Fundam Appl Toxicol* 1989;12:281-290.
161. Brownstein S, Liszaner AD, Jackson WB. Ocular complications of a topical methylene blue-vasoconstrictor-anesthetic preparation. *Can J Ophthalmol* 1989;24:317-324.
162. Mozingo DW, Smith AA, McManus WF, Pruitt BA Jr, Mason AD, Jr. Chemical burns. *J Trauma* 1988;28:142-147.
163. Baranowski-Dutkiewicz B. Skin absorption of phenol from aqueous solutions in men. *Int Arch Occup Environ Health* 1981;49:99.
164. Anon. Final report on the safety assessment of zinc phenolsulfonate. *J Am Coll Toxicol* 1986;5:373-390.
165. Hopkins J. Hexachlorophene: more bad news than good. *Food Cosmet Toxicol* 1979;17:410.
166. Johnstone RT. *Occupational medicine and industrial hygiene* St Louis: C.V. Mosby, 1948;216.
167. Gasset AR. Benzalkonium chloride toxicity to the human cornea. *Am J Ophthalmol* 1977;84:169.
168. Theodore FH. Drug sensitivities and irritations to the conjunctiva. *JAMA* 1953;151:25.
169. Willetts GS. Ocular side-effects of drugs. *Br J Ophthalmol* 1969;53:252.
170. Collin HB. Ultrastructural changes to corneal stromal cells due to ophthalmic preservatives. *Acta Ophthalmol (Copenh)* 1986;64:72-78.
171. Norn MS. Methylene blue (methylthionine) vital staining of the cornea and conjunctiva. *Acta Ophthalmol* 1967;45:347.
172. Anon. p-Toluidine. In: *Documentation of the threshold limit values and biological exposure indices*, 5th ed. Amer Conf Govt Ind Hygienists, 1986;590-591.
173. Anonymous. Final report on the safety assessment of 4-amino-2-hydroxytolene. *J Am Coll Toxicol* 1989;8:569-578.
174. Anonymous. 3,3′-Dichlorobenzidine. In: *Documentation of the threshold limit values of biological exposure indices*, 5th ed. Amer Conf Govt Ind Hygienists, 1986;180.
175. Armaly MF. Ocular tolerance to silicones. *Arch Ophthalmol* 1962;68:390.
176. Setula K, Ruusuvaara P, Punnonen E, Laatikainen L. Changes in corneal endothelium after treatment of retinal detachment with intraocular silicone oil. *Acta Ophthalmol* 1989;67:37-43,
177. Rosengren B. Silicone injection into the vitreous in hopeless cases of retinal detachment. *Acta Ophthalmol* 1969;47:757.
178. De Groot AC, Beverdam EG, Ayong CT, Coenraads PJ, Nater JP. The role of contact allergy in the spectrum of adverse effects caused by cosmetics and toiletries. *Contact Dermatitis* 1988;19:195-201.
179. Passreiter CM, Florack M, Willhua G, Goertz G. Allergic contact dermatitis caused by Asteraceae. Identification of an 8,9-epoxythymol-diester as the contact allergen of *Arnica sachalinensis*. *Derm Beruf Umwelt* 1988;36:79-82.
180. Anon. Final report on the safety assessment of 1-naphthol. *J Am Coll Toxicol* 1989;8:749-768.
181. Wells PG, Wilson B, Lubek BM. *In vivo* murine studies on the biochemical mechanism of naphthalene cataractogenesis. *Toxicol Appl Pharmacol* 1989;99:466-473.
182. Scherling SS, Blondis RR. The effect of chemical warfare agents on the human eye. *Milit Surg* 1945;96:70.

183. Petersen PE, Evans RB, Johnstone MA, Henderson WR Jr. Evaluation of ocular hypersensitivity to dipivalyl epinephrine by component eye-drop testing. *J Allergy Clin Immunol* 1990;85:954–958.
184. Trocme SD, Bonini S, Barney NP, Block KJ, Allansmith MR. Late-phase reaction to topically induced ocular anaphylaxis in the rat. *Curr Eye Res* 1988;7:437–443.
185. Reuhl KR, Rice DC, Gilbert SG, Hallett J. Effects of chronic development lead exposure on monkey neuroanatomy—visual system. *Toxicol Appl Pharmacol* 1989;99:501–509.
186. Niebroj T, Grszczynska M. Reaction of Langerhans cells of the corneal epithelium to topically applied lead. *Klin Oczna* 1989;91:54.
187. Barney NP, Kleinman RE, Trocme SD, Block KJ, Allansmith MR. Attenuation of rat conjunctival response by repeated haptan application. *Curr Eye Res* 1988;7:843–848.
188. Kahn M, Barney NP, Briggs RM, Block KJ, Allansmith MR. Penetrating the conjunctival barrier. The role of molecular weight. *Invest Ophthalmol Vis Sci* 1990;31:258–261.
189. Lemp MA, Zimmerman LE. Toxic endothelial degeneration in ocular surface disease treated with topical medications containing benzalkonium chloride. *Am J Ophthalmol* 1988;105:670–673.
190. Martin G, Draize JH, Kelley EA. Local anesthesia in eye mucosa produced by surfactants in cosmetic formulations. *Proc Soc Sect Toilet Goods Assoc* 1962;37:2.
191. Kennah HE, Hignet S, Laux PE, Dork JD, Barrow CS. An objective procedure for quantitating eye irritation based upon changes in corneal thickness. *Fundam Appl Toxicol* 1989;12:258–268.
192. Anon. Final report on the safety assessment of sodium lauryl sulfate and ammonium lauryl sulfate. *J Am Coll Toxicol* 1983;2:127–181.
193. Anon. Final report on the safety assessment of PEG-2, -6, -8, -12, -20, -32, -40, -50, -100 and -150 stearates. *J Am Coll Toxicol* 1983;2:17–34.
194. Anon. Final report on the safety assessment of benzethonium chloride and methylbenzethonium chloride. *J Am Coll Toxicol* 1985;4:65–106.
195. Booman KA, Caascieri TM, Demetrulias J, et al. *In vitro* methods for estimating eye irritancy of cleaning products phase I. Preliminary assessment. *J Toxicol Cutan Ocular Toxicol* 1988;7:173:185.
196. Gosselin RE, Hodge HD, Smith RP, Gleson MN. *Clinical toxicology of commercial products*, 4th ed. Baltimore: Williams and Wilkins, 1976.
197. *CTFA cosmetic ingredient dictionary*, 2nd ed. Washington, DC: Cosmetic, Toiletry and Fragrance Association, 1976.
198. Kirk RE, Othmer DF, eds. *Encyclopedia of chemical technology*, vol 12, 3rd ed. New York: John Wiley, 1980.
199. Anon. Final report on the safety assessment of hydroquinone and pyrocatechol. *J Am Coll Toxicol* 1986;5:123–165.
200. Anon. Final report on the safety assessment of 2,3-naphthalenediol. *J Am Coll Toxicol* 1988;7:353–357.
201. Anon. Final report on the safety assessment of 1-naphthol. *J Am Coll Toxicol* 1989;8:749–768.
202. Anon. Final report on the safety assessment of 4-amino-2-hydroxytoluene. *J Am Coll Toxicol* 1989;8:569–588.
203. Anon. Final report on the safety assessment of vinyl acetate/cotonic acid copolymer. *J Am Coll Toxicol* 1983;2:125–140.
204. Heine A, Laubstein B. Contact dermatitis from cyclohexanone-formaldehyde resin (L2 resin) in a hair lacquer spray. *Contact Dermatitis* 1990;22:108.
205. Matsunaga K, Hosokawa K, Suzuki M, Arima Y, Hayakawa R. Occupational allergic contact dermatitis in beauticians. *Contact Dermatitis* 1988;18:94–96.
206. Tosti A, Melino M, Bardazzi F. Contact dermatitis due to glyceryl monothioglycolate. *Contact Dermatitis* 1988;19:71–72.
207. Nigam PK, Saxena AK. Allergic contact dermatitis to henna. *Contact Dermatitis* 1988;18:55–56.
208. Gouche R. Hazards of henna. *Anesth Analg* 1989;69:416–417.
209. Natow AJ. Henna. *Cutis* 1986;38:21.
210. Bracher M, Faller C, Spengler J, Reinhardt CA. Comparison of *in vitro* cell toxicity with an *in vivo* eye irritation. *Mol Toxicol* 1987–1988;1:561–570.
211. Pruett RC, Weiter JJ, Goldstein RB. Myopic cracks, angioid streaks and traumatic tears in Bruch's membrane. *Am J Ophthalmol* 1987;103:537–543.
212. De Groot AC, Bruynzeel DP, Bos JD, Van der Meeren HL, Van Joost T, Jagtman BA, Weyland JW. The allergens in cosmetics. *Arch Dermatol* 1988;124:1525–1529.
213. Anon. Final report on the safety assessment of toluenesulfonamide/formaldehyde resin. *J Am Coll Toxicol* 1986;5:471–490.

214. Anon. Final report on the safety assessment of ethyl acetate and butyl acetate. *J Am Coll Toxicol* 1989;8:681-705.
215. Golubovic S, Parunovic A. Cyanoacrylate glue in the treatment of corneal ulcerations. *Fortschr Ophthalmol* 1990;87:378-381.
216. Koo D, Bourier B, Wesley M, Courtwright P, Reingold A. Epidemic keratoconjunctivitis in a university medical center ophthalmology clinic; need for re-evaluation of the design and disinfection of instruments. *Infect Control Hosp Epidemiol* 1989;10:547-552.
217. Kinnunen T, Hannuksela M. Skin reactions to hexylene glycol. *Contact Dermatitis* 1989;21:154-158.
218. Anon. Hexylene glycol. In: *Documentation of the threshold limit values of biological exposure indices*, 5th ed. Amer Conf Govt Ind Hygienists, 1986;309.
219. Anon. Isopropyl alcohol. *Ibid.*, 337.
220. Anon. Final report on the safety assessment of dioctyl adipate and diisopropyl adipate. *J Am Coll Toxicol* 1984;3:101-130.
221. Anon. Final report on the safety assessment of butylene glycol, hexylene glycol, ethoxydiglycol and dipropylene glycol. *J Am Coll Toxicol* 1985;4:223-248.
222. De Respinis PA. Cyanoacrylate nail glue mistaken for eye drops. *JAMA* 1990;263;2301.
223. Siegal JE, Zaidman GW. Surgical removal of cyanoacrylate adhesive after accidental instillation in the anterior chamber. *Ophthalmic Surg* 1989;20:179-181.
224. Arena JM. *Poisoning: toxicology, symptoms, treatment*, 2nd ed. Springfield, IL: Charles C. Thomas, 1970.
225. Hayes WJ. *Toxicology of pesticides*. Baltimore: Williams and Wilkins, 1975.
226. Pullicino P, Aquilina J. Opso clonus in organophosphate poisoning. *Arch Neurol* 1989;46:704-705.
227. Moster MF, Winklerova S, Nemecek R. The toxic effect of organophosphorus compounds on the rabbit eye. I. Ultrastructural changes in the cornea. *Cesk Oftalmol* 1987;43:354-365.
228. Hata S, Bernstein E, Davis LE. Atypical ocular bobbing in acute organophosphate poisoning. *Arch Neurol* 1986;43:185-186.
229. Francis BM. Teratogenicity of bifenox and nitrofen in rodents. *J Environ Sci Health B* 1986;21:303-317.
230. EPA/OTS Doc. #86-870002320. Acute toxicological properties of Dursban 24E insecticide, 1987.
231. Kennedy GL Jr. Acute toxicity studies with oxamyl. *Fundam Appl Toxicol* 1986;6:423-429.
232. Coyes MJ, Barnett PG, Midtling JE, et al. Clinical confirmation of organophosphate poisoning of agricultural workers. *Am J Ind Med* 1986;10:399-409.
233. Anon. Paris green. In: *EPA chemical profiles*. Washington, DC: EPA, 1985.
234. Anon. Chemical hazard information profile draft report. Diethyl phosphorochlorothioate. CAS No. 2524-04-1. Washington, DC: EPA, Office of Toxic Substances, 1981.
235. Ubels JL, Eddhauser HF, Nemioff BJ, Meyer LA, Dicherson CL. Ocular miotic and irritative effects of aerosol and topically applied dichlorvos and propoxur insecticides on rabbit and monkey eyes. *J Toxicol Cutan Ocular Toxicol* 1987;6:61-77.
236. Anand M, Gapal K, Mehrotra S, Chandra SV, Ray PK, Paul AK. Ocular toxicity of organochlorinated pesticides in rabbits. *J Toxicol Cutan Ocular Toxicol* 1987;6:161-171.
237. Anon. Final report on the safety assessment of drometrizole. *J Am Coll Toxicol* 1986;5:455-470.
238. Whorton MD, Obrinsky DL. Persistence of symptoms after mild to moderate acute organophosphate poisoning among 19 farm field workers. *J Toxicol Environ Health* 1983;11:347-354.
239. Olson RJ. Occupational eye disorders. *Environ Occup Med* 1983;367-372.
240. Anon. Information profiles on potential occupational hazards: phthalates. Center for Chemical Hazard Assessment, Syracuse Research Corp, Syracuse, 1982; SCRTR 82-520.
241. Kelly TE. Evaluation of effects of a tick dip on dog's eyes. *J Am Vet Med Assoc* 1981;178:64-65.
242. Anon. Trimethylamine. *Documentation of the threshold limit values of biological exposure indices*, 5th ed. Amer Conf Govt Ind Hygienists, 1986;607.
243. McCormick DP, Davis AL. Injuries in sailboard enthusiasts. *Br J Sports Med* 1988;22:95-97.
244. Rapoza PA, West, SK, Newland HS, Taylor HR. Ocular jellyfish stings in Chesapeake Bay watermen. *Am J Ophthalmol* 1986;102:536-537.
245. Preisova J, Riebel O, Ulkova E, Prokes B, Hnilicka B. Moth fragments as intraocular foreign bodies. *Klin Monatsbl Augenheilkd* 1988;192:30-32.
246. Verin P, Comte P. Emergency treatment of the projection of caterpillar hairs into the cornea. *Bull Soc Ophthalmol Fr* 1987;87:403-404.

247. Martin X, Uffer S, Gaillond C. Ophthalmia nodosa and the oculoglandular syndrome of Parinand. *Br J Ophthalmol* 1986;70:536-542.
248. Marti-Huguet T, Pujol O, Cabiro I, Oteyza JA, Roca G, Marsal J. Endophthalmos caused by intravitreal caterpillar hairs. Treatment by direct photocoagulation with argon lasar. *J Fr Ophthalmol* 1987;10:559-564.
249. Rivand C, Gerault A, Frau E, Faye M. Eye injuries caused by vesicatory insects. *J Fr Ophthalmol* 1990;13:47-50.
250. Surkova VK, Semonov EN. Eye injury caused by bee sting. *Vestn Oftalmol* 1989;105:71-72.
251. Agrawal RK. Traumatic cataract following bee sting. *Indian J Ophthalmol* 1985;33:59-60.
252. Llered RW, Spaulding AG, Sanitato JJ, Wander AH. Ophthalmia nodosa caused by tarantula hairs. *Ophthalmology* 1988;95:166-169.
253. Adams ME. Structure and pharmacology of spider venoms. *FEDRIP database*, National Technical Information Service (NTIS), 1989.
254. Van Tittelboom T, Kuhn D, Strauven A. Eye injuries from toad poison. *J Toxicol Clin Exp* 1988;8:95-99.
255. Kam J, Waron M, Barishak YR, Schachner E, Ishay JS. Intraocular pressure in cats is lowered by drops of hornet venom. *Comp Biochem Physiol [C]* 1989;92:329-331.
256. Waldrep JC, Crosson CE. Induction of keratouveitis by capsaicin. *Curr Eye Res* 1988;7:1173-1182.
257. Agrawal RC, Sarode AV, Lalitha VS, Bhide SV. Chili extract treatment and induction of eye lesion in hamsters. *Toxicol Lett* 1985;28:1-7.
258. Szallasi A, Blumberg PM. Resiniferatoxin, a phorbol-related diterpene, acts as an ultrapotent analog of capsaicin, the irritant constituent of red pepper. *Neuroscience* 1989;30:515-520.
259. Biger Y, Abulafia C. Eye injuries due to cactus thorns. *Harefuah* 1986;110:611-612.
260. Reginella RF, Fairfield JC, Marks JG Jr. Hyposensitization to poison ivy after working in a cashew nut shell oil processing factory. *Contact Dermatitis* 1989;20:274-279.
261. Geller M. Poison ivy, mangoes, cashews and dermatitis. *Ann Intern Med* 1989;110:1036-1037.
262. Yesilada E, Tanaka S, Sezik E, Tabata M. Isolation of an anti-inflammatory principle from the fruit juice of *Ecballium elaterium*. *J Nat Prod* 1988;51:504-508.
263. Baer RL. Poison ivy dermatitis. *Cutis* 1990;46:34-36.
264. Sibony PA, Evinger C, Manning KA. The effects of tobacco smoking on smooth pursuit eye movements. *Ann Neurol* 1988;23:238-241.
265. Kjaergaard SK, Pedersen DF. Dust exposure, eye redness, eye cytology and mucous membrane irritation in a tobacco industry. *Int Arch Occup Environ Health* 1989;61:519-525.
266. Vedal S, Chan Yeung M, Enarson D, Fera T, MacLean L, Tse KS, Langille R. Symptoms and pulmonary function in western red cedar workers related to duration of employment and dust exposure. *Arch Environ Health* 1986;41:179-183.
267. Hansen BM, Brahn G, Tilsley DA. Contact allergy to Australian blackwood (Acacia melanoxylum R. Br.). Isolation and identification of new hydroxyflavin sensitizers. *Contact Dermatitis* 1990;23:33-39.
268. Hinds WC. Basis for particle size-selecting sampling for wood dust. *Appl Ind Hygiene* 1988;3:67-72.
269. de Zotte R, Patussi V, Fiorito A, Larese F. Sensitization to green coffee beans (GCB) and castor bean (CB) allergens among dock workers. *Int Arch Occup Environ Health* 1988;61:7-12.
270. Leads from the MMWR. Mucana pruriens-associated pruitus, New Jersey. *JAMA* 1986;255:313.
271. Subiza J, Subiza JL, Alonso M, Hinojosa M, Garcia R, Jerez M, Subiza E. Allergic conjunctivitis to chamomile tea. *Ann Allergy* 1990;65:127-132.
272. BIBRA Working Group. Carrageenan. In: *Toxicity Profile*. Brit Ind Biol Res Assoc, 1987.
273. Epstein E. Primula contact dermatitis: an easily overlooked diagnosis. *Cutis* 1990;45:411-416.
274. Vache J, Bodnur M. Dieffenbachia and the eye. *Cesk Oftalmol* 1988;44:453-455.
275. Anon. Wood dust. In: *Documentation of the threshold limit values of biological exposure indices*, 5th ed. Amer Conf Govt Ind Hygienists, 1986;635-636.
276. Sussman GL, Dorian W. Psyllium anaphylaxis. *Allergy Proc* 1990;11:241-242.
277. Dugan GM, Gumbmann MR, Friedman M. Toxicological evaluation of jimson weed (Datura stramonium) seed. *Food Chem Toxicol* 1989;27:501-510.
278. Vaishya R. A thorny problem: the diagnosis and treatment of acacia thorn injuries. *Injury* 1990;21:99-100.
279. Vighetto A, Grochowicki M, Juillet-Reitz M. A rare cause of accidental pharmacologic mydriasis. *Presse Med* 1990;19:219.
280. Mozherenko VP. Plants in the treatment of eye disease. *Med Sestra* 1985;44:53-54.

281. Oji EO. Clinical and pathological effects on the rabbits eye of some plant-derived ophthalmic swabs. *Ann R Coll Surg Engl* 1990;72:340-343.
282. Critchfield JW, Calendra AJ, Nesburn AB, Kenney MC. Keratoconus I. Biochemical studies. *Exp Eye Res* 1988;46:953-963.
283. Brooks AM, West RH, Gillies WE. The risks of precipitating acute angle-closure glaucoma with the clinical use of mydriatic agents. *Med J Aust* 1986;145:34-36.
284. Folb PI, Talmud J. Tear gas—its toxicology and suggestions for management of its acute effects in man. *S Aft J Med* 1989;46:295.
285. Fuchs T, in der Wiesche M. Contact allergies to CN and CS ("tear gas") in participants in demonstrations. *Z Hautkr* 1990;65:288-292,295.
286. Leenutaphong V, Goerz G. Allergic contact dermatitis from chloroacetophenone (tear gas). *Contact Dermatitis* 1989;20:316.
287. Petersen KK, Schrder HM, Eiskjaer SP. CS tear gas spray as an injurious agent. Clinical aspects. *Ugeskr Laeger* 1989;151:1388-1389.
288. Goh CL. Allergic contact dermatitis to mace tear gas. *Australas J Dermatol* 1987;28:115-116.
289. Mauchee OM, Strengel R, Schopf E. Chloroacetophenone allergy. *Hautarzt* 1986;37:392-401.
290. Sargent EV, Kirk GD, Hite M. Hazard evaluation of monochloroacetone. *Am Ind Hyg Assoc J* 1986;47:375-378.
291. Jarkman S, Skoog KD, Nilsson SE. The c-wave, the electroretinogram and the standing potential of the eye as highly sensitive measures of effects of low doses of trichloroethylene, methyl chloroform and halothane. *Doc Ophthalmol* 1985;60:375-382.
292. Goldman M, Dacre JC. Lewisite: its chemistry, toxicology and biological effects. *Rev Environ Contam Toxicol* 1989;110:75-115.
293. Pierard GE, Dowlati A. The deleterious effects of vesicant war gases. *Rev Med Liege* 1989;44:133-137.
294. Bake M Ia, Rusakova NE, Emke IA. Gas-chromatographic analysis of carboxide in the air of the work area. *Gig Tr Prof Zabol* 1988;9:46-47.
295. Anon. Chlorine dioxide. In: *Documentation of the threshold limit values of biological exposure indices*, 5th ed. Amer Conf Govt Ind Hygienists, 1986;118.
296. Anon. Chlorine trifluoride. *Ibid.*, 119.
297. Anon. Cyanogen. *Ibid.*, 154.
298. Anon. Dichlorodifluoromethane. *Ibid.*, 181-182.
299. Zeitling GL, Hobin K, Platt J, Woitkoski N. Accumulation of carbon dioxide during eye surgery. *J Clin Anesth* 1989;1:262-267.
300. Stahlbom B, Lundh T, Floren I, Akesson B. Visual disturbances in man as a result of experimental and occupational exposure to dimethylethylamine. *Br J Ind Med* 1991;48:26-29.
301. Akesson B, Bengtsson M, Floren I. Visual disturbances after industrial triethylamine exposure. *Int Arch Occup Environ Health* 1986;57:297-302.
302. Ding YP. Chronic effect of fluorine in the eye. *Chung Hua I Hsueh Tsa Chih* 1989;69:695-697.
303. Weber R, Budmiger H, Siegenthaler W. Chronic formaldehyde exposure—a misunderstood disease? *Schweiz Med Wochenschr* 1988;118:457-461.
304. Krootila K, Uusitalo H, Lehtosalo JI, Palkama A. Effect of topical chemical irritation on the blood-aqueous barrier of the rat eye. *Ophthalmic Res* 1986;18:248-252.
305. Alderman LC, Bergin JJ. Hydrogen selenide poisoning: an illustrative case with review of the literature. *Arch Environ Health* 1986;41:354-358.
306. Bellander T, Hagmar, L. Kriteriengruppen-for-hygieniska-gansvarden. Morfolin. *Arbete Och Halsa* 1982;32:1-32.
307. Abhyankar A, Bhambure N, Kamath NN, et al. Six month follow-up of fourteen victims with short-term exposure to chlorine gas. *J Soc Occup Med* 1989;39:131-132.
308. Dreyfors JM, Jones SB, Sayed Y. Hexamethylenetetramine: a review. *Am Ind Hygiene Assoc J* 1989;50:579-585.
309. Luck J, Kaye SB. An unrecognised form of hydrogen sulfide keratoconjunctivitis. *Br J In Med* 1989;46;748-749.
310. Rabinovitch S, Greyson ND, Weiser W, Hoffstein V. Clinical and laboratory features of acute sulfur dioxide inhalation poisoning: two-year follow-up. *Am J Resp Dis* 1989;139:556-558.
311. Scarborough ME, Ames RG, Lipsett MJ, Jackson RJ. Acute health effects of community exposure to cotton defoliants. *Arch Environ Health* 1989;44:351-360.

312. Anon. Methyl iodide. In: *Documentation of the threshold limit values of biological exposure indices*, 5th ed. Amer Conf Govt Ind Hygienists, 1986;399.
313. Fiore PM. Drug-induced ocular sensitization. *Int Ophthalmol Clin* 1989;29:147-150.
314. ECETOC Working Group. Isophorone. *ECETOC Joint Assessment of Commodity Chemicals* 1989;10:1-55.
315. Anon. Consensus report for nitromethane and tetranitromethane. *Arbete Och Halsa* 1989;32:55-63.
316. Anon. Consensus report for diacetone alcohol. *Arbete Och Halsa* 1989;32:26-33.
317. BIBRA Working Group. Methyl n-amyl ketone. In: *Toxicity profile*. Brit Ind Biol Res Assoc, 1988.
318. NIOSH working group. Occupational exposure to n-alkane monothiols; cyclohexanethiol, benzenethiol. *Criteria for a recommended standard*. NIOSH 78-213, 1978.
319. Anon. Xylene. In: *Documentation of the threshold limit values of biological exposure indices*, 5th ed. Amer Conf Govt Ind Hygienists, 1986;637-638.
320. Anon. VM and P naphtha. *Ibid.*, 631.
321. Anon. Vinyl toluene. *Ibid.*, 630.
322. Anon. 1,2,3-trichloropropane. *Ibid.*, 601-602.
323. Anon. 1,1,2-trichloroethane. *Ibid.*, 594.
324. Anon. Thionyl chloride. *Ibid.*, 572.
325. Anon. Propylene dichloride. *Ibid.*, 501.
326. Anon. n-Propyl alcohol. *Ibid.*, 500.
327. Anon. n-Propyl acetate. *Ibid.*, 500.
328. Anon. Final report on the safety assessment of morpholine. *J Am Coll Toxicol* 1989;8:707-748.
329. Anon. 1-Nitropropane. In: *Documentation of the threshold limit values of biological exposure indices*, 5th ed. Amer Conf Govt Ind Hygienists, 1986;440.
330. Anon. Stoddard solvent. *Ibid.*, 537.
331. Anon. Rubber solvent. *Ibid.*, 516.
332. Anon. Pyridine. *Ibid.*, 507.
333. Anon. Ethyl benzene. *Ibid.*, 244.
334. Anon. Ethyl amyl ketone. *Ibid.*, 243.
335. Anon. Ethyl alcohol. *Ibid.*, 242.
336. Anon. 2-ethoxyethanol. *Ibid.*, 237.
337. Anon. Epichlorohydrin. *Ibid.*, 233.
338. Anon. Dipropylene glycol methyl ester. *Ibid.*, 221.
339. Anon. Dimethylamine. *Ibid.*, 206.
340. Anon. Diisobutyl ketone. *Ibid.*, 203.
341. Anon. Diethylene triamine. *Ibid.*, 199.
342. Anon. Dichloroethyl ether. *Ibid.*, 186.
343. Anon. o-Dichlorobenzene. *Ibid.*, 178.
344. Anon. Diacetone alcohol. *Ibid.*, 171.
345. Anon. Cyclohexanone. *Ibid.*, 159.
346. Anon. Cyclohexane. *Ibid.*, 156.
347. Anon. Cumene. *Ibid.*, 151.
348. Anon. Methyl propyl ketone. *Ibid.*, 408.
349. Anon. Methyl isobutyl ketone. *Ibid.*, 402.
350. Anon. Methyl isobutyl carbinol. *Ibid.*, 401.
351. Anon. Methyl formate. *Ibid.*, 397.
352. Anon. Methyl ethyl ketone. *Ibid.*, 395.
353. Anon. Methylene chloride. *Ibid.*, 391.
354. Anon. Methyl n-butyl ketone. *Ibid.*, 378-379.
355. Anon. Methyl alcohol. *Ibid.*, 372.
356. Anon. Methyl acetate. *Ibid.*, 367.
357. Anon. o-Methylcyclohexanone. *Ibid.*, 386.
358. Anon. Allyl alcohol. *Ibid.*, 18.
359. Anon. Acetylene tetrabromide. *Ibid.*, 9.
360. Anon. Acetone. *Ibid.*, 6-7.
361. Anon. Final report on the safety assessment of n-butyl alcohol. *J Am Coll Toxicol* 1987;6:403-424.
362. Anon. Final report on the safety assessment of butylene glycol, hexylene glycol, ethoxydiglycol and dipropylene. *J Am Coll Toxicol* 1985;4:223-248.
363. NTP Working Group. Toxicology and carcinogenesis studies of benzyl alcohol in F344/N rats and

B6C3F1 mice (gavage studies). National Toxicology Program Technical Report Series 1989;343:1-158.
364. NTP Working Group. Toxicology and carcinogenesis studies of hexachloroethane in F344/N rats (gavage studies). NTP Technical Report Series 1989;361:1-120.
365. Anon. 1,1,2,2-tetrachlorethan. *Beratergremium fuer umweltrelevante Altstoffe (BUA)* 1989;29:1-83.
366. EPA Working Group. An exposure and risk assessment for trichloroethanes. EPA-440/4-85-018, 1982.
367. Illing HPA, Mariscotti SP, Smith AM. Tetrachloroethylene (tetrachloroethene, perchloroethylene). *HSE Toxic Rev* 1987;17:1-81.
368. WHO Working Group. tert-Butanol. *Environ Health Criteria* 1987;65:67-92.
369. ECETOC Working Group. Ethylbenzene. *ECETOC Joint Assessment of Commodity Chemicals* 1986;7:1-39.
370. ECETOC Working Group. Xylenes. *Ibid.*, 6:1-59.
371. NIOSH Working Group. Occupational exposure to 1,1,1-trichloroethane (methyl chloroform). *Criteria for a Recommended Standard*; NIOSH76-184, 1976;1-179.
372. WHO Working Group. Toluene. *Environ Health Criteria* 1985;52:1-146.
373. WHO Working Group. Trichloroethylene. *Ibid.*, 50:1-133.
374. WHO Working Group. Tetrachloroethylene. *Ibid.*, 1984;31:1-48.
375. Merigan WH. Visual indices of neurotoxicity (monkeys). In: *Crisp data base*. Washington, DC: National Institutes of Health.
376. Anon. 2-Methoxyethyl acetate. In: *Documentation of the threshold limit values of biological exposure indices*, 5th ed. Amer Conf Gov Ind Hygienists, 1986;366.
377. Anon. Mesityl oxide. *Ibid.*, 361.
378. Anon. Isopropyl ether. *Ibid.*, 339.
379. Anon. Isopropyl alcohol. *Ibid.*, 337.
380. Anon. Isopropyl acetate. *Ibid.*, 336.
381. Anon. Isobutyl acetate. *Ibid.*, 330.
382. Anon. Isoamyl alcohol. *Ibid.*, 329.
383. Anon. Hexylene glycol. *Ibid.*, 309.
384. Anon. sec-Hexyl acetate. *Ibid.*, 308.
385. Anon. Hexane isomers. *Ibid.*, 307.
386. Anon. Hexane. *Ibid.*, 305-306.
387. Anon. Furfural. *Ibid.*, 280.
388. Anon. Ethyl ether. *Ibid.*, 259.
389. Anon. Ethylene glycol. *Ibid.*, 259.
390. Anon. Final report on the safety assessment of methylene chloride. *J Am Coll Toxicol* 1988;7:741-835.
391. Anon. Final report on the safety assessment of amyl acetate and isoamyl acetate. *J Am Coll Toxicol* 1988;7:705-719.
392. Anon. 3-methylbutanol-1. *Toxikologische Bewertungen* 1988;95:1-17.
393. Anon. n-Butylmercaptan: In: *Documentation of the threshold limit values of biological exposure indices*, 5th ed. Amer Conf Govt Ind Hygienists, 1986:83.
394. Anon. n-Butyl alcohol. *Ibid.*, 76.
395. Anon. Sec-butyl acetate. *Ibid.*, 73.
396. Anon. Sec-amyl acetate. *Ibid.*, 29.
397. Reutter S. Trichloroethane: a summary of the toxicological data. *Government Reports Announcements & Index*, Issue 18, 1989.
398. Anon. Trichlorofluoromethane. Paris: Institut National de Recherche et de Securite, 1988.
399. Ansell JM, Fowler JA. The acute oral toxicity and primary ocular and dermal irritation of selected n-alkyl-2-pyrrolidones. *Food Chem Toxicol* 1988;25:475-479.
400. Ballantyne B, Myers RC. The comparative acute toxicity and primary irritancy of the monohexyl ethers of ethylene and diethylene glycol. *Vet Hum Toxicol* 1987;29:361-366.
401. Lundberg I. Methylene chloride. *Arbete Och Halsa* 1987;40:75-120.
402. Haley TJ. Solvents and chemical intermediates. In: Haley TF, Berndt, eds. *Handbook of toxicology*. New York: Hemisphere Publishing, 1987;504-554.
403. O'Donoghue JL. Alkanes, alcohols, ketones and ethylene oxide. In: O'Donoghue JF, ed. *Neurotoxicity of industrial and commercial chemicals*, vol 1. Boca Raton, FL: CRC Press, 1985;61-97.
404. Von Burg R. Toxicology updates. Xylene. *J Appl Toxicol* 1982;2:269-271.

405. Macewen CJ. Eye injuries: a prospective survey of 5,671 cases. *Br J Ophthalmol* 1989;73:888-894.
406. Schein DD, Hibberd PL, Shingleton BJ, et al. The spectrum and burden of ocular injury. *Ophthalmology* 1983;95:300-305.
407. Micovic V, Milenkovic S, Opric M. Acute aseptic panophthalmitis caused by a copper foreign body. *Fortschr Ophthalmol* 1990;87:362-363.
408. Good P, Gross K. Electrophysiology and metallosis: support for an oxidative (free radical) mechanism in the human eye. *Ophthalmalogica* 1988;196:204-209.
409. Sneed SR, Weingeist TA. Management of siderosis bulbi due to a retained iron-containing intraocular foreign body. *Ophthalmology* 1990;97:375-379.
410. Zagorski Z, Palae O, Grabowski J, Lang GK, Naumann GO. Comparative studies in chronic ocular chalcosis. *Klin Oczna* 1989;91:73-75.
411. Adams HA, Hossemer V, Jacobi KW, Kempelmann G. Plasma level of lidocaine and adrenaline in local anesthesia with addition of colloid in eye surgury. *Fortschr Ophthalmol* 1990;87:209-213.
412. Kanai A, Alba RM, Takano T, et al. The effect on the cornea of alpha cyclodextrin vehicle for cyclosporin eye drops. *Transplant Proc* 1989;21:3150-3152.
413. Karcioglu ZA, Aran AJ, Holmes DL, Kapiciglu Z, Lopez J. Inflammation due to surgical glove powders in the rabbit eye. *Arch Ophthalmol* 198;106:808-811.
414. NIOSH Working Group. Occupational exposure to coal tar products. *Criteria for a Recommended Standard.* NIOSH 78-107, 1978;189.
415. Thomson SA. Toxicology of carbon fibers. *Appl Ind Hygiene* 1989;special issue:29-33.
416. BIBRA Working Group. Carbon black. In: *Toxicity profile*. Brit Ind Biol Res Assoc, 1986.
417. Anon. Eye safety: irritants exposure effects and protective devices. Jan 1976-June 1989. (Citations from the Energy Department Base.) *Government Reports, Announcements & Index*, Issue 16, 1989.
418. Algvere P, Wallow IH, Martini B. The development of vitreous membranes and retinal detachment induced by intravitreal carbon microparticles. *Graefes Arch Clin Exp Ophthalmol* 1988;226:471-478.
419. BIBRA Working Group. Acetic acid and its common salts. In: *Toxicity profile*. Brit Ind Biol Res Assoc, 1987.
420. Anon. Acetic acid. In: *Documentation of the threshold limit values of biological exposure indices*, 5th ed. Amer Conf Govt Ind Hygienists, 1986;4.
421. NIOSH Working Group. Occupational exposure to chromic acid. NIOSH HSM 73-11021, 1973;83.
422. Passi S, Picardo M, Mingrone G, Breathnach AS, Nazzaro-Porro M. Azelaic acid—biochemistry and metabolism. *Acta Derm Venereol Suppl (Stockh)* 1989;143:8-13.
423. Ormerod LD, Abelson MB, Kenyon KR. Standard models of corneal injury using alkali-immersed filter discs. *Invest Ophthalmol Vis Sci* 1989;30:2148-2153.
424. Chung JH. Experimental corneal alkali wound healing. *Acta Ophthalmologica* 1988;66(suppl) 187:5-35.
425. Mattax JB, McCulley JP. Corneal surgery following alkali burns. *Int Ophthalmol Clin* 1988;28:76-82.
426. Anon. Ammonia. In: *Documentation of the threshold limit values of biological exposure indices*, 5th ed. Amer Conf Govt Ind Hygienists, 1986;28.
427. Anon. Ammonia. In: *Medical and biological effects of environmental pollutants*. National Research Council, 1979;354.
428. WHO Working Group. Ammonia. *Environ Health Criteria* 1986;54:1-210.
429. Millen TP, Kucan JO, Smoot EC 3rd. Anhydrous ammonia injuries. *J Burn Care Rehabil* 1989;10:448-453.
430. Wrong O. Ammonia burns to the eye. *Br Med J Clin Res* 1988;296:1263.
431. BIBRA Working Group. Calcium hydroxide. In: *Toxicity profile*. Brit Ind Biol Res Assoc, 1988.
432. Kriteriegruppen for hygieniskagransvarden. Consensus report for some aliphatic amines. *Arbete Och Halsa* 1983;36:19-34.
433. Anon. Diisopropylamine. In: *Documentation of the threshold limit values of biological exposure indices*, 5th ed. Amer Conf Govt Ind Hygienists, 1986;204.
434. Anon. Nine toxicity studies on diisopropylamine with cover letter. EPA/OTS Doc #89-880000108, 1988.
435. Chung JH. Healing of rabbit corneal alkali wounds *in vitro*. *Cornea* 1990;9:36-40.
436. BIBRA Working Group. Ethanolamine. In: *Toxicity profile*. Brit Ind Biol Res Assoc, 1989
437. Anon. Diaminotoluenes. In: *Environmental health criteria 74*. IPCS (International Programme on Chemical Safety), Geneva: World Health Organization, 1987.

438. Sutton WL. Aliphatic and alicyclic amines. In: Fassett DW, Iris DD eds. *Industrial hygiene and toxicology*, vol 2, 2nd ed. New York: Wiley Interscience, 1963;2037-2067.
439. Warren DW Jr, Selchan DF. An industrial hygiene appraisal of triethylamine and dimethylethylamine exposure limits in the foundry industry. *Am Ind Hygiene Assoc J* 1988;49:630-634.
440. Albrecht WN, Stephenson RL. Health hazards of tertiary amine catalysts. *Scand J Work Environ Health* 1988;14:209-219.
441. Deschamps D, Garnier R, Savoye J, Chabaux CH, Fethymiou ML, Fournier E. Allergic and irritant contact dermatitis from diethyl-beta-chloroethylamine. *Contact Dermatitis* 1988;18:103-105.
442. Fernandex-Durango R, Trivino A, Ramirez JM, et al. Immunoreactive atrial natriuretic factor in aqueous humor: its concentration is increased with high intraocular pressure in rabbit eyes. *Vision Res* 1990;30:1305-1310.
443. Shearer TR. Calcium activated proteases in cataract formation. In: *Crisp data base*. Washington, DC: National Institutes of Health, 1989.
444. Gondorowa RA, Bordjugowa GG, Choroschilowa-Maselewa IP, Tschesnokowa NB, Ilatowskaja LW, Sosulina NE. Treatment of eye burns with a polyvalent proteolytic inhibitor. *Klin Monatsbl Augenheikld* 1990;197:1-5.
445. Ji YJ, Cui MZ. Toxicological studies on safety of rare earths used in agriculture. *Biomed Environ Sci* 1988;1:270-276.
446. Wald PH. Review of the literature on the toxicity of rare-earth metals as it pertains to the engineering demonstration surrogate test. Revision 1. *Government Reports, Announcements & Index*, Issue 17, 1990.
447. London JE. Toxicological study of gadolinium nitrate. *Government Reports, Announcements & Index*, Issue 23, 1988.
448. Yamashita M, Nakamura K, Naito H et al. Acute blasticidin-s poisoning. *Vet Human Toxicol* 1987;29:8-11.
449. Vale JA, Meredith TJ, Buckley BM. Paraquat poisoning: clinical features and immediate general management. *Human Toxicol* 1987;6:41-47.
450. Kennedy GL Jr. Acute and environmental toxicity studies with hexazinone. *Fundam Appl Toxicol* 1987;4:603-611.
451. Scarborough ME, Ames RG, Lipsett MJ, Jackson RJ. Acute health effects of community exposure to cotton defoliants. *Arch Environ Health* 1989;44:355-360.
452. Hoffer E, Taitelman U. Exposure to paraquat through skin absorption: clinical and laboratory observations of accidental splashing on healthy skin of agricultural workers. *Hum Toxicol* 1989;8:483-485.
453. Hart TB. Paraquat—a review of safety in agricultural and horticultural use. *Hum Toxicol* 1987;6:13-18.
454. Anon. Calcium cyanamide. *Cahiers de medecine interprofessionnelle* 1981;21:43.
455. *American hospital formulary service*, vol 2. Washington, DC: American Society of Pharmacists 1976;40:28.
456. Hughes WF Jr. Alkali burns to the eye. I. Review of literature and summary of present knowledge. *Arch Ophthalmol* 1946;35:423.
457. Hughes WF Jr. Alkali burns to the eye. II. Clinical and pathological course. *Arch Ophthalmol* 1946;36:189.
458. Stanley J. Strong alkali burns to the eye. *N Engl J Med* 1965;273:1265.
459. Ebert E, Leist KH, Mayer D. Summary of safety evaluation toxicity studies of glufosinate ammonium. *Food Chem Toxicol* 1990;28:339-349.
460. Wrong O. Ammonia burns to the eye. *Br J Med Clin Res* 1988;296:1263.
461. Douglas RB, Coe JE. The relative sensitivity of the human eye and lung to irritating gases. *Ann Occup Hyg* 1987;31:265-267.
462. Anon. Eye safety: irritants, exposure effects, and protective devices. *Government Reports, Announcements & Index*, Jan 1976-May 1987.
463. Brands A. Asphyxiant gases. In: Haley TJ, Berndt WO, eds. *Handbook of toxicology*. New York: Hemisphere Publishing, 1987;472-503.
464. Mozingo DW, Smith AA, McManus WF, Pruitt BA Jr, Mason AD Jr. Chemical burns. *J Trauma* 1988;28:642-647.
465. Nesterova MF. Evaluation of soil fumigants from the standpoint of nutrition. *Gig Sanit* 1988;6:83-84.
466. Van Joost T, de Jong G. Sensitization to DD soil fumigant during manufacture. *Contact Dermatitis* 1988;18:307-308.

467. Anon. Arsenic trioxide. In: *Arbetarskyddsnamnden*. Stockholm, 1987.
468. Anon. Arsenous oxide. In: EPA chemical profiles. Washington, DC: EPA, 1985.
469. Stern GA, Knapp A. Iatrogenic peripheral corneal disease. *Int Ophthalmol Clin* 1986;26:77-89.
470. Anon. *Arsenic and its compounds (except arsine)*. Toronto: Industrial Accident Prevention Assoc., 1986.
471. Pashley EL, Birdsong NL, Bowman K, Pashley DH. Cytotoxic effects of NaOCl on vital tissue. *J Endod* 1985;11:525-528.
472. Jessen HJ. Improving the quality of bathing water by oxygen releasing substances. *Z Gesamte Hyg* 1989;35:376-380.
473. Vigoli J, Whitehead B, Marcus SM. Oven-cleaner pads: new risk for corosive injury. *Am J Emerg Med* 1985;3:412-414.
474. Barbee SJ, Thackara JW, Rinehart WE. Acute inhalation toxicology of nitrogen trichloride. *Am Ind Hyg Assoc J* 1983;44:145-146.
475. McDonnell F, Horstman DH, Hazucha MJ, Seal E Jr, Haak Ed, Salaam SA, House DE. Pulmonary response during exposure to low concentrations of ozone. *Adv Med Environ Toxicol* 1983;5:139-144.
476. Rowes MD, Nowak KM, Moskowitz PD. Health effects of oxidants. *Environ Int* 1983;9:515-528.
477. Ng TP, Tsin TW, O'Kelly FJ. An outbreak of illness after occupational exposure to ozone and acid chlorides. *Br J Ind Med* 1985;42:686-690.
478. Anon. Sulfamic acid. Cahiers de notes documentaires. *Securite et Hygiene du Travail 3rd Qtr* 1985;120:393-396.
479. Anon. Sulfamic acid. *Cahiers de Medecine Interprofessionnelle*. 1982;22:11.
480. Anon. *Sodium hydroxide*. Hamilton, Ontario; Canadian Centre for Occup. Health and Safety, 1987.
481. Nelson JD, Kopietz LA. Chemical injuries to the eyes. Emergency, intermediate and long-term care. *Postgrad Med* 1987;81:62-75.
482. Flynn WJ, Manger TF, Hill RM. Corneal burns: a quantitative comparison of acid and base. *Acta Ophthalmol (Copenh)* 1984;62:542-548.
483. Moon ME, Robertson JF. Retrospective study of alkali burns of the eye. *Aust J Ophthalmol* 1983;11:281-286.
484. Chung JH, Fagerholm P. Endothelial healing in rabbit corneal alkali wounds. *Acta Ophthalmol (Copenh)* 1987;65:648-656.
485. DeGroot AC, Beverdam EG, Ayong CT, Coenraads PJ, Nater JP. The role of contact allergy in the spectrum of adverse effects caused by cosmetics and toiletries. *Contact Dermatitis* 1988;19:195-201.
486. Morgan RL, Sorenson SS, Castles TR. Prediction of ocular irritation by corneal pachymetry. *Food Chem Toxicol* 1987;25:609-613.
487. Freeberg FE, Nixon GA, Reer PJ, Weaver JE, Bruce RD, Griffith JF, Sanders LW 3rd. Human and rabbit eye responses to chemical insult. *Fundam Appl Toxicol* 1986;7:626-634.
488. Peer J, Ben Ezra D. Corneal damage following the use of the pediculocide A 200 pyrinate. *Arch Ophthalmol* 1988;106:106-107.
489. Clarke JS. Corneal abrasions following the use of A-200 pyrinate shampoo. *Pediatr Emerg Care* 1986;2:65.
490. Del Palacio Hernanz A, Delgado Vincente S, Menendez Kamos F, Rodriguez-Noriega-Belanstegai A. Randomized comparative clinical trial of itraconazole and selenium sulfide shampoo for the treatment of pityriasis versicolor. *Rev Infect Dis* 1987;9(suppl 1):S121-S127.
491. Carlson AN, Wilhelmus KR. Giant papillary conjunctivitis associated with cyanoacrylate glue. *Am J Ophthalmol* 1987;104:437-438.
492. Report on eye irritation in rabbits using Elmer's plastic resin cascamite glue. EPA/OTS Doc. #878213874, 1983.
493. Haley TJ. Solvents and chemical intermediates. In: Haley TJ, Berndt WO, eds. *Handbook of toxicology*. New York: Hemisphere, 1987;504-514.
494. Rabbit eye irritation test with liquid urea-formaldehyde resin. EPA/OTS Doc. #868600010, 1986.
495. McGuiness R, Beaumont P. Gold dust retinopathy after the ingestion of canthaxanthine to produce skin-bronzing. *Med J Aust* 1985;143:622-623.
496. Fowler JF Jr. Selection of patch test materials for gold allergy. *Contact Dermatitis* 1987;17:23-25.
497. *AMA drug evaluations*, 4th ed. New York: John Wiley, 1980;104-106,1092.
498. Grubb BR, Matthews DO, Bentley PJ. Ocular chrysiasis: accumulation of gold in the rabbit eye. *Curr Eye Res* 1986,5:891-893.
499. McCormick SA, DiBartolomeo AG, Raju VK, Schwab IR. Ocular chrysiasis. *Ophthalmology* 1985,92:1432-1435.

500. Estrig WJ, Cavalieri SA, Wald P, Becker CE, Jones JR, Cone JE. Evidence of neurologic dysfunction related to long-term ethylene oxide exposure. *Arch Neurol* 1987;44:1283-1286.
501. BIBRA Working Group. Hydroquinone. In: *Toxicity profile*. Brit Ind Biol Res Assoc, 1986.
502. NIOSH Working Group. Occupational exposure to hydroquinone. In: *Criteria for a recommended standard*. NIOSH 78-155, 1978.
503. Ballantyne B, Myers RC. The comparative acute toxicity and primary irritancy of the monohexyl ethers of ethylene and diethylene glycol. *Vet Human Toxicol* 1987;29:361-366.
504. BIBRA Working Group. Ethylene glycol. In: *Toxicity profile*. Brit Ind Biol Res Assoc, 1988.
505. Anon. Ethylene glycol. In: *Documentation of the threshold limit values of biological exposure indices*, 5th ed. Amer Conf Govt Ind Hygienists, 1986;253.
506. Siegel E, Watson S. Mothball toxicity. *Pediatr Clin North Am* 1986;33:369-374.
507. Anon. p-Dicholorobenzene. In: *Documentation of the threshold limit values of biological exposure indices*, 5th ed. Amer Conf Govt Ind Hygienists, 1986;179.
508. Shapkin-Gunko VA, Leus NF, Drozhzhina GI. Characteristics of the development of cataract models against a background of poisoning. *Oftalmal Zh* 1989;2:116-119.
509. Martin G, Draize JH, Kelley EA. Local anesthesia in eye mucosa produced by surfactants in cosmetic formulations. *Proc Sci Sect Toilet Goods Assoc* 1962;37:2.
510. Hezemans-Boer M, Toonstre J, Meulenbelt J, Zwaveling JH, Sangster B, van Vloten WA. Skin lesions due to exposure to methyl bromide. *Arch Dermatol* 1988;124:917-921.
511. Anon. Chlorobromomethane. In: *Documentation of the threshold limit values of biological exposure indices*, 5th ed. Amer Conf Govt Ind Hygienists, 1986;125-126.
512. Illing HPA, Mariscotti SP, Smith AM. Tetrachloroethylene (tetrachloroethane, perchloroethylene). *HSE Toxic Rev* 1987;17:1-81.
513. WHO Working Group. Tetrachloroethylene. *Environ Health Criteria* 1984;31:1-48.
514. Miller NR. *Walsh and Hoyt's clinical neuro-ophthalmology*, 4th ed. Baltimore: Williams and Wilkins, 1982.
515. Wirtschafter ZT. Toxic amblyopia and accompanying physiological disturbances in carbon tetrachloride intoxication. *Am J Public Health* 1933;23:1035.
516. Smith AR. Optic atrophy following inhalation of carbon tetrachloride. *Arch In Hyg* 1950;1:348.
517. Ng SK, Goh CL. Contact allergy to sodium hypochlorite in Insol. *Contact Dermatitis* 1989;21:281.
518. Huang AJ, Belldegrun R, Hanninen L, Kenyon KR, Tseng SC, Refojo MF. Effects of hypertonic solutions on conjunctival epithelium and mucinlike glycoprotein discharge. *Cornea* 1989;8:15-20.
519. Kruger RA, Higgins J, Rashford S, Fitzgerald B, Land R. Emergency eye care. *Aust Fam Physician* 1990;19:934-938.
520. Fassihi AR, Naidoo NT. Irritation associated with tear-replacement ophthalmic drops: a pharmaceutical and subjective investigation. *S Afr Med J* 1989;75:233-235.
521. WHO Working Group. Ammonia. *Environ Health Criteria* 1986;54:1-210.
522. Anon. Ammonium chloride. In: *Documentation of the threshold limit values of biological exposure indices*, 5th ed. Amer Conf Govt Ind Hygienists, 1986;21.
523. Anon. Final report on the safety assessment of hydroquinone and pyrocatechol. *J Am Coll Toxicol* 1986;5:123-165.
524. Willis CM, Stephens CJM, Wilkinson JD. Experimentally-induced irritant contact dermatitis. Determination of optimum irritant concentrations. *Contact Dermatitis* 1988;18:20-24.
525. Finger PT, Ho TK, Fastenberg DM, Hyman RA, Stroh EM, Packer S, Perry HD. Intraocular radiation blocking. *Invest Ophthalmol Vis Sci* 1990;31:1724-1730.
526. Refojo MF. Synthetic hydrophylic polymers for eye surgery (rabbits). In: *Crisp data base*. Washington, DC: National Institutes of Health, 1988.
527. Schuchereba ST, Clifford CB, Vargas JA, Bunch D, Bowman PD. Morphological alterations in rat retina after hypervolemic infusion of cross-linked hemoglobin. *Biometer Artif Cells Artif Organs* 1990;18:299-307.
528. Anon. Catechol. In: *Documentation of the threshold limit values of biological exposure indices* 5th ed. Amer Conf Govt Ind Hygienists, 1986;112.
529. Anon. Pentoborane. *Ibid.*, 459.
530. Anon. Consensus report for nitroethane and tetranitromethane. *Arbete Och Halsa* 1989;32:55-63.
531. Yarbrough BE, Garrettson LK, Zolet DI, Cooper KR, Kellaher AB, Steele MH. Severe central nervous system damage and profound acidosis in persons exposed to pentoborane. *J Toxicol Clin Toxicol* 1985-1986;23:519-536.

532. Logai JM, Guseva OG, Kalvinsh IIa. The use of lysomotropic preparations in treating some experimental chemical burns. *Oftalmol Zh* 1989;8:497-500.
533. O'Grady TC. Mass eye casualties at sea. *Milit Med* 1989;154:596-598.
534. BIBRA Working Group. Calcium hydroxide. In: *Toxicity profile*. Brit Ind Biol Res Assoc, 1988.
535. Anon. Calcium hydroxide. In: *Documentation of the threshold limit values of biological exposure indices*, 5th ed. Amer Conf Govt Ind Hygienists, 1986;92.
536. Anon. Calcium oxide. *Ibid.*, 92.
537. Wang Y, Xia J, Wang QW. Clinical report on 62 cases of acute dimethyl sulfate intoxication. *Am J Ind Med* 1988;13:455-467.
538. Anger WK, Moody L, Burg J, et al. Neurobehavioral evaluation of soil and structural fumigation using methyl bromide and sulfuryl fluoride. *Neurotoxicology* 1986;7:137-156.
539. Hezemans-Boer M, Toonstra J, Meulenbelt J, Zwavaling JH, Sangster B, van Vloten WA. Skin lesions due to exposure to methyl bromide. *Arch Dermatol* 1988;124:917-921.
540. Anon. Methyl chloride. In: *Documentation of the threshold limit values of biological exposure indices*, 5th ed. Amer Conf Govt Ind Hygienists, 1986;380-381.
541. Anon. Methyl iodide. *Ibid.*, 399.
542. Anon. Methylamine. *Ibid.*, 373.
543. Anon. Thionyl chloride. *Ibid.*, 572.
544. Sharir M, Chen V, Blumenthal M. Red phosphorus as a cause of corneal injury. A case report. *Ophthalmologica* 1987;194:204-208.
545. Kriteriegruppen for Hygienisksa-gransvarden. Consensus report for some aliphatic amines. *Arbete Och Halsa* 1983;36:19-34.
546. Albrecht WN, Stephenson RL. Health hazards of tertiary amine catalysts. *Scand J Work Environ Health* 1988;14:209-219.
547. BIBRA Working Group. Acetic anhydride. In: *Toxicity profile*. Brit Ind Biol Res Assoc, 1987.
548. Anon. Acetic anhydride. In: *Documentation of the threshold limit values of biological exposure indices*, 5th ed. Amer Conf Govt Ind Hygienists, 1986;5.
549. Anon. Boron tribromide. *Ibid.*, 5.
550. Anon. Occupational safety and health guidelines for chemical hazards. Division of Standard Development and Technology Transfer, NIOSH, Cincinnati, OHHS (NIOSH) Publ #89-104 Suppl 12-OHG, 1988.
551. Anon. Phosphorus trichloride. In: *Documentation of the threshold limit values of biological exposure indices*, 5th ed. Amer Conf Govt Ind Hygienists, 1986;486.
552. Anon. Phosphorus pentachloride. *Ibid.*, 485.
553. Shichi H. Glutathione-dependent detoxification of peroxides in bovine ciliary body. *Exp Eye Res* 1990;50:813-818.
554. BIBRA Working Group. Calcium chloride. In: *Toxicity profile*. Brit Ind Biol Res Assoc, 1989.
555. Hightower KR, Farnum R. Calcium induces opacities in cultured human lenses. *Exp Eye Res* 1985;41:565-568.
556. Krootila K, Uusitalo H, Lehtosalo JI, Palkama A. Effect of topical chemical irritation on the blood-aqueous barrier of the rat eye. *Ophthalmic Res* 1986;18:248-252.
557. Singh G, Bohnke M, Vom Domarus D, Draeger J, Linstrom RL, Doughman DJ. Vital staining of corneal epithelium. *Cornea* 1985-1986;4:80-91.
558. Takahasi WK, Saito TR, Amao H, Kosaka T, Obata M, Umeda M, Shirazu Y. Acute reversible cataract due to nitro compounds in Japanese quail Cornutix cornutix japonica. *Jikken Dobutsu* 1988;37:239-243.
559. BIBRA Working Group. Lactic acid. In: *Toxicity profile*. Brit Ind Biol Res Assoc, 1990.
560. BIBRA Working Group. Methyl cyclopentadienyl manganese tricarbonyl. In: *Toxicity profile*. Brit Ind Biol Res Assoc, 1987.
561. Anon. 2-methylcyclopentadienyl manganese tricarbonyl. In: *Documentation of the threshold limit values of biological exposure indices*, 5th ed. Amer Conf Govt Ind Hygienists, 1986;387-388.
562. NIOSH-Working Group. Occupational exposure to nitric acid. Criteria for a recommended standard. NIOSH Pub. # 76-141, 1976;78.
563. Anon. Oxalic acid. In: *Documentation of the threshold limit values of biological exposure indices*, 5th ed. Amer Conf Govt Ind Hygienists, 1986;451.
564. BIBRA Working Group. N,N'-diphenyl-para-phenylenediamine. In: *Toxicity profile*. Brit Ind Biol Res Assoc, 1989.

565. Anon. Final report on the safety assessment of 2-nitro-p-phenlyenediamine and 4-nitro-0-phenylenediamine. *J Am Coll Toxicol* 1985;4:161-202.
566. Anon. Phthalic anhydride. In: *Documentation of the threshold limit values of biological exposure indices*, 5th ed. Amer Conf Gov Ind Hygienists, 1986;487.
567. Venables KM. Low molecular weight chemicals, hypersensitivity and direct toxicity. The acid anhydrides. *Br J Ind Med* 1989;46:222-232.
568. Anon. Quinone. In: *Documentation of the threshold limit values of biological exposure indices*, 5th ed. Amer Conf Govt Ind Hygienists, 1986;509.
569. Anson SW. Mechanisms of chemically induced photosensitivity. In: *Crisp data base*. Washington, DC: National Institute of Health, 1988.
570. Anon. Aniline. Commission of the European Communities. International Programme on Chemical Safety (IPCS) WHO, Geneva, Switzerland, 1990.
571. Anon. *Aniline*. Chicago: National Safety Council, 1988.
572. Anon. Ethyl benzene. In: *Documentation of the threshold limit values of biological exposure indices*, 5th ed. Amer Conf Govt Ind Hygienists, 1986;244.
573. Anon. Divinyl benzene. *Ibid.*, 228.
574. Ladefoged O. Industribensin. *Arbete Och Halsa* 1982;21:1-54.
575. Anon. *Benzene*. Hamilton, Ontario: Canadian Centre for Occupational Health and Safety, 1989.
576. Anon. Soluble barium compounds (as barium). *Noticias de seguridad*, 1989;51;insert 4.
577. Vevchenko MS, Vysochin VI. Detection of occupational trinitrotoluene cataract. *Vrach Delo* 1988;2:108-109.
578. WHO Working Group. Photochemical oxidants. *Environ Health Criteria* 1978;7:1-110.
579. Anon. Tetryl. In: *Documentation of the threshold limit values of biological exposure indices*, 5th ed. Amer Conf Govt Ind Hygienists, 1986;568.
580. Anon. 1,1-dimethylhydrazine. *Ibid.*, 210.
581. Anon. Hydrazine. *Ibid.*, 310.
582. Anon. Hydrazine. *Environ Health Criteria*. Geneva: WHO, 1987;68.
583. Anon. *Hydrazine hydrate and aqueous solutions*. Paris: Institut National de Recherche et de Securite, 1989.
584. Anon. *Soluble barium compounds (as barium)*. Paris: Institut National de Recherche et de Securite, 1989.
585. Bennett SR, Abrams GW. Band keratopathy from emulsified silicone oil. *Arch Ophthalmol* 1990;108:1387.
586. Suzuki M, Okada T, Takeuchi S, Ishii Y, Yamashita H, Hori S. The effect of silicone oil on the ocular tissues. *Nippon Ganka Gakkai Zasshi* 1990;94:160-166.
587. Setula K, Ruusuvaana P, Punnonen E, Laatsikainen L. Changes in corneal endothelium after treatment of retinal detachment with intraocular silicone oil. *Acta Ophthalmol (Copenh)* 1989;67:37-43.
588. Butcher BT, Bernstein IL, Schwartz JH. Guidelines for the clinical evaluation of occupational asthma due to small molecular weight chemicals. *J Allergy Clin Immunol* 1989;84:834-838.
589. Adenis JP, Leboutet MJ, Salomon JL, Duprat F, Loubet R. Experimental and clinical study of conjunctival-scleral tolerance of PTFE (Goretex) suture compared to polyglactine (Vicryl). *Ophtalmologie* 1989;3:231-232.
590. Steinkogler FJ. Polytetrafluoroethylene in enucleation surgery. *Fortschr Ophthalmol* 1988;85:321-322.
591. Johnson RN, Flynn HW Jr, Parel JM, Portugal LM. Transcient hypopyon with marked anterior chamber fibrin following pars plana vitrectomy and silicone oil injection. *Arch Ophthalmol* 1989;107:683-686.
592. Robert Y, Gloor B, Wachsmuth ED, Herbst M. Evaluation of the tolerance of the intraocular injection of hydroxypropyl methyl cellulose in animal experiments. *Klin Monatsbl Augenheilkd* 1988;192:337-339.
593. Anon. *Phosphoric acid*. Paris: Institute National de Recherche et de Securite, 1988.
594. Booman KA, Cascieri TM, Demetrulias J, et al. *In vitro* methods for estimating eye irritancy of cleaning products phase I: preliminary assessment. *J Toxicol Cutan Ocular Toxicol* 1988;7:173-185.
595. Anon. Final report on the safety assessment of triethanolamine, diethanolamine and monoethanolamine. *J Am Coll Toxicol* 1983;2:183-235.
596. Rabbit eye irritation after introduction of approximately 10 mg of solid or 0.1 mg of liquid into the conjunctival sac, with cover letter dated 060789. EPA/OTS Doc #86-890000314, 1989.

597. Acute oral LD50 and subacute feeding (28 days) in albino rats and acute dermal LD50, primary skin irritation and acute eye irritation in albino rabbits, with attached cover sheets and letter. EPA/OTS Doc #86-890000524S, 1989.
598. EPA Working Group. Health assessment document for acrylonitrile. Final report. EPA-600-8-82-007F, 1983.
599. Anon. Methyl acrylate. *IARC Monographs on the Evaluation of the Carcinogenic Risks of Chemicals to Humans* 1986;39:99-112.
600. BIBRA Working Group. Dibutyl phthalate. In: *Toxicity profile*. Brit Ind Biol Res Assoc, 1987.
601. BIBRA Working Group. Ethyl acrylate. In: *Toxicity profile*. Brit Ind Biol Res Assoc, 1988.
602. Anon. Furfural. In: *Documentation of the threshold limit values and biological exposure indices*, 5th ed. Amer Conf Govt Ind Hygienists, 1986;280.
603. Nielsen J, Fahraens C, Bensryd I, Akesson B, Welinder H, Linden K, Skerfving S. Small airways function in workers processing polyvinyl chloride. *Int Arch Occup Environ Health* 1989;61:427-430.
604. Anon. Toluene 2,4-diisocyanate. In: *Documentation of the threshold limit values of biological exposure indices*, 5th ed. Amer Conf Govt Ind Hygienists, 1986;580-581.
605. Anon. Tributyl phosphate. *Ibid.*, 591.
606. Anon. Vinyl acetate. *Ibid.*, 621.
607. Maki-Paakkanen J, Norppa H. *Vinyl acetate. Arbete Och Halsa* 1988;33:77-113.
608. BIBRA Working Group. Acetophenone. In: *Toxicity profile*. Brit Ind Biol Res Assoc, 1987.
609. Keimig DG, Castellan RM, Kullman DG, Kinsley KB. Respiratory health status of gilsonite workers. *Am J Ind Med* 1987;11:287-296.
610. Anon. Arsenic and arsenic compounds. *IARC Monographs on the Evaluation of the Carcinogenic Risk of Chemicals to Humans* 1980;23:39-141.
611. BIBRA Working Group. Menthol. In: *Toxicity profile*. Brit Ind Biol Res Assoc, 1986.
612. Anon. Methylal. In: *Documentation of the threshold limit values of biological exposure indices*, 5th ed. Amer Conf Govt Ind Hygienists, 1986;371.
613. Anon. n-Propyl acetate. *Ibid.*, 500.
614. Anon. Final report on the safety assessment of 1-naphthol. *J Am Coll Toxicol* 1989;8:749-768.
615. ECETOC Working Group. Methyl isobutyl ketone. *ECETOC Joint Assessment of Commodity Chemicals*, 1987;8:29.
616. Anon. Lithium hydride. In: *Documentation of the threshold limit values of biological exposure indices*, 5th ed. Amer Conf Govt Ind Hygienists, 1986;349.
617. BIBRA Working Group. Cyclohexylamine. In: *Toxicity profile*. Brit Ind Biol Res Assoc, 1986.
618. Anon. Cyclohexylamine. In: *Documentation of the threshold limit values of biological exposure indices*, 5th ed. Amer Conf Govt Ind Hygienists, 1986;161-162.
619. Anon. Beta-chloroprene. *Ibid.*, 135.
620. BIBRA Working Group. Diethanolamine. In: *Toxicity profile*. Brit Ind Biol Res Assoc, 1988.
621. Anon. Diethanolamine. In: *Documentation of the threshold limit values of biological exposure indices*, 5th ed. Amer Conf Govt Ind Hygienists, 1986;197.
622. BIBRA Working Group. Diethylamine and its hydrochloride. In: *Toxicity profile*. Brit Ind Biol Res Assoc, 1989.
623. Anon. Diethylamine. In: *Documentation of the threshold limit values of biological exposure indices*, 5th ed. Amer Conf Govt Ind Hygienists, 1986;197.
624. Anon. Dimethylamine. *Ibid.*, 206.
625. Ogawa Y, Kamata E, Suzuki S, et al. Toxicity of 2-mercaptobenzothiazole in mice. *Eisei Shikenjo Hokoku* 1989;107:44-50.
626. Anon. Alpha-methyl styrene. In: *Documentation of the threshold limit values of biological exposure indices*, 5th ed. Amer Conf Govt Ind Hygienists, 1986;410.
627. Kennah HE, Hignet S, Laux PE, Dorko JD, Barrow CS. An objective procedure for quantitating eye irritation based upon changes of corneal thickness. *Fundam Appl Toxicol* 1989;12:258-268.
628. Fielder RJ, Lowing R. Styrene. *HSE Toxic Rev* 1981,1:42.
629. Anon. Sulfur monochloride. In: *Documentation of the threshold limit values of biological exposure indices*, 5th ed. Amer Conf Govt Ind Hygienists, 1986;545.
630. Anon. Thiram. *Ibid.*, 573.
631. Dalvi RR. Toxicity of thiram (tetramethylthiuram disulfide). A review. *Vet Human Toxicol* 1988;30:480-482.
632. BIBRA Working Group. 2-mercaptobenzothiazol and its sodium salt. In: *Toxicity profile*. Brit Ind Biol Res Assoc, 1986.

633. Anon. Final report on the safety assessment of oleic acid, lauric acid, palmatic acid, myristic acid and stearic acid. *J Am Coll Toxicol* 1987;6:321-401.
634. Anon. Final report on the safety assessment of sodium sesquicarbonate, sodium bicarbonate, and sodium carbonate. *J Am Coll Toxicol* 1987;6:121-138.
635. Babaian Ea, Nazerotian RA, Khachatrian RR. Toxicological characteristics and hygienic standardization of the levels of sodium hydrocarbonate and potassium carbonate in the air of the work place. *Gig Tr Prof Zabol* 1989;5:30-32.
636. Anon. Potassium hydroxide. In: *Documentation of the threshold limit values of biological exposure indices*, 5th ed. Amer Con Govt Ind Hygienists, 1986;495.
637. Burns FR, Paterson CA. Prompt irrigation of chemical eye injuries may avert severe damage. *Occup Health Saf* 1989;58:33-36.
638. BIBRA Working Groups. Methyl silicate. In: *Toxicity profile*. Brit Ind Biol Res Assoc, 1988.
639. Anon. Methyl silicate. In: *Documentation of the threshold limit values of biological exposure indices*, 5th ed. Amer Conf Govt Ind Hygienists, 1986;409.
640. Anon. Ethyl silicate. *Ibid.*, 264.
641. Anon. Thioglycolic acid. *Ibid.*, 521.
642. BIBRA Working Group. 1,2-dihydro-2,2,4-trimethylquinoline (monomer and polymer). In: *Toxicity profile*. Brit Ind Biol Res Assoc, 1989.
643. Anon. Final report on the safety assessment of toluenesulfonamide/formaldehyde resin. *J Am Coll Toxicol* 1986;5:471-490.
644. BIBRA Working Group. Maleic acid. In: *Toxicity profile*. Brit Ind Biol Res Assoc, 1985.
645. Anon. Maleic anhydride. In: *Documentation of the threshold limit values of biological exposure indices*, 5th ed. Amer Conf Govt Ind Hygienists, 1986;353.
646. Dreyfors JM, Jones SB, Sayed Y. Hexamethylene tetramine: a review. *Am Ind Hygiene Assoc J* 1989;50:579-585.
647. Venables KM. Low molecular weight chemicals, hypersensitivity and direct toxicity: the acid anhydrides. *Br J Ind Med* 1989;46:222-232.
648. Schwartz CS. Toxicity of advanced composite matrix materials. *Appl Ind Hygiene* 1989;Special issue:23-28.
649. Vale PT, Rycroft RJG. Occupational irritant contact dermatitis from fibreboard containing urea-formaldehyde resin. *Contact Dermatitist* 1988;19:62.
650. Anon. Eye safety: irritants, exposure effects and protective devices Jan 1976-June 1989. *Government Reports, Announcements & Index*, Issue 16, 1989.
651. Peters AC. Toxicity tests of 1,6-hexanediamine (rats, mice). NIH Proposal, 1986.
652. Anon. Vinylidene chloride. *IARC Monographs on the Evaluation of the Carcinogenic Risk of Chemicals to Humans* 1986;39:195-226.
653. Morgan EW, Hiatt GF, Korte DW. Primary ocular irritation potential of Ball Powder (trade name) in male rabbits. *Government Reports, Announcements & Index*, Issue 01, 1990.
654. NIOSH Working Committee. Occupational exposure to fibrous glass. *Criteria for a recommended standard*. NIOSH 77-152, 1977.
655. Watanabe H, Shearer TR. Lens crysallins in aqueous and vitreous humor in selenite overdose cataract. *Curr Eye Res* 1989;8:979-986.
656. David LL, Takemoto LJ, Anderson LS, Shearer TR. Proteolytic changes in main intrinsic polypeptide (MIP26) from membranes in selenite cataract. *Curr Eye Res* 1988;7:411-417.
657. Anon. Rosin core solder pyrolysis products. In: *Documentation of the threshold limit values of biological exposure indices*, 5th ed. Amer Conf Govt Ind Hygienists, 1986;514.
658. Anon. Fluorides. *Ibid.*, 272-273.
659. Anon. *Zinc Chloride*. Calcutta: Indian Chemical Manufacturers Association, India Exchange Place, 1986.
660. Ding YP. Chronic effect of fluorine on the eye. *Chung Hua I Hsueh Tse Chic* 1989;69:695-697.
661. Anon. *Inorganic fluorides*. Chicago: National Safety Council, 1988.
662. Cremers PM, Hofstee AW. Dangers of batteries. *J Toxicol Clin Exp* 1989;9:11-19.
663. Anon. *Aniline*. Chicago: National Safety Council, 1988.
664. Anon. Pyridine. In: *Documentation of the threshold limit values and biological exposure indices*, 5th ed. Amer Conf Govt Ind Hygienist, 1986;507.
665. Dutertre-Catella H, Phu-Lich N, Huyen VN, Olivier L, Truhaut R, Claude JC. Eye and skin irritation induced by picolines. *Arch Toxicol* 1989;suppl 13:428-432.

666. Anon. Formaldehyde. In: *Documentation of the threshold limit values of biological exposure indices*, 5th ed. Amer Conf Govt Ind Hygienists, 1986;276-277.
667. Fielder RJ. Formaldehyde. *HSE Toxic Rev* 1981;2:1-18.
668. Burns FR, Paterson CA. Prompt irrigation of chemical eye injuries may avert severe damage. *Occup Health Safety* 1989;58:33-36.
669. Emmett EA. Occupational skin disease. *J Allergy Clin Immunol* 1983;72:649-656.
670. NIOSH Working Committee. Occupational exposure to fibrous glass. NIOSH 77-152, 1977.
671. Caravata EM. Acute hydrofluoric acid exposure. *Am J Emerg Med* 1988;6:143-150.
672. Flood S. Hydrofluoric acid burns. *Am Fam Physician* 1988;37:175-182.
673. Anon. Yttrium and compounds. In: *Documentation of the threshold limit values of biological exposure indices*, 5th ed. Amer Conf Govt Ind Hygienists, 1986;641.
674. London JE. Preliminary toxicological study of yttrium barium copper oxide. *Government Reports, Announcements & Index*, Issue 10, 1989.
675. Anon. Indium and compounds. In: *Documentation of the threshold limit values of biological exposure indices*, 5th ed. Amer Conf Govt Ind Hygienists, 1986;322.
676. BIBRA Working Group. Cobalt naphthenate. In: *Toxicity profile*. Brit Ind Biol Res Assoc, 1988.
677. Anon. Toxicity of cobalt. *Government Reports, Announcements & Index*, Issue 05, 1990.
678. Merigan WH. Visual indices of neurotoxicity. In: *Crisp data base*. Washington, DC: National Institutes of Health, 1989.
679. Anon. Silver and compounds. In: *Documentation of the threshold limit values of biological exposure indices*, 5th ed. Amer Conf Govt Ind Hygienists, 1986;529-531.
680. Pifers JW, Friedlander BR, Kintz RJ, Stockdale DK. Absence of toxic effects in silver reclamation workers. *Scand J Work Environ Health* 1989;15:210-221.
681. Illing HPA, Shillaker RO. 1,3-butadiene and related compounds. *HSE Toxic Rev* 1985;11:1-34.
682. Anon. Diepoxybutane. *IARC Monographs on the Evaluation of the Carcinogenic Risk of Chemicals to Humans*, 1971;11:115-123.
683. Anon. Diazomethane. In: *Documentation of the threshold limit values of biological exposure indices*, 5th ed. Amer Conf Govt Ind Hygienists, 1986;173.
684. Anon. Tantalum. *Ibid.*, 554.
685. Clark CR, Ferguson PW, Katchen MA, Dennis MW, Craig BK. Comparative toxicity of shale and petroleum-derived distillates. *Toxicol Ind Health* 1989;5:1005-1016.
686. BIBRA Working Group. Alpha-methylstryene. In: *Toxicity profile*. Brit Ind Biol Res Assoc, 1989.
687. Fielder RJ, Lowing R. Styrene. *HSE Toxic Rev* 1981;1:1-42.
688. Parke A, Bhattacherjee P, Palmer RM, Lazarus NR. Characterization and quantification of copper sulfate-induced vascularization of the rabbit cornea. *Am J Pathol* 1988;138:123-128.
689. Yu HS, Pastor SA, Lam KW, Yee RW. Ascorbate-enhanced copper toxicity on bovine corneal endothelial cells *in vitro*. *Curr Eye Res* 1990;9:177-182.

Ophthalmic Toxicology, edited by
George C. Y. Chiou. Raven Press, Ltd.,
New York © 1992.

8

Air Pollution and Ocular Toxicity

James L. Way, Lynn Baxter, Elizabeth P. Cannon, and Luqi Pei

*Department of Medical Pharmacology and Toxicology,
Texas A & M University, College of Medicine, College Station, Texas 77843*

AIR POLLUTION

The air that we breathe consists of a mixture of gases. This gaseous mixture is considered polluted when gaseous particles or energy forms are added and alter this gaseous mixture to have either a direct or an indirect adverse effect on humans. Most of our concerns about air pollution are usually focused on carbon monoxide, nitrogen oxides, sulfur oxides, hydrocarbons, and particular matter, as most studies are concerned with ambient air pollution, i.e., air in the outdoor environment. Air pollution, however, is not confined solely to the outdoor environment. There is a significant amount of air pollution of our indoor environment, e.g., homes, offices, and other workplaces (1). The pollution of our air is not solely due to man, as natural causes such as the volcano at Mt. St. Helens in Washington, forest fires, ozone from electrical storms, etc., are natural phenomena that contribute significantly to our air pollution problems. However, in this chapter our primary emphasis will be ocular toxicity of ambient air pollutants.

Probably the greatest contribution to air pollution is the incomplete combustion of organic matter. This dates from prehistory, when the cavemen began burning wood for warmth and cooking, to the use of coal in homes and industries, and, more recently, to the incomplete combustion of various organic compounds by internal combustion engines.

There are some air pollution terms that warrant precise definition prior to our discussion of air pollution. *Smog* is frequently used to describe severe pollution conditions of ambient air and is derived from the words *smoke* and *fog*. Smog usually implies a pollution situation where there is a severe decrease in visibility as frequently occurs in Los Angeles, London, and Tokyo. Very often, smog is characterized in more detail such as *photochemical smog*, which indicates that there is a sequence of photochemical reactions occurring among the pollutant gases, where an abundance of sunlight leads to the formation of strongly oxidizing products. *Haze* is a term often used in air pollution discussions, and it differs from smog predominantly in degree, as reduction of visibility occurring with haze is not as severe as with smog. Whereas haze occurs more frequently along the eastern seaboard and the midwestern United States, smog occurs predominantly in California. Gases and particles are frequently referred to in air pollution studies. *Particles* usually represent both solid and liquid phases and these two phases are dispersed in the ambient air, resulting in a suspension of particles called an aerosol. The type of smog produced by gas condensation and concomitant photochemical reactions can reduce visibility.

The predominant air pollutants are gases, and they account for 90% of the air pollution on a weight basis. Major sources of pollution are transportation (cars, trains, ships), electricity generation, fossil fuels, industrial processes, and solid waste disposal. The major contributor to air pollution is the automobile, as it accounts for about 75% of all pollutant emission. Some of the primary pollutants are carbon monoxide, sulfur oxide, nitrogen oxides, hydrocarbons, and particulate matters.

Gaseous Pollutants

The concentration of gases in air pollution investigations are expressed as mixing ratios as parts per million (ppm) where one part per million is equal to a volume of gas mixed in a million volume of air:

$$1 \text{ ppm} = \frac{1 \text{ volume ml gas}}{1 \times 10^6 \text{ volume of air}}$$

In other words, 1 µl of a gas in a liter of air would be a concentration of one part per million. Depending on the mixing ratios, this concentration can be expressed as parts per billion (ppb), parts per trillion (ppt), etc.

Recently, there has been increasing interest in using the metric system to express concentrations of air pollutants. These measurements are made in microgram per cubic meter ($\mu g/m^3$). These two terms, *ppm* and $\mu g/m^3$, are inconvertible, as

$$\mu g/m^3 = \text{ppm} \times \text{molecular weight} \times 40.9 \text{ and ppm} = \mu g/m^3 \times \frac{2.45 \times 10^{-2}}{\text{molecular weight}}$$

The use of the metric system clearly has some advantages; however, it also has disadvantages, as it is influenced by temperature and pressure. There are reviews available on air pollution and its effect on human health (1-3).

There are probably thousands of gaseous pollutants, and over 400 already have been identified in automobile exhaust alone. Many more result from photochemical reactions in the atmosphere.

Particulates

Particulate matter usually refers to small particles (0.005 to 500 µm) that are solids or liquids. Solid or liquid particulates vary in size and chemical composition. These particulates are derived primarily either from fuel combustion or from industrial sources. Secondary particulates are derived from various chemical and physical transformations in the atmosphere. The more common secondary aerosol particulates are sulfates, nitrates, and oxygen-containing hydrocarbons (2). Particulate air pollutants are solids or liquids and usually are expressed in very specific terms, e.g., dust, fumes, mist, smoke, or spray (14). The largest particles are dust (100+ μm). They are solids formed by mechanical processes and include coal and ash cement. Sprays (10+ μm) are liquids, usually water, formed by atomization of another liquid. Mists (0.5 to 3 μm) are liquid particulates formed by vapor condensation, i.e., sulfuric acid mist. The smallest particles are fumes (0.03–0.3 μm) and smoke (0.05–1.00 μm). Fumes are solids formed by vapor condensation, i.e., zinc and lead oxides. Smoke is a solid formed by incomplete combustion of hydrocarbons, e.g., cigarette smoke. Usually, the larger the particle the more irritating to the eye. For example, during Mt. St. Helens' eruption in 1980 less than 20% of those who received emergency care had retained foreign bodies in the cornea or conjunctiva.

EFFECT ON HUMAN HEALTH

Air Pollution Casualties

There have been a series of episodes of epidemic proportion when ambient air was polluted to such a magnitude that it caused serious public health problems. Death and illness have been reported where persistent thermal inversions resulted in high pollutant concentrations. Such incidents occurred in the Muse Valley, Belgium (1930), Donora, Pennsylvania (1948), London (1952), and Tokyo (1970). The illnesses resulting from episodes were characterized by a series of predominantly pulmonary disturbances; however, the most frequent sensory component complaint was irritation of the eyes.

Although eye irritation it usually cited, there is a paucity of major investigative efforts focusing on eye irritation by air pollutants. This is rather surprising, as eye irritation is one of the most frequently cited effects of air pollutants and usually is attributed to various photochemical oxidants or aldehyde derivatives, such as formaldehyde and peroxyacyl nitrate (PAN), and, surprisingly, not to the principal oxidants, such as ozone or nitrogen dioxide. Although there also are various cardiovascular and deleterious effects on the respiratory and pulmonary systems from these air pollutants, the emphasis of this chapter is on effects of air pollution on the eye.

Pollutant categories are regulated by the federal government to minimize adverse effects on public health. These pollutants are included in the National Ambient Air Quality Standard and are regulated under the National Emissions Standard for Hazardous Air Pollutants. Air pollutants that are regulated and included in air quality standards are carbon monoxide, sulfur oxides, particulate matter, ozone, hydrocarbons, nitrite oxides, and lead. The Hazardous Emissions Standard includes asbestos, beryllium, mercury, vinyl chloride, and benzene. The ocular irritants in the air are usually focused on formaldehyde, acrolein, and PAN, the eye irritants in photochemical smog. Eye irritation threshold for these agents ranges from 0.25 ppm for acrolein, which causes eye irritation, to 20 ppb for PAN. The consensus appears that the eye irritation resulting from photochemical smog can be attributed to these hydrocarbons and some of their derivatives.

Air Pollution—Outdoors

With regard to these large numbers of pollutants, only a few actually reach sufficient concentration to pose possible adverse effects on the human eye. Some of these are discussed below.

Carbon Monoxide

Carbon monoxide (CO) is the major air pollutant in the atmosphere. It is a colorless, odorless, gas and is derived primarily from the incomplete combustion of coal, oil, and natural gases. Carbon monoxide is effectively removed from the atmosphere by soil bacteria, which oxidizes it to carbon dioxide. In spite of this natural oxidative pathway, carbon monoxide does attain sufficient concentration as an air pollutant to exert toxic effects on the eye.

Sulfur Compounds

The predominant sulfur compounds occurring in polluted air are sulfur oxides. Of the various forms of sulfur oxides, sulfur dioxide (SO_2) is the chief species that attains sufficient concentrations to produce adverse effects on humans. This is a colorless gas that can usually be detected by taste and odor in concentrations of 0.3 to 1 ppm. In concentrations higher than 3 ppm, it has a pungent odor and is quite irritating to the eyes and respiratory system. Also, after it reaches the atmosphere it undergoes further oxidation by various pathways, i.e., photochemical processes, etc., to be ultimately converted to sulfate (SO_4-). The amount of SO_2 in the air usually is relatively low. The ambient SO_2 concentration in urban areas has been reduced due to recent regulatory measures; however, near metal smelters, the concentration of SO_2 can reach high levels. Sulfur dioxide is effectively removed from the atmosphere by natural processes. For example, because of its high water solubility, it is readily removed during rain.

Nitrogen Compounds

There are various gaseous species of nitrogen in our air. The major gases of concern found in the stratosphere are nitrous oxide (N_2O), nitric oxide (NO), and nitrogen dioxide (NO_2). These gases are even more important pollutants in the lower atmosphere.

Nitric oxides are a colorless, odorless, and tasteless gas that is minimally irritating to the eye. Nitrogen oxides are formed in large amounts in automobile exhaust and in the generation of alternative energy, from coal to oil. Its predominant adverse effect on the eye is attributed to its oxidation, as it is involved in various photochemical reactions with hydrocarbons, ozones, and formaldehyde.

Nitrogen dioxide is yellowish to reddish in color and has a rather pungent, irritating property. This is probably the worst of the nitrogen gases observed and is quite irritating to the eye. It can be produced by the oxidation of NO, particularly on a sunny day. The concentration of NO and NO_2 are frequently referred together as NO_X. The resident time of NO_X in the atmosphere has been estimated at 3 to 4 days. NO is oxidized to NO_2, and NO_2 is ultimately oxidized to nitrate.

Photochemical Oxidants

Organic nitrite compounds are formed by photochemical reactions involving a series of hydrocarbons and NO_X. Organic nitrite compounds such as peroxyacyl nitrate (PAN), peroxypropionyl nitrate (PPN), and peroxybuteryl nitrate (PBN) are formed in the atmosphere by photochemical reactions. The one that is of concern in this chapter is PAN as it can cause eye irritation. Hydrocarbons are important primary pollutants because they enter into these photochemical atmospheric reactions. The chemicals involved are the aliphatic hydrocarbons, olefins, and polyunsaturated hydrocarbons such as acetylene, as they are precursors to forming aromatic hydrocarbons such as benzopyrene, benzene, etc. Photochemical oxidants usually are referred to as chemicals that can easily oxidize chemicals not readily oxidized by oxygen. These photochemical oxidants are usually formed by chemical reactions of organic compounds with NO_X, oxygen, and sunlight. They are usually referred to in air pollution research as ozone (O_3), nitrogen dioxide (NO_2), peroxyacyl nitrate (PAN), and related compounds. These reactions occur in sunlight, and the secondary hydrocarbons of these organic compounds occur in severe smog. These reactions can raise the concentration of primary pollutants such as formaldehyde, olefinic hydrocarbons, and various organic formaldehydes.

Ozone is the most widely distributed and is one of the most important of the photochemical oxidants. It is found in high concentrations in the stratosphere, and it is of value because it absorbs ultraviolet radiation. Ozone in the troposphere is obtained from photochemical reactions of nitrogen oxides and the hydrocarbons. The concentration of oxidants has been decreasing in the atmosphere in California primarily due to greater efforts to institute an effective motor vehicle emission control system.

Air Pollution—Indoors

Most of the emphasis on air pollution is placed on our ambient air outdoors, although air inside factories, business offices, and homes also can be polluted by a large variety of pollutants. Since the exposure indoors is often of long duration, there have been serious public health problems associated with both public office buildings and residential homes. The air pollutants associated with the outdoors are predominately sulfur dioxide, ozone, and various hydrocarbons, whereas the indoor pollutants usually include formaldehyde, acrolein, various hydrocarbons, and biological organisms. Some pollutants that are common to both the indoor and outdoor environment are nitrogen oxides, carbon monoxide, particulate matters, and various hydrocarbons.

Building Pollutants and Associated Illnesses

Occupants of offices, public buildings, and schools have reported outbreaks of illnesses, and in some buildings the number affected exceeded 40% to 50% of the occupants (1). Among the various signs and symptoms associated with these building-related illnesses, eye irritation is the most frequent symptom reported.

Building Materials, Furnishings, and Contents

Formaldehyde is probably the most prominent causal factor associated with indoor pollutant complaints, as formaldehyde is a common material used in wall paneling and pressed wood insulation. Other indoor polluting chemicals are solvents that are associated with paint products, e.g., xylene and toluene. Other sources of contamination are building furnishings such as furniture, carpeting, wood panels, etc. Carpet adhesives using cyclopentadine have been associated with irritation, and dimethyl acetamide in plastic office dividers is a potent irritant. Also, formaldehyde is present in the various wood-related products used in paneling. Of course, the use of office equipment can present problems such as signature machines using methacrylate and duplicators using methyl alcohol. Photocopying machines produce high concentrations of ozone and are associated with volatile hydrocarbon emissions.

Pyrolytic End Products

Ever since the caveman burned wood inside his cave for warmth and comfort, man has been forever plagued with combustion by-products. Indoor air pollution associated with the use of open fires fueled by wood, charcoal, straw, dung, kerosene, and petroleum products has always been in our midst. Gas stoves release various carbon monoxides, nitrogen oxides, formaldehydes, and hydrocarbon particles that can produce eye irritations as well as other adverse effects on health. One of the greatest concerns with indoor combustion is the accumulation of carbon monoxide. Although this is a health concern, carbon monoxide itself is usually not an eye irritant. To place the problem in proper perspective, with a wood burning stove one can measure various emissions of CO, NO_X, SO_2, formaldehydes, particulate matters, and a series of volatile hydrocarbon pollutants, some of which have been identified as known carcinogens. However, one of the indoor pollutants of greatest concern is tobacco smoke. The concerns here are not only in the liberation of formaldehyde, acrolein, and cyanide, but also in carcinogens like nitrosamine and polycyclic aromatic hydrocarbons. These products, particularly acrolein and formaldehyde, can cause eye irritation, as they frequently occur in smoke-filled rooms. It should be emphasized again that the adverse health effects of tobacco smoke are not only on the eyes, but also on other systems, e.g., cardiovascular, pulmonary, and central nervous system.

Formaldehyde

Formaldehyde is a widely used chemical in industry and appears in various chemical products; therefore, its distribution in the indoor environment is widespread. Formaldehyde is very irritating not only to the eyes, but also to the upper respiratory tract and skin. The Committee on Toxicology at the National Academy of Sciences has reported that approximately 10% of the United States population may be hypersensitive to the irritating effects of formaldehyde, and one of the most prominent sites of irritation is the eye. The primary source of this chemical in the indoor environment is its use as a urea-formaldehyde foam insulation, which is frequently used in mobile as well as in conventional homes. In addition to irritation of the eyes, formaldehyde also produces irritation of the respiratory tract causing dyspnea, chest pain, etc. Further signs and symptoms include insomnia, headaches, memory loss, dizziness, fatigue, nausea, diarrhea, skin rashes, and abdominal pains.

Some commercial products that liberate sufficient formaldehyde to contaminate the indoor air at a high level are wood products, particularly particleboard, foam insulation, and other building materials that use urea-formaldehyde or resin, especially as adhesives. The rationales for the formaldehyde liberation are the following: (a) The instability of urea-formaldehyde resins: as they degrade, free formaldehyde is liberated from the foam insulation, particleboard subflooring, etc. (b) In recently installed materials, urea is the limiting reagent. Formaldehyde is used in excess to drive the polymerization reaction; therefore, the excess formaldehyde is slowly liberated.

Under these conditions formaldehyde liberation is directly proportional to the temperature and humidity of the home. As the temperature and humidity increases, the formaldehyde concentration also will increase. Government regulation of potentially health-threatening indoor pollution is rather complex, as it includes several federal agencies such as the Consumer Products Safety Commission, Environmental Protection Agency, Department of Housing and Urban Development, Department of Energy, National Institute of Safety and Health, and Office of Safety and Health Agency. Unfortunately, no single federal agency has complete regulatory authority over air pollution problems to control indoor air quality. Standards have been set for acceptable thresholds for indoor air quality, and some of these guidelines cover air contaminants that cause eye irritation and include sulfur dioxide, particulate matters, photochemical oxidants, formaldehyde, phenol, and acrolein.

IMPACT OF AIR POLLUTION ON CALIFORNIA RESIDENTS

Because of the abundance of sunshine, copious production of nitrogen oxides and sulfur oxides, and its unique topography, the endemic persistence of serious air pollution problems continues to exist in California. Research on smog probably has its focal point in California because of the persistence of smog in such geographic areas as Los Angeles, and, to a lesser extent, the San Francisco Bay region (3). The California Health and Mobility Survey studied the influence by air pollution. Questions such as how many were affected, what geographic areas were affected, and in what manner were they affected have been discussed at length. One of the major surprises revealed by this survey was that the air pollution problem is not limited to Los Angeles County or the San Francisco Bay region, as almost half (45%) of the adult population indicated that they were bothered by air pollution, with the most frequent adverse health effect reported being referable to the eye (79%). This study indicated that over 35% of the population of California suffers from eye irritation as a result of air pollution. With respect to Los Angeles County, approximately 67% of the population is bothered by air pollution, and 89% of the affected individuals indicated that the most frequent adverse effect of air pollution is eye irritation. This would indicate that at least 60% of the general population of Los Angeles County suffers from eye irritation as a direct result of air pollution.

Questions on this health survey regarding the effect of air pollution on the eye warranted such responses as watery eyes, burning eyes, inability to see well because of irritated eyes, constant wiping of the eyes because they were watery, and smarting of the eyes as one drove through certain localized areas. These complaints occur more frequently during the summer months (July, August, September). This correlates with the time period when smog reaches its highest concentration. The seriousness of air pollution is becoming more apparent, as one out of five people surveyed who had formerly lived in an air-polluted area indicated that the pollution had some influence on their decision to move.

Eye irritation appears to be the sign and symptom most frequently associated with air pollution in California, as a major portion of the population surveyed reported eye complaints. This is not to suggest that the state of California is not attempting to ameliorate this problem, as in the past two decades the air pollution has leveled off in spite of the continued increase in population density. This survey makes it apparent that the ocular effects of air pollution represent a condition of epidemic proportion since it is affecting a major segment of the population. From a public health viewpoint, it should be considered an alarming health problem of epidemic proportion that has not been investigated. The occurrence of eye irritation from air pollutants warrants serious investigative efforts to attempt to reduce the frequency of this toxic effect.

When one takes into account additional toxic effects of other chemicals on the eye, besides air pollution, the issue of ocular toxicity becomes of major importance. For example, various other toxicants, such as methanol, can affect the visual areas in the central nervous system, causing a decrease in visual acuity, papilledema, scotomas, optic atrophy, and tobacco amblyopia. In addition, there are other ocular toxins associated with papilledema, such as cortical steroids, ethylene glycol, nalidixic acid, and tetracycline. Numerous other substances have been associated with optic neuropathies, producing damage to the optic nerve and thereby causing visual loss or impairment, alteration of color vision, and centrocecal scotomas, e.g., chloramphenicol, isoniazid, and lead.

IMPACT OF AIR POLLUTION ON THE EYE

General

The eye is an organ that is quite vulnerable to the effects of air pollution. Although it is generally recognized that eye irritation is *the* most frequently reported toxic sign associated with exposure of humans to air pollution, this ocular effect is frequently overlooked (4). Eye irritants can be formed in our atmosphere by the interaction of hydrocarbons with sulfur oxides and nitrogen oxides. Some of the potent irritants formed in synthetic smog systems includes formaldehyde, peroxybenzol nitrate (PBzN) (5), peroxyacetyl nitrate (PAN), and acrolein. For pragmatic reasons most of the investigative efforts of air pollution have focused on synthetic rather than natural smog. This synthetic smog usually is produced from automobile exhaust or from olefin-nitrogen oxide mixtures, or by ultraviolet (UV) irradiation of aromatic hydrocarbons and nitrogen oxides. Chemical species usually found in this synthetic smog are formaldehyde, acrolein, and PAN, with the addition of aromatic hydrocarbon PBzN. The relationship of these irritants formed in synthetic smog to those formed in natural smog still remains to be established. Therefore, the investigation of mechanisms of eye irritation from smog must await the identification of the chemical species involved in producing this toxic effect. Investigation of eye irritants would be facilitated if there were some good objective methods and standards for measuring eye irritation (4,6).

In recent years, the composition and production of tears from exposure to eye irritants has been intensely investigated. Tears are rather complex fluids that are derived from the secretion of lacrimal glands and from accessory glands. Tears from lacrimal glands contain lysozyme, whereas tears derived from accessory glands, the goblet cells of the conjunctiva, do not contain lysozyme (7). Most studies on lysozyme were on the protein components. One protein of interest is a specific tear protein (STP) that does not correspond to any protein in serum (8). The role of STP has not been clearly elucidated. There have been suggestions of an inverse relationship between a decrease in lysozyme concentration with an increase in STP. Chemical analyses of tears have probably been limited in the past due to sample size. Recent introduction of capillary electrophoresis where the sample size requirements have been dramatically reduced may afford the opportunity to gain more insight on the alteration of chemical composition of tears during exposure to various eye irritants. New technology may provide greater opportunities to obtain more objective biomarkers to establish some relationship among the specific chemicals that produce eye irritation.

Another approach to the measurement of eye irritation in response to specific chemicals is electrophysiological measurement of neuronal responses subsequent to stimulation of the sensory receptors in the cornea (9). Studies in which electrodes are attached to the long ciliary nerves in decerebrate cats to record the impulses after mechanical or thermal stimulation also have been conducted (10). Other recordings have been made from the trigeminal nerve complex. These studies show neurons that are capable of responding to chemical stimulation of the cornea (11,12). There have been attempts to record action potentials resulting from chemical irritants in smog with measurements made on the eye *in situ* and on cats. When placed on the cornea, chemical irritants such as acrolein can evoke bursts of spike potentials. Due to animal welfare concerns, these types of studies of eye irritation from smog will be limited in the future (13).

One of the limitations on investigations of eye irritants is the lack of methods for consistent quantitation of the degree of eye irritation. Current methods often include subjective evaluation of the degree of irritation. An objective measurement of eye irritation still needs to be developed to allow correlation of the degree of eye irritation to the concentration of the irritant. Changes in lysozyme concentration is a presently used biomarker. Dose-response relationship measurements have been attempted in the past to relate degree of irritation with the concentration of smog. Presently these measurements have not been as satisfactory as one would desire, particularly when natural smog is employed. However, a more satisfactory dose-response relationship has been established when synthetic smog is employed.

Since the composition of photochemical smog depends on atmospheric conditions, only a limited number of these chemical mixtures have been investigated. Sensitive objective methods of quantification of eye irritation, coupled with improved methods of analyses of these complex photochemical mixtures, would permit accurate correlation of the degree of eye irritation with the chemical irritants. Subjective evaluation of eye irritation is a valuable approach and does provide a somewhat toxicological assessment of the effects of eye irritation, which is invaluable. However, the addition of more precise chemical objective methods to measure eye irritation with biomarkers would provide an important contribution to obtaining greater understanding of what is happening in the use of these photochemical irritants.

The determination of lysozymes and pH value of tears are a useful initial approach; moreover, the introduction of capillary electrophoresis (where only microliter samples are required), coupled with sensitive detectors, e.g., laser-induced fluorescent detectors, may provide an approach that would be worth exploring and that would permit development of a more precise relationship between the concentration of the irritant and the degree of eye irritation produced.

The assessment of photochemical irritants on the atmosphere involves very complex pharmacological-toxicological problems. The first problem arises in dealing with an atmospheric oxidant mixture of varying composition and the assessment of these irritants on a dose-response relationship. Because no standard of composition for the irritant exists and because there is no objective measure of irritation, such a relationship is difficult to establish precisely. This problem becomes even more complex when coupled with biological variations of sensitivity and resistance of some members of the population to these various photochemical oxidants. Attempts to assess these responses could be improved if precise objective methods were available to quantitate the concentration of the photochemical eye irritants with a precise biomarker response. These problems have limited progress in assessing the biological effect of atmospheric photochemical eye irritants derived from smog on man, especially with respect to the eye. A major investigative effort needs to be made to establish methods of assessing eye irritants. This research is warranted as eye irritation from smog is without question one of the most frequently recorded toxic complaints. In a heavily polluted area, this public health issue has reached epidemic proportion as it affects a high percentage of the population.

Clinical

The most frequently reported environmental complaints concern the adverse effects of air pollution on the ocular system, especially eye irritation (14). These are not only the most frequently reported complaints, but are one of the earliest signs and symptoms, as eye irritations usually precede other health problems such as asthma, nasal and throat irritation, sinus difficulties, allergies, bronchitis, coughing, and headaches associated with air pollution (1,3). The gases involved in air pollutants have been discussed earlier.

Acute exposure to primary pollutants causes complaints of eye irritation including foreign body sensation, hyperemia, and chemosis of the conjunctival tissue. With the secondary air pollutants from photochemical oxidants, such as formaldehyde, acrolein, and PAN (15), the symptoms usually observed are hyperemia, tearing, chemosis, and dry sensation of the eye (5). Of all these air pollutants, PAN was found to be 200 times more irritating to the eye than formaldehyde (5), whereas ozone was found not to be an important eye irritant (16,17).

There have been increasing concerns about indoor pollution, especially in the home environment, as, unlike the industrial setting, there have been only recent federal or state guidelines for threshold limit values or maximal allowable concentrations for exposure to these pollutants in the home. Outdoor air pollutants can be concentrated in the indoor environment because of a diminished air exchange. In the indoor commercial environment, some buildings contain endogenous air pollutants sufficient to cause adverse toxic effects on the personnel. The resultant symptoms have been ascribed to a "sick building syndrome." The World Health Organization has included eye irritation and erythema among the signs and symptoms of this syndrome, with eye irritation being the first physical sign and symptom to occur (18). Some of the symptoms manifested by sick building syndrome, in addition to irritation to the eye, nose, and throat, are dry mucus membranes and skin, erythema, mental fatigue, headaches, increased frequency of respiratory infection, coughing, nausea, and dizziness. Other complaints of subjects exposed to smog eye irritation are watery eyes, burning eyes, stinging eyes, foreign body sensation, and rubbing and itching of the eyes.

OCULAR TOXICITY

Carbon Monoxide

Carboxyhemoglobin levels of 5%, such as would occur in slow, heavy traffic (30 ppm of CO), can cause a decreased sensitivity to light, particularly at night (19). At 500 ppm, retinal hemorrhage and papilledema occur. Of course, duration of CO exposure is critical to the manifestation of this pathology. Carbon monoxide intoxication also produces neuro-ophthalmic findings of cortical blindness, visual field constriction, nystagmus, optic neuritis, optic atrophy, and pupillary abnormality (20).

Halperin et al. (19) investigated the effects of carbon monoxide on visual thresholds and were able to differentiate between hypoxic hypoxia and CO hypoxia by using gas mixtures containing low partial pressure of oxygen to carbon monoxide ratios. Recovery of visual discrimination was prolonged after exposure to carbon monoxide, whereas the visual effects of hypoxic hypoxia were rapidly reversed by the administration of 100% oxygen. The prolonged carbon monoxide effect on vision is consistent with the lesion observed upon clinical and histological examinations of the central nervous system after carbon monoxide poisoning. Using a visual discriminometer, the clinical measurement employed was visual sensitivity to differences in light intensity as an index of the effect of carbon monoxide versus hypoxic hypoxia by breathing air, oxygen, and carbon dioxide mixtures (21). These studies showed that carbon monoxide caused a decreased visual sensitivity, and these effects not only persisted much longer than that of hypoxic hypoxia due to oxygen deprivation, but continued long after carbon monoxide was eliminated from the blood. This suggested that carbon monoxide exerted a pharmacological effect on vision receptors in the central and/or peripheral visual system that combines with oxygen and carbon monoxide. In other words, carbon monoxide is binding and is exerting a pharmacologic effect on central visual receptors in addition to producing hypoxia by combining with hemoglobin to form carboxyhemoglobin to decrease the oxygen-carrying capacity of the blood.

Ophthalmic examination during carbon monoxide intoxication indicated a reversible ischemic retinopathy that is presumed to be attributed to carbon monoxide (20). This ophthalmic pathology of the retina reveals retinal hemorrhage, retinal edema, and papilledema, which are consistent with retinal toxicity induced by carbon monoxide. In carbon monoxide poisoning, the neuro-ophthalmological findings include cortical blindness (22), constriction of the visual field (23), disturbances of the optic nerve including optic neuritis and atrophy, extraocular palsies (24), and pupillary abnormalities. There also have been occasional reports of retinal venous congestion, hyperemia of the papilla, and fine retinal hemorrhage. Visual acuity also has been reported to be markedly impaired by exposure to carbon monoxide.

Volcanic Eruption of Mt. St. Helens

In a random telephone survey 6 weeks after the volcanic eruption of Mt. St. Helens in southwest Washington, the Washington Department of Social Health and Service reported that 4% to 8% of urban populations in the high ash fallout area complained of ocular irritation (25). A survey to evaluate the ocular effects of this volcanic eruption was conducted among residents of four northwestern states, on loggers exposed to high concentrations of the volcanic ash, and to a control group not exposed to the ash. The most commonly documented ocular problem was a foreign body sensation. Approximately half of the exposed individuals had irritative conjunctivitis, resulting from the volcanic ash, but less than 20% had conjunctival or corneal foreign bodies that required removal. Individuals who wore contact lenses or who had sicca syndrome were bothered most by the volcanic ash exposure, and hard contact lens wearers had more problems than wearers of soft contact lenses. Loggers working in the ash environment suffered from ocular hyperemia and foreign body sensation. The ocular symptoms usually subsided in 1 to 2 days after leaving the ash environment. In general, the volcanic ash caused minimal ocular mucosal damage other than chemical irritation, which resulted in hyperproduction and secretion of mucus. The toxic effect of the volcanic pollutants was less than expected. It has been conjectured that this may be attributed to the small size of the particulate matter, which permits elimination through the nasolacrimal duct. Also, the ash was chemically inert and contained only 4% to 6% free silica (14).

Bhopal Disaster

This incident represents one of the few air pollutant disasters where the chemical can be well defined. The chemical was methylisocyanate (26). On the first day after the Bhopal disaster, the Department of Ophthalmology at Ghandi Medical College examined victims with eye injury (26), and found signs and symptoms of streaming eyes, photophobia, profuse lipidema, and superficial corneal ulcerations. More variable findings included inferior punctate keratopathy, conjunctival chemosis, and pigmentary deposition on the central inferior aspect of the cornea. The most frequent symptoms reported by these victims were burning of the eyes and throat. No case of blindness could be attributed to the exposure. In a subsequent follow-up, some cases of unilateral corneal scars were observed that could ultimately impair vision, but there were no cases of blindness detected among these victims.

SUMMARY

The mechanism of toxicity of air pollutants is not well defined as these are complex and variable mixtures. Attempts to mimic air pollutant models under laboratory conditions have met with only limited success. Biomedical investigations of the effects of air pollutants on the ocular system have been hampered by the lack of good microanalytical approaches to attain objective biochemical markers. This limits our understanding of the biochemical mechanisms of ocular toxicity resulting from air pollution, which may be resolved in the near future as more sophisticated analytical methods are developed.

REFERENCES

1. Godish T. *Air quality*. Chelsea, MI: Lewis Publishers, 1985;1-328.
2. Patterson RG. Particulate pollutant characteristics. In: Calvert S, Englund H, eds. *Handbook of air pollution technology*. New York: John Wiley, 1984;97-134.
3. Hausknect R. *Air pollution: effect reported by California residents*. Berkeley, CA: California State Department of Health, 1959.
4. Wilson KW. Survey of eye irritation and lachrymation in relation to air pollution. Report proposed for the NY Coordination Research Council, Inc. by the Copley International Corp. 1974;1-45.
5. Heuss JM, Glasson A. Hydrocarbon reactivity and eye irritation. *Environ Sci Tech* 1968;2:1109-1116.
6. Wilson WE, Levy A, McDonald EH. Role of SO_2 and photochemical aerosol in eye irritation from photochemical smog. *Environ Sci Tech* 1972;6:423-427.
7. McEwen WK, Goodner EK. Secretion of tears and blinking. In: Davson H, ed. *The eye*, vol 3. New York: Academic Press, 1969;27-38.
8. Bonavida B, Sapse T, Sercarz E. Specific tear albumin: a unique lachrymal protein absent from serum and other secretions. *Nature* 1969;221:375-376.
9. Tower S. Unit for sensory reception in cornea. *J Neurophysiol* 1940;3:486-500.
10. Lele PP, Weddell G. Sensory nerves of the cornea and cutaneous sensibility. *Exp Neurol* 1959;1:334-359.
11. Mosso JA, Kruger L. Spinal trigeminal neurons excited by noxious and thermal stimuli. *Brain Res* 1972;38:206-210.
12. Mosso JA, Kruger L. Receptor categories represented in spinal trigeminal nucleus caudalis. *J Neurophysiol* 1973;26:472-488.
13. McEwen K. A proposed objective test of eye irritation. *Proceedings of the Fourth Air Pollution Medical Research Conference*, San Francisco, CA. Sponsored by the California State Department of Public Health, 1960;76-97.
14. Klopfer J. Effects of environmental air pollution on the eye. *J Clin Rev* 1989;60:773-778.
15. Orcutt JA. Relative eye-irritation potency of acrolein, formaldehyde and irradiated auto exhaust hydrocarbons in air as measured by the quantal response in humans. *The Pharmacologist* 1969;11:2.
16. Schuck EA, Doyle GJ. Photooxidation of hydrocarbons in mixtures containing oxides of nitrogen and sulfur dioxide. *Air Pollution Foundation Report*. San Marino, CA 1959;29:104-112.
17. Hamming WJ, MacBeth WG, Chass RL. The photochemical air pollution syndrome. *Arch Environ Health* 1967;14:137-149.
18. Nero AV Jr. Controlling indoor air pollution. *Sci Am* 1988;258;42-48.
19. Halperin MN, McFarland RA, Niven J. The time course of effects of carbon monoxide on visual thresholds. *J Physiol* 1959;86:142-144.
20. Bilchik RC, Muller-Bergh HA. Ischemic retinopathy due to carbon monoxide poisoning. *Arch Ophthalmol* 1971;86:142-144.
21. Crozier WJ, Holway AH. Theory and measurement of visual mechanisms. I. A visual discriminometer. *J Gen Physiol* 1939;22:341-364.
22. Grimsdale H. A case of gas poisoning with unusual ophthalmological complications. *Br J Ophthalmol* 1934;18:443-446.
23. Fink AI. Carbon monoxide asphyxia with visual sequelae. *Am J Ophthalmol* 1951;34:1024-1027.
24. Walsh FB, Hoyt WF. *Clinical neuro-ophthalmology*. Baltimore: Williams Wilkins, 1969;69-91.
25. Fraunfelder FT, Kalina RE, Buist AS, Berstein RS, Johnson DS. Ocular effects following the volcanic eruptions of Mount St. Helens. *Arch Ophthalmol* 1983;101:373-378.
26. Andersson N, Kermuir M, Salmon AG. Bhopal disaster: eye followup and analytical chemistry. *Lancet* 1985;761-762.

Ophthalmic Toxicology, edited by
George C. Y. Chiou. Raven Press, Ltd.,
New York © 1992.

9

Occupational Hazards and Ocular Toxicity

James L. Way, Lynn Baxter, David McGuinn,
Ann Hawkins Zitzer, and Ilona Petrikovics

*Department of Medical Pharmacology and Toxicology,
Texas A & M University, College of Medicine, College Station, Texas 77843*

Although occupational medicine has become of increasing importance, the toxicologic hazards to the eye are frequently overlooked and are not included in some textbooks on occupational medicine. This is somewhat of a paradox as Bernardino Ramazzini (1), who is generally regarded as the father of occupational medicine, described eye injuries in detail in the first book on occupationally related disease of the eye. His concerns were the toxic injuries, by a noxious gas, to the eyes of individuals who worked in the sewer systems. It was noted that these workers had red, inflamed eyes and complained of a burning sensation. This irritant effect prompted these workers to rinse their eyes frequently with water throughout the work period. Prognosis for these workers was rather poor, as they ultimately lost their sight. The irritant gas that caused these injuries, of course, was hydrogen sulfide, which can be present in relatively high concentrations in septic pools, sewers, and underground passages. This gas is quite toxic and its irritant properties can cause severe conjunctivitis and keratitis (1). Occurrence of toxic insult to the eye due to chemicals is presently widespread, especially in high smog areas, such as Los Angeles, where eye irritation as a result of air pollution occurs quite frequently. One of the pioneering texts on occupationally related diseases and injuries to the eye was written by Minton (2). A more recent textbook on the effects of chemicals on the eye is the classic work of Grant (3). This discipline has now matured, and an International Society of Ocular Toxicology has been formed. This group met in Toronto, Ontario, in 1988 as the First Congress of the International Society of Ocular Toxicology (4).

Occurrence of eye injury caused by hazardous chemicals in the workplace is rather common and widespread. Damage to the eye results from topical injuries or from systemic absorption of these chemicals. These effects on the eye may occur immediately or may occur insidiously. Although at times the injury to the eye is obvious, e.g., nystagmus and decreased visual acuity, often the effect on the eye is very subtle and is easily overlooked. An extensive list of chemicals that can have injurious effects on the eye has been compiled by Grant (4) and Anger and Johnson (5). This chapter concentrates on a few particularly relevant chemicals, emphasizing chemical agents, rather than physical agents, that can produce ocular toxicity. Moreover, many of the chemicals that could have been included herein already have been discussed in the chapter by Way, Baxter, and Cannon.

CHEMICALS

Ammonia

Inadvertent release of ammonia gas from accidents or defective agricultural and industrial equipment accounts for many deaths and injuries. Exposure to ammonia should never be underestimated and special attention must be addressed to the eye (and also the skin and pulmonary system) since ammonia gas is quite hygroscopic. Ammonia is a colorless gas that has a characteristic pungent odor. It combines easily with water to form ammonium hydroxide. Severity of the damage to the tissue is attributed to the dissociation of ammonium hydroxide into hydroxyl ion. This strong base causes saponification and liquefaction of exposed mast epithelial surfaces of the moist surfaces of the eye. The eye is especially sensitive to these caustic burns. Such injuries are usually associated with an increase in intraocular pressure and the destruction of tissues, and frequently result in blindness.

Increase in intraocular pressure after ammonia exposure has been reported by Highman (6). The clinical course after ammonia exposure is similar to that seen in individuals with acute-angle closure glaucoma and is associated with corneal edema and semidilated fixed pupil. Birken et al. (7) have reported on the exposure to ammonia gas causing tissue damage to the eyes, skin, and respiratory tract. This report indicated that the most important factor to minimize the toxic effects from exposure to ammonia is prompt, vigorous ocular irrigation with water. These researchers suggest that severe injury to the eye resulting from ammonia exposure should be treated with topical steroid cream applied to the eyes, and that prophylactic antibiotics should be given. Even with vigorous and timely treatment, severe exposure to ammonia can cause total destruction of the cornea, resulting in blindness.

The predominant uses of ammonia are as fertilizers, detergents, and as an intermediate in the manufacture of other chemicals. Workers who are involved in the manufacture and transport of ammonia are at risk of toxic exposure primarily because of the potential for accidental leaks and spills. In addition to its use as a fertilizer, it also is used industrially in the manufacture of nitric acid, urea, synthetic fibers, dyes, plastics, chemicals, and pharmaceuticals.

The characteristic odor of ammonia is readily detectable by smell well below the toxic level. Ammonia odor usually can be detected at 30 ppm, and eye irritation occurs at 50 ppm (8). Ammonium hydroxide is usually available in solutions of 10% and 29%; the commercial household ammonia is approximately 7%.

Carbon Disulfide

Carbon disulfide is a volatile, colorless, flammable liquid. In its pure form, it has an ethereal odor; however, it usually is encountered in a technical grade that has a rather unpleasant odor because of other sulfide contaminants. Global production of carbon disulfide is estimated at over 1 million metric tons (9). Carbon disulfide is used primarily to produce viscose rayon and cellophane, and this accounts for over 50% of the industrial uses of carbon disulfide. Another 25% of carbon disulfide is used as a raw material in the industrial production of carbon tetrachloride. Other commercial uses of carbon disulfide are grain and soil fumigants, polymerization for vinyl chloride, electroplating solutions, corrosion inhibitors, and in the production of rubber accelerators. Estimates by the National Institute of Occupational Safety and Health (NIOSH) (10) indicate that over 20,000 workers in the United States are exposed to carbon disulfide annually. Carbon disulfide previously was used as an anesthetic agent, but was discontinued because of its toxicity (11) and explosive properties.

Federal regulation for a permissible level of carbon disulfide exposure is 20 ppm as an 8-hr TWA (time weighted average) concentration, 30 ppm as a 30-min ceiling standard, and 100 ppm as the maximum peak. Recommendations were made by NIOSH (12) of a standard of 1 ppm (3 mg/m^3) as a TWA concentration for up to a 10-hr work shift and a 40-hr work week; also a 15-min ceiling concentration of 10 ppm (30 mg/m^3). The threshold limit value (TLV) presently suggested for occupational exposure is 10 ppm in the United States. This TLV was recommended to protect against cardiovascular toxicity, but this concentration also is assumed to protect against neurotoxicity (13).

The effects of carbon disulfide on the ocular system have been reviewed (12). Goto and Hottar (14) examined workers exposed to carbon disulfide in rayon plants by direct ophthalmoscopy and reported small retinal hemorrhages or microaneurysms. Goto et al. (15) examined individuals exposed to carbon disulfide in Japan and Yugoslavia by fluorescein angiography and reported an enhanced occurrence of microaneurysms. The frequency of microaneurysms was found to be directly related to the extent of carbon disulfide exposure. These toxic manifestations of carbon disulfide are rarely reported in Finland but are quite common in Japan and Yugoslavia (16). These researchers also used hemodynamic studies with ocular pulse-waves and fluorescein angiography to observe delayed peripapillary filling.

Most of the reports on the ocular toxicological effect of carbon disulfide on the eye were obtained from workers in the viscose rayon industry. This presents some difficulties in the interpretive evaluation of these data, as it is not possible to dissociate carbon disulfide and hydrogen sulfide toxicities. Both of these toxic compounds are present in the rayon factory atmosphere at a ratio of 10:1. Szymankowa (17) reported conjunctival inflammation and disturbed color vision from carbon disulfide at an exposure level not exceeding 3 ppm. However, there are some controversies concerning these findings, as the reporting of the air concentration of carbon disulfide has been questioned. Maugeri et al. (18) suggested the use of ophthalmodynamography as a diagnostic test for detecting early signs of carbon disulfide–induced cerebral involvement, as this method can detect cerebral circulatory disturbances. Delayed peripapillary filling has been reported as the first indication of chronic carbon disulfide poisoning, followed by behavioral deterioration and, lastly, coronary heart disease (19).

In his summary of the toxicity to the eye by carbon disulfide, Grant (20) indicated that the peripheral and central signs and symptoms were quite varied. In severe chronic poisoning, visual disturbances would suggest retrobulbar neuritis, which is characterized by central scotoma, decreased visual acuity, and impaired color discrimination of red and green. Permanent, complete blindness rarely occurs. Although irritation of the eye and keratitis epithelialis have been attributed to carbon disulfide, these symptoms are more likely due to the concomitant release of hydrogen sulfide.

In addition to the effects on the ocular system, carbon disulfide exposure in humans has major toxic effects on other systems (21). Central nervous system involvement frequently is reported from carbon disulfide poisoning. The encephalopathy begins insidiously with signs and symptoms of paresthesia, motor defects, spastic paralysis, fatigue, headaches, irritability, somnolence, memory deficit, and personality changes (22). There also are other neuropathic changes, as there is a slowing of sensory nerve conduction velocity (23) and EEG changes (24). Carbon disulfide toxicity, if not severe, can lead to delayed partial or complete recovery (22). Besides the nervous system, toxicity has been noted in the cardiovascular system where there is an increase in mortality from coronary heart disease and a higher prevalence of hypertension, elevated cholesterol and lipoprotein. Other toxic effects can occur on the reproductive system, where there is a lower sperm count with an increased frequency of abnormal spermatozoa. Loss of libido and impotence do occur. Also, in exposed women there are increased menstrual abnormalities and higher instances of spontaneous abortions and premature births.

Concerning the mechanism of toxicity, carbon disulfide behaves similarly to other electrophiles; therefore, there is an affinity for nucleophilic groups such as hydroxyl, sulfhydryl, and amino groups. For example, carbon disulfide reacts with the amino group of amino acids and proteins and participates in cyclization reactions with the formation of thiazolidine compounds. Carbon disulfide also can form metal chelates by complexing with zinc and copper. Two proposed mechanisms of action of carbon disulfide toxicity are as follows: (a) depletion of copper in the nervous system by the formation of a thiazolidine ring structure; and (b) a high affinity of carbon disulfide for sulfhydryl groups, which can cause inhibition of various enzymatic reactions. The mechanism of toxicity of carbon disulfide also has been shown to interfere with catecholamine metabolism (25). This effect may be due to the inhibition of dopamine β-hydroxylase, which is responsible for the conversion of dopamine to norepinephrine since this enzyme is copper-requiring, and carbon disulfide may chelate this metal and inhibit the enzyme (25).

Carbon disulfide has also been reported to inhibit liver microsomal oxidative drug metabolizing enzymes (26). Carbon disulfide will decrease cytochrome P-450 activity in phenobarbital-induced animals. Carbon disulfide exposure in human males also leads to a decrease of liver microsomal drug metabolizing enzymes as noted by a decrease in oxidative demethylation of amidopyrine (27). Another toxicity reported for carbon disulfide is on the endocrine system. There is an impairment of sexual function, especially impotence and decreased libido, in chronic carbon disulfide toxicity (22). The pathology in humans shows scattered necrosis of the brain and peripheral neuropathy. Lastly, nephrosclerosis has been reported in autopsies of humans exposed to carbon disulfide (15).

Ethylene Oxide

Ethylene oxide is a reactive compound that is used quite extensively in the United States. It is one of the top twenty-five chemicals produced in the United States, and over 4 billion pounds are consumed annually. Peripheral neuropathy is one of the major toxic lesions of ethylene oxide (28). There appears to be a correlation between ethylene oxide exposure and cataract formation (29). These toxic effects of ethylene oxide have become of increasing concern, as hospital workers are exposed routinely to high levels of ethylene oxide. The chemical and biological properties of ethylene oxide have been reviewed (30).

This reactive gas is colorless at room temperature and has a characteristic ethereal odor. Ethylene oxide is a potent alkylating agent and acts directly on nucleophiles such as -OH, -SH, $-NH_2$, and -COOH groups; therefore, it would be expected to react with the nitrogen atoms of purines, pyrimidines, and amino acids. Ethylene oxide binds covalently to DNA predominately at *N*-7 of guanosine to form *N*-7-hydroxyethyl guanine. This reaction may be the basis of the mutagenicity of ethylene oxide (31). It also binds to the histidine moiety in hemoglobin to form *N*-3-(2-hydroxyethyl)-histidine. This provides the basis for biological monitoring of exposures to ethylene oxide (32). In aqueous solutions, ethylene oxide degrades to ethylene chlorohydrin and ethyleneglycol.

Exposure to high concentrations of ethylene oxide results in lacrimation, conjunctival inflammation, and clouding of the cornea. Ethylene oxide is irritating to the respiratory tract and skin. Headaches, nausea, vomiting, diarrhea, lymphocytosis, and central nervous system depression have been reported. At one time, ethylene oxide was used as a general anesthetic, but was abandoned because of its inherent toxicity. Ethylene oxide in solution can cause burns with blisters (33). Peripheral neuropathy has been reported on acute exposure (34) and usually occurs on chronic exposure. Nerve conduction can be affected. This reactive compound is mutagenic (35) and is regarded as a potential human carcinogen. Epidemiological studies indicate that exposure to ethylene oxide increases the risk of developing leukemia (36). It would be desirable to reduce the exposure of workers to ethylene oxide (37).

Formaldehyde

Formaldehyde is a reactive gas with an acrid odor. In an aqueous concentration of 30%, it is called formalin. It is not surprising that it is used as a compressed gas, because formaldehyde has a tendency to polymerize in the gaseous form. Formaldehyde is an intermediate that is used widely in many occupations; over 225 occupations encounter formaldehyde (38). Some of the industries where there are high formaldehyde concentrations in the ambient air are iron foundries and plywood and particleboard industries, as formaldehyde-base resins are extensively employed. These formaldehyde-base resins are the primary components of particleboards, fiberboards, plywood, and insulating materials.

With formaldehyde concentrations of 0.05 ppm eye irritation is detectable, and lacrimation occurs at concentrations of 20 ppm in air. Exposure to formaldehyde in the ambient air causes irritation of the eye, skin, and respiratory tract. Irritation of the eyes in humans has been the most frequent complaint due to formaldehyde released from urea-formaldehyde and phenol-formaldehyde resins used in various wood paneling. If a 40% formalin solution is accidentally splashed in the eye, it is immediately painful but the eye appears uninjured for the first few hours. However, in the next 12 hr all areas of the cornea will show damage and edema and the interior segment will undergo degeneration. In the following few days, the cornea undergoes degeneration and opacification, and the victim suffers from photophobia, swelling of the lid, and chemosis, and ecchymosis becomes evident. The treatment of such eye exposure should consist of immediate irrigation with water (39).

There is a latent period of a few hours postexposure where the eye appears to be normal (40). This period of apparent toxic grace could provide an opportunity for major investigative effort to interrupt the interaction of formaldehyde with various tissue components. It seems that it should be possible to attempt to sequester formaldehyde or its biotransformation product by binding formaldehyde immediately to an agent with a higher affinity for formaldehyde than the tissue proteins. Inspired formaldehyde was found to be mutagenic and carcinogenic in Fisher rats by the Chemical Industry Institute of Toxicology (CIIT) (38). More importantly, exposure of Fisher rats to concentrations that may be encountered by humans was manifested by the development of nasal carcinoma.

The panel that was convened by CIIT to evaluate their studies indicated that formaldehyde should be regarded as posing a cancer risk to man even though no studies have demonstrated a direct carcinogenic effect of formaldehyde in man. These studies were of concern from a human health viewpoint, as many homes use a urea-formaldehyde type of insulation, and some mobile homes built with particleboard and plywood also have a high indoor formaldehyde concentration. These homes can have concentrations of formaldehyde that range up to 1.77 ppm (41,42). The indoor air in these homes with high concentrations of formaldehyde has been reported to cause irritation of the eyes and the upper respiratory tract and increased incidence of cough, headaches, memory lapse, and drowsiness (43). Also of increasing concern is that formaldehyde and hydrogen chloride can interact in moist air to form bis-(chloromethyl) ether, a known carcinogen for humans.

n-Hexane and Methyl *n*-Butyl Ketone

The aliphatic alkanes form a class of compounds that has wide commercial applications and the annual consumption runs into billions of pounds. Exposure to most alkanes or ketones even in high concentrations usually results in narcosis or anesthesia, but does not produce neurotoxic signs. The exceptions to this are *n*-hexane and methyl *n*-butyl ketone, as these compounds do produce neurotoxicity in humans. *n* Hexane is still widely used industrially and both *n*-hexane and methyl *n*-butyl ketone are biotransformed by a pathway that forms a common neurotoxic metabolite that is more toxic than the starting compounds. Japanese researchers first reported the development of peripheral neuropathy resulting from exposure to *n*-hexane found in printing plants and pharmaceutical firms (44). Actual peripheral neuropathy resulting from *n*-hexane exposure also has been reported in Italy, France, Spain, Morocco, Portugal, Japan, and the United States (45). These two solvents are used in adhesives, lacquer thinner, paints, and in many other commercial products. Neuropathology usually occurs at high concentrations and/or from repetitive use (or abuse) over a prolonged period. The most severe cases reported are usually due to glue sniffing (46).

Hexane is well absorbed in the inhalation route, and occupational exposure is primarily due to inhalation of the toxic vapors. Some of the toxicity referable to the ocular system are blurred vision, polyneuropathy, optic atrophy, and retrobulbar neuritis. In experimental animals, visual loss, abnormal pupillary reflexes, and nystagmus have been reported (47,48). Raitta et al. (49) indicated that retinal toxicity and macular damage are important aspects of *n*-hexane toxicity, as these cause color discrimination defects. High concentration exposure is usually associated with central effects such as vertigo and alteration of touch perception. In many cases, there are skeletal motor weaknesses, which ultimately involve the musculature of the pelvis and thigh. Usually, there is also central and peripheral axonal degeneration. Studies by Schaumberg and Spencer (48) reported hexane neuropathy is associated with axonal swelling, nerve fiber degeneration, and subsequent demyelination. Color vision loss has been correlated with solvent exposure (50). This chromatic discrimination loss increases with exposure level. Also, an increased incidence of diminished foveal reflex and incipient lens opacification was noted to occur with solvent exposure.

Cyanide

This compound has become well known for its rapid lethal action. Since the cyanide ion has a pKa of 9.2, it is readily liberated from solution as a gas (hydrogen cyanide). Cyanide is widely distributed with regard to its industrial use, as over 1 billion pounds of sodium cyanide are consumed annually in the United States. This toxicant has wide distribution with regard to its application, as it is used in manufacturing steel, electroplating industries, and photographic films. It is also present in many poisonous plants and in a variety of fruit pits, such as apricot kernels, and in range grasses. Cyanide has actually been advocated as a putative cancer cure in the form of the drug, Laetrile, and has caused problems in drugs used to treat malignant hypertension, such as sodium nitroprusside, which liberates large quantities of cyanide.

With regard to the mechanism of acute poising, cyanide is believed to exert its toxic effect by the inhibition of the terminal oxidase, cytochrome oxidase. With regard to the acute effects on vision, cyanide characteristically produces a dilated pupil, and can cause blindness and damage the optic nerves and retina (51). Marked central retinal edema has been reported. In experimental animals, lesions in the retina and optic nerve, degeneration in the optic nerve, optic chiasma, and changes in the electroretinogram have been reported.

Cyanide wastes have contaminated our waterways and our drinking water. These wastes are produced by the electroplating, steel, aluminum and paint industries, and by certain mining operations. A series of litigations have been introduced in an attempt to control environmental contamination with cyanide. Regulation of discharge of cyanide wastes into our waterways is included in the Federal Water Pollution Act (BL 92-500). The Environmental Protection Agency (EPA) filed a Refuse Acts suit against the Armco Steel Co. for the discharge of cyanide into the shipping channel in Houston, Texas, and successfully prosecuted this company (CA 70-H-1335). Presently, there are other litigations pending against an aluminum company for allegedly contaminating the aquifer in Washington. Unlike in surface water, cyanide in the underground water table is not easily dissipated.

One of the sources of hydrogen cyanide air pollution is the petrochemical industry. Recently, automobiles equipped with malfunctioning catalytic platinum converters have been reported by Bell Laboratories to produce hydrogen cyanide (52). Another source of hydrogen cyanide in the air is from home fires because of the increase in plastic contents in homes. Various plastics, such as polyurethane, liberate hydrogen cyanide upon pyrolysis (53). Lastly, one of the major sources for the inhalation of hydrogen cyanide affecting man is tobacco smoke. The use of low-tar, low-nicotine, or filter cigarettes does not reduce the hydrogen cyanide concentration in cigarette smoke.

With regard to the chronic exposure to cyanide, e.g., tobacco smoking (54) and cassava ingestion, various optic neuropathies and Leber's optic atrophy have been observed (55). It has been proposed that ingestion of cassava, which has a high cyanide content, can cause optic neuritis (56) and tobacco amblyopia (57). In both of these cases, it has been suggested that the biotransformation of cyanide to the less toxic thiocyanate was altered. The evidence suggesting that tobacco ambylopia can be attributed to cyanide is that the administration of hydroxocobalamin, a cyanide antidote and chelator, lowers blood cyanide level and rapidly reverses the tobacco amblyopia. The disease, Leber's optic atrophy, has been attributed to a deficiency in the enzyme thiosulfate sulfurtransferase, better known as rhodanese (55). Individuals with this enzyme deficiency cannot metabolize cyanide to the less toxic thiocyanate.

Questions have been raised with regard to the differences in expression of cyanide toxicity with the route of administration. Cassava ingestion and tobacco smoking cause optic neuropathy, whereas chronic industrial inhalation exposure usually is not expressed in this manner. Part of the explanation for this disparity may be different physiological dispositions of cyanide when it is inhaled rather than ingested. With regard to the association of tobacco smoking with tobacco amblyopia, the pulse of cyanide in tobacco smoke would be relatively high and in industrial exposure it would be low. A high, spiking cyanide exposure is more apt to produce an optic lesion. The effect of cyanide on the cornea of humans is of interest, as during fumigation with hydrogen cyanide the development of edema of the cornea with residual effects has been reported (58). No similar corneal disturbances have been produced in the eyes of laboratory animals exposed to cyanide.

There appears to be a difference in the selectivity of hydrogen cyanide and hydrogen sulfide in their respective reactions on the corneal epithelium. Although both compounds appear to inhibit organometallo enzymes (specifically cytochrome oxidase), hydrogen sulfide has become notorious for highly selective toxicity to the corneal epithelium, whereas the effect of hydrogen cyanide on the eye usually is more diffuse. The mechanism of cyanide toxicity and its antagonism have been reviewed (59).

Treatment of cyanide poisoning should be immediate and should include symptomatic treatment as well as the use of cyanide antidotes. The treatment of cyanide poisoning in the United States is available in commercial kits (Eli Lilly). These kits consist of ampules of amyl nitrite which can be inhaled to form methemoglobin from hemoglobin while the intravenous administration of sodium nitrite is being prepared. Sodium nitrite and sodium thiosulfate are then subsequently administered. The mechanism for this antidotal combination is that nitrite is employed to sequester cyanide as cyanomethemoglobin and thiosulfate is employed as a sulfur donor to convert cyanide to the less-toxic thiocyanate in the presence of the enzyme rhodanese. In Europe, there are two different cyanide antidotes. The first is cobalt ethylenediamine teraacetate (CoEDTA) (60). In Germany, a different antidotal combination is used, dimethylaminophenol (DMAP) and sodium thiosulfate. DMAP was developed because it formed methemoglobin much more rapidly than sodium nitrite. Questions have been raised that the mechanism of action of sodium nitrite in antagonizing the lethal effect of cyanide may be due in part to an alternative mechanism, a vasogenic action, rather than methemoglobin formation.

Hydrogen Fluoride

Hydrogen fluoride usually is used as an aqueous 49% or 79% stock solution, hydrofluoric acid. The number of commercial uses for hydrofluoric acid is rapidly increasing (61). It is widely used in the etching of silica products, e.g., in the production of semiconductors. It also is used in the manufacture of aluminum fluoride, in electroplating, in the manufacture of high-performance plastics, and as an alkylating agent for production of high-octane gasoline. Fluoride salts also are used in the fluoridation of drinking water to minimize dental cavities. Hydrofluoric acid is irritating to the mucous membrane, conjunctiva, and skin, and concentrations as low as 5 ppm can cause irritation to the eyes. Hydrogen fluoride presence in the industrial air can cause conjunctival hyperemia in the palpebral fissure, but corneal disturbance is rare (62). Hydrofluoric acid in the ambient air causes not only irritant effects in the ocular system, but also may cause pulmonary edema in the respiratory system. Some of the toxicity is referable to the gastrointestinal tract, causing nausea, vomiting, and anorexia. When absorbed systemically, a severe hypocalcemia occurs with associated changes in the Q-T segment on the EKG (63). Metabolic acidosis and hypomagnesemia have been reported.

The mechanism of toxicity of hydrogen fluoride is not fully understood. Fluoride can be complexed with a divalent ion, particularly with calcium and magnesium. An alternative explanation is related to the observation that ocular burn with hydrofluoric acid is more severe than with any other halogenated acids. With direct contact of hydrofluoric acid solution in the eye, there is immediate coagulation and eventual sloughing of the corneal surface, with moderate conjunctival inflammation developing. Also, chemosis and mild corneal opacity can develop. The difference in relative toxicity between hydrochloric acid and hydrofluoric acid may be due to the increased penetration of the fluoride ion into the corneal stroma and underlying ocular structure.

Injuries resulting from hydrofluoric acid burns are somewhat unique as is the treatment of these injuries. Hydrofluoric acid splashed in the eye should be treated immediately and vigorously (61). With minimal exposure to hydrofluoric acid, a delayed ocular toxicity is noted. A case report indicated that when the eye was irrigated after initial exposure to hydrofluoric acid, there was subsequent delayed toxicity that became manifested 4 days after exposure. Attempts have been made to extrapolate the treatment of hydrofluoric acid burns to the skin to similar treatment for the eye. In both cases, immediate steps should be taken to remove the excessive acid and to dilute the acid present in the tissue. In an attempt to minimize the penetration of hydrofluoric acid and to bind the dissociated fluoride ion, irrigation solutions for skin burn usually contain soluble calcium salts and, more recently, quaternary ammonium detergents (63). Although these solutions have been shown to be appropriate for washing the skin, some difficulties were encountered when these solutions were used to irrigate the eye. The use of 10% calcium gluconate and benzalkonium detergent solutions causes injury to the eye by themselves (64). Since the use of these additional chemicals in the irrigating solution can cause further corneal alteration their use does not seem reasonable. Irrigation solutions that can be employed for hydrofluoric acid contact are water and isotonic sodium chloride. These were found to be the most effective treatment for ocular hydrofluoric burns. Speed of irrigation is most important to the removal of the hydrofluoric acid and to prevent its penetration to ocular structure. Also, the use of isotonic calcium chloride irrigation was not as toxic as calcium gluconate, but there was increased frequency of corneal ulceration. The quaternary ammonium detergents are effective in treating hydrofluoric acid skin burns; however, these solutions are unacceptable for use in the eye because they, too, can alter the cornea.

Hydrogen Sulfide

Hydrogen sulfide is a gas that is widely used in various industrial processes and that poses a hazard of exposure in a variety of conditions. This highly toxic gas is found in natural gas, volcanoes, and in certain natural spring waters. It is used widely in the manufacture of cellophane, depilatories, dyes, felt, fertilizers, adhesives, silk, rayon, and various synthetic petroleum products. It is also encountered in the processing of sugar beets, mining where sulfide ores are present, in sewers and sewer treatment plants, and in wells and caissons. There is a great degree of concern in Texas and Edmonton, Canada, where hydrogen sulfide is encountered in the drilling of gas wells, which results in high morbidity and mortality among workers associated with this occupation. Hydrogen sulfide exposure also is encountered in tanneries, breweries, slaughterhouses, and in lithography and photoengraving processes.

Hydrogen sulfide is a rapidly acting poison with an extremely high knockdown potency. There have been a series of cases reported where the rescuer becomes the victim in areas of high sulfide contamination. This gas is colorless, heavier than air, and has a well-recognized odor of rotten eggs. Although this gas can be easily detected at very low concentrations, this should not be relied upon as an indication of danger, as olfactory fatigue rapidly occurs at 100 to 150 ppm. This fatigue leads to the false impression that the hydrogen sulfide gas is diminishing in concentration whereas it may be actually increasing (65).

Hydrogen sulfide was one of the first chemicals to spark interest in industrial medicine. Its toxic properties were described by Ramazzini (1) in the first textbook on industrial medicine. The patients he observed were sewer workers laboring in a high hydrogen sulfide concentration. These workers suffered from severe chronic irritation to their eyes and eventually lost their sight. This was one of the first observations of the conceptual importance of occupational medicine as it related the etiology of disease to the workers' occupations. The effect of hydrogen sulfide on the eye is of considerable importance, as this ocular effect occurs at concentrations that provide no other observable systemic effect. At higher concentrations of hydrogen sulfide, collapse, coma, and death from respiratory failure can occur in a few seconds (66).

The effect of hydrogen sulfide in producing injury to the cornea and conjunctiva at low concentration is of interest with reference to occupational workers. At concentrations of 200 ppm hydrogen sulfide, workers have reported pain in the eyes, visual blurring, and superficial cornea turbidity (67). At lower concentrations of hydrogen sulfide, workers were aware of the unpleasant odor, and ocular symptoms usually developed a few hours later. Usually, there is a gradual onset of ocular symptoms, i.e., scratchy, irritating sensation, tearing, and burning. Slit-lamp biomicroscopic examination of the eye at these concentrations reveals only a conjunctival hypermia and keratitis. This exposure can lead to increasing burning discomfort, photophobia, and color halos (rings around lights). As exposure becomes more severe, the corneal surface may become lusterless and eroded from death and loss of epithelial cells.

Although there are many antidotes reported for hydrogen sulfide to protect against these toxic effects, at the present time there are no really effective antidotes.

The effect of hydrogen sulfide on the eyes has been reported (68). After acute exposure to hydrogen sulfide, at the point of recovery, it has been generally presumed that elimination of the gas is complete, and resumption of normal activity occurs. However, recent studies suggest that, after acute knockdown from hydrogen sulfide, there may be subtle residual damage.

Hydrogen sulfide toxicity in humans has been summarized by the EPA (67). In acute intoxication at 2,000 ppm, the worker becomes unconscious within a few seconds (termed "knockdown") followed almost immediately by respiratory paralysis. Death will occur unless the victim is removed from the contaminated site and artificial ventilation instituted. The lethal effects of hydrogen sulfide are believed to be directly on the central nervous system as the respiratory center of the brain ceases functioning and breathing terminates. In lower lethal concentrations (500 to 1,000 ppm), it is believed that cellular fixation occurs. Hydrogen sulfide is thought to exert its toxic effect by inhibition of cytochrome oxidase, thereby inhibiting tissue utilization of oxygen. In acute poisoning, permanent neurological damage occurs and is associated with prolonged comas, convulsions, increased tonus with extension muscle spasm, and a positive Babinski's sign (69). Toxicity referable to the heart also has been reported (70). Studies by computerized tomography (CT) scan (69) and postmortem examination of brain tissue suggest that the hydrogen sulfide lesion is not really a specific neurotoxic lesion, but is characterized by cerebral anoxia (71).

Toluene Diisocyanate

Toluene diisocyanate is a reactive chemical that is employed in the production of polyurethane foam. This foam is used in mattresses, upholstery, packaging material, and various automobile parts. Polyurethane is formed by the reaction of polyols and isocyanate in the presence of water to yield a polymeric foam. The primary toxicity from toluene diisocyanate is associated with respiratory health complications precipitating occupational asthma (72). It has been reported to be a potent inducer by sensitization reaction (73). Exposure to toluene diisocyanate vapors occurs primarily when it is used to form polyurethane. The toxicity of toluene diisocyanate to the eye has been reported by Luckenback and Kielar (74). Some of the toxicities reported by workers exposed to toluene diisocyanate vapors are decreased visual acuity, red irritated eyes, blurred or foggy vision, mild edema of the corneal epithelium, and conjunctival infection. These signs and symptoms are gradually alleviated in a few days.

REFERENCES

1. Ramazzini B. Diseases of workers. (Translated by Wright WC.) From *De Morbis Artificum Diatriba, 1713*. New York: Hafner, 1964.
2. Minton J. *Occupational eye diseases and injuries*. New York: Grune & Stratton, 1949;39–110.
3. Grant WM. Toxicology of the eye. In: Thomas CC, ed. *Drug, chemicals, plants and venom*. Springfield, IL: Charles C. Thomas, 1974;1–1201.

4. Lerman C, Tripathi RC. *Ocular toxicology, proceedings of the First Congress of the International Society of Ocular Toxicology*. New York, Basel: Marcel Dekker, 1990.
5. Anger WK, Johnson BL. Chemicals affecting behavior. In: O'Donoghue JL, ed. *Neurotoxicology of industrial and commercial chemicals*. Boca Raton, FL: CRC Press, 1985;51-148.
6. Highman VN. Early rise in intraocular pressure after ammonia burns. *Br Med J* 1969;2:259-260.
7. Birken GA, Fabri PJ, Carey LC. Acute ammonia intoxication complicating multiple trauma. *J Trauma* 1981;33:820-822.
8. Rom WN. *Environmental and occupational medicine*. Boston: Little, Brown, 1983;273-274.
9. Timmerman W. Carbon disulfide. In: Bushey GJ, Campbell L, Klingsberg A, van Nes EJ, eds. *Kirk-Othmer encyclopedia of chemical technology*, vol 4, 3rd ed. New York: John Wiley-Interscience, 1978;742-748.
10. National Institute of Occupational Safety and Health. *Occupational exposure to carbon disulfide*. Publication Number 77-156. Washington, DC: Department of Health, Education and Welfare. 1977.
11. Simpson JY. Notes on the anesthetic effects of chloride hydrocarbon, nitrite of ethyl, benzene aldehyde and bisulphurate of carbon. *Mo J Med Sci* 1848;8:740-745.
12. Health effects of occupational exposure to carbon disulfide. NIOSHTIC Number 00135185 Chapter 7. 1984;1-15.
13. Carbon disulfide. In: *Documentation of the threshold limit values for substances in work room air*, 4th ed. Cincinnati: American Conference of Governmental Industrial Hygienist, 1980;70.
14. Goto S, Hottar R. The medical and hygiene of carbon disulfide poisoning in Japan. In: Briber, Teisinger, eds. *Toxicology of carbon disulfide*. Amsterdam: Excerpta Medica Foundation, 1967;219-230.
15. Goto S, Hottar R, Sugimoto K. Studies on chronic carbon disulfide poisoning—pathogenesis of renal microaneurysm due to carbon disulfide with special reference to a subclinical defect of carbohydrate metabolism. *Int Arch Arbitsmed* 1971;28:115-126.
16. Sugimoto K, Goto S, Taniguchi H, Craitta B, Tolonen M. Ocular fundus photography of workers exposed to carbon disulfide. A comparative of epidemiological studies between Japan and Finland. *Int Arch Occup Environ Health* 1977;39:97-101.
17. Szymankowa G. Observation of the effects of carbon disulfide on vision engaged in the manufacture of synthetic fibers. *Klin Oczna* 1968;38:41-44 (Polish).
18. Maugeri U, Cavalleia VL. Ophthalmodynamography in occupational carbon disulfide poisoning. *Med Lav* 1966;57:730-740 (Italian).
19. Tolonen M. Chronic subclinical carbon disulfide poisoning. *Work Environ Health* 1974;11:154-161.
20. Grant WM. *Toxicology of the eye*. Springfield, IL: Charles C. Thomas, 1974;231-235.
21. Spencer PS, Schaumberg HH. Experimental and clinical neurotoxicology. In: Seppalainen AM, Holtia M. *Carbon disulfide*. 1980;356-372.
22. Vigliani EC. Carbon disulphide poisoning in viscose rayon factories. *Br J Ind Med* 1954;11:235-241.
23. Vasilescu C. Sensory and motor conduction in chronic carbon disulphide poisoning. *Eur Neurol* 1976;14:447-455.
24. Styblova V. Die Elektroencephalographie in de Diagnostik der frühzeitigen Hirnschädigung durch Schwefelkohlenstoff. *Int Arch Occup Environ Health* 1977;38:263-271.
25. Magos L, Jarvis J. The effects of carbon disulfide exposure on brain catechols in rats. *Br J Pharmacol* 1970;39:26.
26. Freundt KJ, Liebaldt GP, Sieber K. Effect of barbiturates on the liver of rats exposed to carbon disulfide vapour. *Int Arch Occup Environ Health* 1974;32:297-304.
27. Mack T, Freundt KJ. Inhibition of oxidative N-demethylation in man by low doses of inhaled carbon disulfide. *Biochem Pharmacol* 1974;3:607-613.
28. Greenberg MK, Swift TR. Ethylene oxide peripheral neuropathy: four year followup. *Muscle Nerve* 1982;557.
29. Jay WM, Swift TR, Hull DS. Possible relationship of ethylene oxide to cataract formation. *Am J Ophthalmol* 1982;93:727-732.
30. Rom WN. Environmental and occupational medicine. In: Casey KR, ed. *Ethylene oxide*. Boston: Little, Brown, 1983;663-666.
31. Ehrenberg L, Hiesche KD, Osterman-Golkar S, et al. Evaluation of genetic risks of alkylating agents: tissue doses in the mouse from air contaminated with ethylene oxide. *Mutat Res* 1974;24:83-91.
32. Calleman CJ, Ehrenberg L, Jansson B, et al. Monitoring and risk assessment by means of alkyl groups in hemoglobin in persons occupationally exposed to ethylene oxide. *J Environ Pathol Toxicol* 1978;2:427-436.

33. Sexton RJ, Henson EV. Experimental ethylene oxide human skin injuries. *Arch Ind Hyg Occup Med* 1950;2:549-557.
34. Gross JA, Haas ML, Swift TR. Ethylene oxide neurotoxicity. Report of four cases and review of literature. *Neurology* 1979;29:978-983.
35. Nolman SR. Mutational consequences of exposure to ethylene oxide. *J Environ Pathol Toxicol* 1979;2:1289-1293.
36. Hogstedt C, Malmquist N, Wadman B. Leukemia in workers exposed to ethylene oxide. *JAMA* 1979;241:1132-1139.
37. National Institute of Occupational Safety and Health. *Ethylene oxide*. Current intelligence bulletin #35, DHEW Publication No. (NIOSH) 81-130. Washington, DC: U.S. Government Printing Office, 1981.
38. National Institute of Occupational Safety and Health, U.S. Department of Health and Human Services. *Formaldehyde: evidence of carcinogenicity*. Current intelligence bulletin 34. Washington, DC: U.S. Government Printing Office, 1981.
39. Clark RP. Formaldehyde in pathology departments. *J Clin Pathol* 1983;36:839-846.
40. Grant WM, Thomas CC. *Toxicology of the eye*, 2nd ed. Springfield, IL: Charles C. Thomas, 1974;502-507.
41. Forni A, Cappelline A, Pacifico E, et al. Chromosome changes and their evolution in subjects with past exposure to benzene. *Arch Environ Health* 1971;23:385-388.
42. Breysse PA. The health cost of "tight" homes (editorial). *JAMA* 1981;245:267-273.
43. Bander JR, Mullin L, Graepel GJ, et al. Eye irritation response of humans to formaldehyde. *Am Ind Hyg J* 1983;46:463-465.
44. Yamada S. Intoxication in polyneuritis in workers exposed to *n*-hexane. *Jpn J Ind Health* 1967;9:651-659.
45. Allen N, Mendell JR, Billmaier DJ, et al. Toxic polyneuropathy due to methyl *n*-butyl ketone. *Arch Neurol* 1975;32:209-217.
46. Korobkin R, Asbury AK, Sumner AJ, et al. Glue sniffing neuropathy. *Arch Neurol* 1975;32:158-167.
47. Spencer PS, Schaumberg HH. Neurotoxic properties of certain allophatic hexacarbons. *Proc R Soc Med* 1977;70:37-39.
48. Schaumberg HH, Spencer PS. Degeneration in central and peripheral nervous system produced by pure *n*-hexane: an experimental study. *Brain* 1976;99:183.
49. Raitta C, Seppalainen AM, Houskonen MS. *n*-Hexane maculopathy in an industrial worker. *Arch Klin Exp Ophthalmol* 1978;209:99-110.
50. Mergler D, Blain L, Lagace JP. Solvent related colour vision loss: an indication of neural damage. *Arch Occup Environ Health* 1987;59:313-321.
51. Grant WM. Toxicology of the eye. In: Thomas CC, ed. *Drug, chemicals, plants, and venom*. Springfield, IL: Charles C. Thomas, 1974;333-337.
52. Voorhoeve RJH, Patel CKN, Trimble LE, et al. Hydrogen cyanide production during reduction of nitric acid over platinum catalysts. *J Catalyst* 1978;54:102-105.
53. Jellinek HAG, Takata K. Toxic gas evolution from polymers: evolution of hydrogen cyanide from polyurethanes. *J Polymer Sci* 1977;15:2269-2288.
54. Smith ADM, Duckett S. Cyanide, vitamin B_{12}, experimental demyelination and tobacco amblyopia. *Br J Exp Pathol* 1965;46:615-622.
55. Wilson J. Leber's hereditary optic atrophy—a possible disorder of cyanide detoxication. *Excerpta Med Int Congr Series* 1967;154:70-73.
56. Osuntokun BO. An ataxic neuropathy in Nigeria. *Brain* 1968;91(part II):215-248.
57. Darby PW, Wilson J. Cyanide smoking and tobacco amblyopia. *Br J Ophthalmol* 1967;51(5):336-338.
58. Robbie WA, Leinfelder PJ, Duane TD. Cyanide inhibition of corneal respiration. *Am J Ophthalmol* 1947;30:1381-1387.
59. Way JL. Cyanide intoxication and its mechanism of antagonism. *Annu Rev Pharmacol Toxicol* 1984;451-481.
60. Paulet G. Intoxication cyanhydrique et chelates de cobalt. *J Physiol* 1958;438-442.
61. Hatai JK, Weber JN, Doizaki K. Hydrofluoric acid burns of the eye: report of possible delayed toxicity. *Toxicol Cutan Ocular Toxicol* 1986;5:79-184.
62. Grant WM. *Toxicology of the eye*, 2nd ed. Springfield, IL: Charles C. Thomas, 1974;557-559.
63. McCully JP, Whiting DW, Lauber SE. Hydrofluoric acid burn of the eye. *J Occup Med* 1983;25:447-449.

64. Wetherhold JM, Sheppard FP. Treatment of hydrofluoric acid burns. *J Occup Med* 1965;7:193-196.
65. Rom WN. *Environmental and occupational medicine*. Boston: Little, Brown, 1983;225-276.
66. National Institute of Occupational Safety and Health. *Occupational exposure to hydrogen sulfide salts*. DHEW Publications number (NIOSH). 77-158. Washington, DC: U.S. Government Printing Office, 1976.
67. Environmental Protection Agency. *Health assessment document for hydrogen sulfide*. Report number EPA/600/8-86/026A. Washington, DC: Office of Health and Environmental Assessment, 1986.
68. Beasley RW. The eye and hydrogen sulfide. *Br J Med* 1963;20:32-40.
69. Matsuo F, Cummins JW, Anderson RE. Neurologic sequelae of massive hydrogen sulfide inhalation. *Arch Neurol* 1979;36:451-452.
70. Arnold IMF, Dufresne RM, Alleyne BC, et al. Health implications of occupational exposure to hydrogen sulfide. *J Occup Med* 1985;27:373-376.
71. Lund OE, Wieland H. Pathologic anatomical findings in experimental hydrogen sulfide poisoning (H_2S). A study on rhesus monkeys (German). *Int Arch Gewerbepathol Gwewebehyg* 1966;22:46-65.
72. Zapp JA Jr. Hazards of isocyanates in polyurethane foam plastics production. *Arch Industr Health* 1957;15:324-330.
73. Schrenk HH. Industrial hygiene. *Industr Engin Chem* 1955;47:107A-108A.
74. Luckenback M, Kielar R. Toxic corneal epithelial edema from exposure to high atmosphere concentration of toluene diisocyanate. *Am J Ophthalmol* 1980;90:682-686.

Ophthalmic Toxicology, edited by
George C. Y. Chiou. Raven Press, Ltd.,
New York © 1992.

10

Treatment of Chemical Ocular Injury

Linda C. Epner

Private Practice
Baltimore, Maryland 21224

GENERAL PRINCIPLES

Immediate and copious irrigation of the injured eye with a bland irrigating solution is the key element in the treatment of any chemical injury to the eye. Irrigation must begin on-site within seconds after the injury and continue en route to, and at, the emergency facility. The victim should not wait until arrival at the emergency room for irrigation to begin (1–3). To begin irrigation, the victim's eyelids should be spread open with a lid retractor (Desmarres), or even with the fingertips if a retractor is not available, and flooded with a bland solution such as water or Ringer's intravenous fluid (4,5). Remove any goggles, glasses, or contact lenses that may interfere with irrigation (6). The victim should be asked to roll the eyes in all directions to improve irrigation of ocular surfaces, including conjunctival cul-de-sacs. The eyes should be examined carefully, including sweeping of the conjunctival fornices, to remove any foreign particles such as solid chemicals that, if retained, will continue to leak chemicals into the eyes despite irrigation. Any foreign particles may be gently lifted off the conjunctiva of the cornea with a clean tissue or cotton tip applicator. Alternatively, foreign particles, once identified, may be irrigated off the ocular surface as well.

Irrigation after arrival at the medical facility continues using suspended bags of pH balanced intravenous fluid connected by sterile tubing with or without a scleral contact lens on the injured eye. Depending on the nature of the insult, irrigation must continue for a minimum of 1 l irrigation fluid for a mild injury to several hours of irrigation for a severe alkali injury. Periodically, the pH of the conjunctival cul-de-sac should be checked with litmus paper, and irrigation must continue until the pH is normal again. Alkalies cause deeper ocular damage and may remain deep in ocular tissue acting as a reservoir of base. They can continue to produce ocular damage despite irrigation. Alkali injuries, therefore, require prolonged irrigation, until the pH is normal and remains normal with repeated checks.

After irrigation, the eye should be examined at the slit lamp with fluorescein stain to look for any epithelial defects and for the depth of the anterior chamber. Once it is determined that the patient will tolerate mydriasis without risk of angle closure, a strong cycloplegic agent, such as atropine 1%, should be started twice daily. Topical antibiotic eyedrops also are indicated, four times a day, to prevent infection. If possible, an attempt should be made to measure the intraocular pressure. Secondary glaucoma especially develops in alkali burns due to collagen shrinkage. Acetazolamide (an oral carbonic anhydrase inhibitor) may be started to control intraocular pressure. In severe alkali burns, normalization of the pH of the aqueous by anterior chamber paracentesis with reformation with balanced salt solution or phosphate buffer may be useful, but this procedure is controversial (2,3,7).

The role of topical steroids also is controversial. They may be used safely during the first week after injury whether the corneal epithelium is intact or not. Beyond the first week, experimental data suggests they may contribute to corneal ulceration, and even perforation, due to interference with new collagen synthesis which is necessary in the reparative process (8). If topical steroids are used at all, they should be discontinued after the first week until the corneal epithelium is again intact.

There is an outpouring of collagenase after chemical burns, which leads to corneal ulceration. Various collagenase inhibitors have been advocated in the treatment of alkali burns. These agents include acetylcysteine (Mucomyst 10% or 20%), cysteine, penicillamine 0.15 M, calcium ethylenediaminetetraacetic acid (EDTA), and medroxyprogesterone (2,7,9). Collagenase inhibitors act to either reversibly or irreversibly inhibit collagenase action or synthesis.

Ascorbate levels in the aqueous humor are normally 15 to 20 times the plasma level (1). Alkali injuries cause a dramatic and prolonged drop in ascorbate levels (10). Since ascorbate is necessary for fibroblast collagen synthesis and critical for postinjury corneal repair, it has been used to treat alkali burns (1). Either topical 10% solution or high oral dosages (2 g four times a day) may be used to maintain high aqueous ascorbate levels to minimize ulceration.

Severe alkali injuries, in particular, may result in vision and even eye-threatening scarring. Symblepharon formation should be minimized by symblephara rings, scleral contact lenses, and lysis of early conjunctival adhesions as they form. Once symblephara are fixed, however, surgical measures are required to release them. These include conjunctival autografts if a normal conjunctiva is available and buccal mucosal grafts if it is not (11,12).

Often, despite very aggressive treatment of alkali and other chemical burns to the eye, severe scarring of the cornea, eyelids, and intraocular tissues occurs. Any rehabilitative surgery, such as penetrating keratoplasties, lid repairs, etc., should be delayed for as long as possible, preferably for at least 1 year postinjury (1). This allows inflammation to clear, and improves the success rate of rehabilitative surgery (13–16). Other issues that must be addressed in a timely fashion include continued treatment of any glaucoma and any formed cataracts. Keratoprosthesis is reserved for the most difficult of cases where lid function cannot be restored and penetrating keratoplasties have failed (17,18).

EXPERIMENTAL ANIMAL TREATMENT MODELS

Paracentesis/Anterior Chamber Irrigation with Phosphate Buffer

Bennett et al. (19) designed an experimental model using albino rabbits to determine the effect of phosphate buffer irrigation of the anterior chamber in alkali-burned corneas in rabbits. Alkali burns were produced by using one drop of 0.5 N NaOH placed on an 8-mm filter paper disk that was applied to the rabbit cornea for 40 sec. The rabbits were divided into five experimental groups. Groups 1 and 2 served as controls, receiving either corneal burns with no irrigation (group 2) or phosphate irrigation with no burn (group 1). Groups 3, 4, and 5 all received corneal burns, but phosphate buffer irrigation was instituted at varying times: immediate treatment, 15 min later, and 30 min later. After 6 weeks, eyes were examined clinically and histologically to determine the amount of corneal opacification and cataract formation. Burned corneas not receiving buffer irrigation uniformly developed extensive corneal vascularization and cataract formation. In contrast, burned corneas receiving phosphate buffer irrigation within 15 min developed less corneal vascularization and cataract formation. All eyes developed cataracts if buffer irrigation occurred at 30 min. Control eyes were unaffected by buffer irrigation, either clinically or histologically. This study suggests that early paracentesis and normalization of aqueous pH with phosphate buffer in alkali-burned corneas may decrease the degree of injury to the eye.

Treatment of Hydrofluoric Acid Burns

Hydrofluoric (HF) acid is used commonly in a variety of industrial settings. Eye injuries involving HF acid result in more serious damage compared with other acids, due to the ability of the fluoride ion to penetrate and cause liquefactive necrosis. McCulley et al. (20) investigated the benefit of various irrigation solutions and topical ointments in treating HF corneal burns in rabbits. Some of the irrigating solutions investigated included $MgCl_2$, NaCl, lanthanum chloride ($LaCl_3$), 0.2% Hyamine, and Zephiran. Magnesium oxide or $MgSO_4$ topical petrolatum ointments also were tried. Many of the above proved unsuitable for treatment due to toxicity in normal rabbit eyes. The study revealed that the best treatment for HF burns remains immediate irrigation with water, isotonic saline (NaCl), or $MgCl_2$. Repetitive irrigation was found to be less effective than single irrigation with increased risk of corneal ulceration. Since water and isotonic saline are the most immediately available irrigation solutions at the time of injury, they remain the gold standard for treatment of HF and other acid ocular burns.

Evaluation of Hypertonic Saline and Glucose on Alkali Corneal Burns

Alkali burns to the cornea produce edema, which is thought to be a precondition for revascularization (21). An inadequate glucose supply to the cornea also is implicated in stromal ulceration (22). These observations prompted evaluation of hypertonic saline and glucose ointment on rabbit corneal burns by Korey et al. (23). Corneal burns were produced by applying 0.5 N NaOH soaked filter paper for 30 sec with the rabbit under general anesthesia, followed by 60-sec lavage with distilled water. The rabbits were divided into three groups and treated with either vehicle, 40% glucose, or 5% NaCl ophthalmic ointment. Eyes were examined at 3 weeks and 6 weeks, both clinically and histologically, for corneal neovascularization, corneal ulceration, lenticular clouding, and red reflex. The results of this study demonstrate that treatment of corneal alkali burns with hypertonic glucose and saline ointments in rabbits resulted in much less corneal ulceration and neovascularization. Notably, there was no difference between hypertonic glucose and saline in the degree of corneal ulceration, and corneal clarity was better with hypertonic NaCl. Histologically, NaCl-treated rabbit eyes demonstrated more endothelium regeneration.

Ascorbic Acid for Corneal Burns

Levinson, Patterson, and Pfister found that ascorbate levels in the aqueous dramatically drop after alkali injury to rabbit cornea. They hypothesized that treating alkali-burned eyes with topical or subconjunctival injections of ascorbate to normalize aqueous ascorbate levels may help corneal healing. In their studies (10,24,25), New Zealand rabbits were anesthetized with pentobarbital sodium. Uniform-sized corneal burns were produced by filling a 6-mm or 12-mm lucite well with 1 N NaOH placed on the proptosed cornea. The NaOH was pipetted out after 20 sec, and the lucite well and cornea were rinsed with saline for 5 sec. Control rabbits received no treatment, while the remainder of the rabbits received daily injections of ascorbate either subcutaneously or topically. The researchers discovered that ascorbate-treated rabbits were less likely to develop descemetoceles and corneal perforation. Their findings have been confirmed by others (26,27). Ascorbate's mechanism of action remains unclear. It is known that ascorbate is necessary for new collagen synthesis, but it also may act to inhibit collagenase activity (26). Others feel it works as a superoxide radical scavenging agent (27).

Investigational Use of Tissue Adhesive for Corneal Perforations

Descemetocele formation leading to corneal perforation is a formidable treatment challenge. CHC tissue adhesive (carbohexoxymethyl 2-cyanoacrylate monomer) produced by Ethicon has been used on an investigative basis for treatment of corneal perforations. Investigators at the Wilmer Institute have been studying its use since 1974 (28). The glue is applied under microscopic control with topical anesthetic. After meticulously drying the perforation site, the anterior chamber is partially reformed with a small air bubble at the perforation site. A small drop of the tissue adhesive is then placed at the perforation site. After the glue has dried, it may be covered with a bandage-style soft contact lens, or a more definitive surgery may be performed once the anterior chamber is fully reformed. The tissue adhesive may be left in place for up to a year if it does not dislodge spontaneously sooner. It may be removed easily, if necessary, with a pair of sterile fine-toothed forceps. Investigators at Wilmer have found in a retrospective study that the incidence of enucleation after corneal perforation had decreased from 19% to 6% since initiation of tissue adhesive treatment, and 29% compared to 19% of the patients achieved visual acuities of 20/200 or better (28).

Medroxyprogesterone for Prevention of Alkali-Burn Perforations

Newsome and Gross (9) examined the effects of a known collagenase synthesis inhibitor, medroxyprogesterone, on collagenase activity in alkali-burned rabbit cornea. Albino rabbits were anesthetized with intravenous sodium pentobarbital, and uniform-sized alkali burns were induced by 1 N NaOH-soaked gauze disks. Rabbits were separated into control and treatment groups. Treated rabbits were further subdivided by mode of medroxyprogesterone administration: (a) topical drops consisting of 0.5% suspension of medroxyprogesterone in 1% methylcellulose daily or twice daily, (b) subconjunctival depot injections of 10 mg Depo-Provera repeated at weekly intervals, and (c) 200 mg intramuscular injections of Depo-Provera into the hind leg of rabbits at 7- to 8-day intervals.

All three modes of administration were effective in preventing corneal perforation. Only 4 out of 85 untreated corneas healed, compared with 51 out of 87 treated corneas that reepithelialized without perforation. There was a three- to four-fold decrease in collagenolytic activity in the treated animals compared to the controls. The rates of corneal ulceration were similar, approximately one-quarter in each group ulcerated but did not perforate. Of note, far fewer medroxyprogesterone-treated animals developed corneal perforation (8 out of 87) compared with a greater than 50% perforation rate in untreated corneas (49 out of 85 eyes). Further studies are necessary to delineate minimum effective dosages that may be as effective as the large doses used in this study.

Epidermal Growth Factor in Alkali Corneal Reepithelialization

Treatment of poorly reepithelializing corneas and recurrent corneal erosions is a major therapeutic challenge in alkali-burned corneas. Currently available treatment modalities, including bandage contact lenses, ascorbate, topical corticosteroids, etc., often fail. Epidermal growth factor (EGF) is a polypeptide known to stimulate corneal epithelial cell proliferation. It is isolated from mouse submaxillary glands. EGF was studied in a double-masked fashion to evaluate its effect on corneal reepithelialization in alkali-burned rabbit corneas (21). Rabbits were anesthetized with intravenous sodium pentobarbital and topical 0.5% proparacaine eyedrops. Ten-millimeter circular corneal alkali burns were produced by placing 1 N NaOH-soaked 10 mm-diameter Whatman filter paper disks on central corneas for 1 min.

Eyes were rinsed with distilled water, and methylene blue (0.5%) was used to confirm the area of epithelial loss. Mouse EGF eyedrops were produced by suspending 0.05 μg/ml EGF in phosphate buffer saline. Rabbits were randomly assigned to three treatment groups. Groups A and B received either EGF drops or placebo drops four times a day, beginning 16 hr after the alkali injury; then drops were reversed, and those receiving placebo drops received EGF, and vice versa, beginning on day 6 after the alkali injury. Group C served as control receiving no treatment drops at all. The results showed increased corneal epithelial wound healing in eyes receiving EGF. When EGF drops were discontinued, the corneal epithelium broke down again centrally. Those rabbits receiving placebo drops initially showed incomplete reepithelialization; however, once EGF was started, the wound closed completely. Histopathological studies revealed poorly adherent epithelium growing over no basement membrane and alkali-burned cornea stroma. The authors conclude that although EGF enhances epithelial growth in alkali-burned rabbit corneas, it has no effect on adherence of the epithelium to its underlying damaged stroma and, thus, has no effect in preventing the well-known complication of recurrent erosions. The authors suggest that a combination of EGF and other factors that may enhance epithelial attachment to underlying stroma may prove to be helpful therapeutic modalities in the future (21).

Conservative Management of Symblephara

One of the most difficult complications of alkali burns is shortening of the conjunctival fornices from scarring and the formation of adhesions between raw deepithelialized conjunctival surfaces (symblephara). Since treatment of extensive, formed symblephara is quite difficult, many different techniques have been tried to prevent their formation in the first place. Treatment modalities include symblephara rings, a scleral conformer fitted to prevent shortening of conjunctival fornices, or scleral contact lens. Other modalities that have been tried with limited success include plastic wrap and eggshell membrane lining of conjunctival fornices (29). A standard prophylactic treatment is daily sweeping of conjunctival fornices to lyse any forming symblepharon with a glass rod (30).

Platelet Activating Factor Antagonism

In addition to prostaglandins (PGs) and leukotrienes (LTs), platelet activating factor (PAF) is considered to be involved in the inflammatory reaction. It follows that PAF antagonists could be used as anti-inflammatory agents after alkali burns (31). PAF stimulates release of arachidonic acid and production of hydroxyeicosatetraenoic acid (HETE). In this study, a PAF antagonist, BN 52021, was applied topically to NaOH-burned corneas of New Zealand white rabbits in which 6 μl of labeled arachidonic acid were injected into the anterior chamber. The PAF antagonist was applied according to three experimental designs varying the spacing and frequency of drops. Postmortem analysis of corneal buttons were analyzed to measure levels of PGs and HETEs. Results showed that the PAF antagonist significantly inhibited production of radiolabeled cyclooxygenase and lipoxygenase products (HETEs) after alkali injury, especially when applied in an uninterrupted manner during the immediate postinjury period every 30 min for a total of nine times. No effect was noted, however, in the amount of protein content in aqueous humor with PAF antagonist.

Corticosteroid Use on Ulceration in Alkali Burns

A study was done by Donshik et al. (8) to evaluate the effect of topical corticosteroid drops on ulcerated alkali-burned corneas. The study was performed on albino rabbits. The results show that topical steroids given during postinjury weeks 2 and 3 resulted in increased severity of corneal ulcerations. The mechanism for this still is unclear, but may be related to inhibition of new collagen synthesis, rather than steroid enhancement of collagenase enzyme activity. Generally, if topical steroids are to be used at all after severe alkali corneal ulceration, it should be used only during the immediate postinjury period, days 1 through 6, then discontinued until the cornea is intact again. If, at any time during steroid use, corneal melting begins, steroids should be discontinued immediately.

SURGICAL TREATMENT

Surgical transplantation of conjunctiva and cornea are frequently done to relieve symptoms of eye injury for therapeutic or cosmetic benefit. Details of surgical techniques are not covered here. Readers are encouraged to consult the original literature or surgical texts if interested.

Conjunctiva

Conjunctival Transplantation

Unilateral chemical injuries in which there is severe conjunctival scarring may benefit from autologous conjunctival transplantation from the normal fellow eye. The scarred abnormal conjunctiva is dissected free, and the normal graft conjunctiva is then sutured in place either as a single doughnut-shaped graft or as multiple, smaller islands of conjunctiva.

Conjunctival Flap

A Gunderson conjunctival flap is another technique that has been used in eyes with nonhealing epithelium and poor visual potential. A variation on the Gunderson technique has been described by Paton and Milauskas (12). The keys to a successful flap include (a) no buttonholes, (b) an absence of traction from the flap base, and (c) thinness of the flap. It is important to remove Tenon's capsule from the undersurface of the dissected flap prior to securing on the cornea. The free margin of the flap is sutured to the episclera and the eye patched for 12 to 24 hr postoperatively. Most patients experience pain relief. Vision is limited by density of the central corneal scar and the thickness of the conjunctival flap.

Cornea

Pressure Patch

Mild contact thermal burns to the cornea, such as those from curling irons, may cause opacification of the corneal epithelium. Conservative management of such injuries include topical cycloplegia, antibiotic eyedrops, and pressure patching the injured eye with a soft sterile eye pad over the closed eyelid. The injured cornea usually reepithelializes within 24 to 72 hr, depending on the size of the epithelial defect (32).

Therapeutic Contact Lenses

Hydrophilic contact lenses can be used in patients with delayed healing of corneal and conjunctival injuries after chemical or thermal burns (33,34). Any necrotic tissue from the injured site should be gently debrided prior to placement of the bandage contact lens. These lenses allow regeneration of the epithelium and patient comfort. Hydrophilic contact lenses also have been used as a mode of therapy for descemetoceles. The cornea in a descemetocele is reduced in the involved area to only Descemet's membrane with no overlying stroma or epithelium.

Keratoplasty

Keratoplasty has been used as a surgical treatment for a variety of ocular conditions. It may be used in the late treatment of alkali burns, although the prognosis is not as favorable as penetrating keratoplasties performed for other ocular disorders, such as keratoconus or corneal stromal dystrophies. Postcorneal transplants performed after severe chemical injuries may be complicated by poor wound healing, severe dry eye, recurrent epithelial breakdown, and glaucoma. These complications can be minimized by pre- and postoperative glaucoma control, preservation of donor epithelium, and control of postoperative inflammation (30).

Corneal Perforation

Corneal Perforation Repair

When a full-thickness corneal defect occurs, it may be repaired by several techniques. A peripheral corneal perforation away from the visual axis may be repaired with a scleral or corneal patch graft (35). As sclera is opaque, this technique is not suitable for corneal defects that are within the visual axis. Donor cornea tissue may be used as a lamellar patch graft (15,16) for central perforations. Sutures should be placed away from the visual axis, and deep corneal bites should be used to avoid "cheese-wiring" of sutures through edematous corneal tissue. In some cases, very tiny corneal perforations may seal themselves spontaneously. Techniques used to plug a perforation include bandage soft contact lenses, autogenous Tenon's capsule, and cyanoacrylate adhesive glue. Cyanoacrylate adhesives provide a relatively simple means of closing a corneal perforation that is small (< 2 mm) or temporizing until penetrating keratoplasty may be performed with a formed anterior chamber. Since the polymerized adhesive leaves an irregular surface, a bandage contact lens should be placed over the site after placing the glue plug. The glue plug usually dislodges spontaneously within several weeks or is removed at the time of the corneal transplant (36).

Keratoprosthesis

When ocular scarring is so severe that penetrating keratoplasty techniques have failed, prosthokeratoplasty may be considered as a last resort. Keratoprosthesis may provide a limited amount of sight in the end stages of severe scarring disorders, such as cicatricial pemphigoid, erythema multiforme (Stevens-Johnson syndrome), and severe chemical burns. Various types of keratoprostheses have been tried with limited success. Polack and Heimke (18) designed a two-piece ceramic keratoprosthesis. It consists of an aluminum oxide, 10-mm-long optical cylinder, and an 8.5 mm in diameter retaining disk with 12 suture holes and a central 3-mm opening (17). Complications of keratoprostheses include infection, extrusion of implant, glaucoma, and retinal detachment (37).

REFERENCES

1. Pfister RR, Koski J. Alkali burns of the eye: pathophysiology and treatment. *South Med J* 1982;75:417–422.
2. Pfister RR. Chemical injuries of the eye. *Ophthalmology* (Rochester) 1983;90:1246–1253.
3. Campochiaro PA, Fogle JA, Spyker DA. Chemical and drug injury to the eye. In: Haddad LM, Winchester JF eds. *Chemical management of poisoning and drug overdoses*. Philadelphia: W.B. Saunders, 1990,370–378.
4. Nelson JD, Kopietz LA. Chemical injuries to the eye. Emergency, intermediate and long-term care. *Postgrad Med* 1987;81:62–66,69–71,75.

5. Burns FR, Paterson CA. Prompt irrigation of chemical eye injuries may avert severe damage. *Occup Health Saf* 1989;58:33-36.
6. Pyramid Films Corp. Preserving eyesight through quick response. *Occup Health Saf* 1981;50:70-73.
7. Deutsch TA, Feller DB. *Paton and Goldberg's management of ocular injuries*, 2nd ed. Philadelphia: W.B. Saunders, 1985;93-100.
8. Donshik PC, Berman MB, Dohlman CH, Gage J, Rose J. Effect of topical corticosteroids on ulceration in alkali-burned corneas. *Arch Ophthalmol* 1978;96:2117-2120.
9. Newsome NA, Gross J. Prevention of medroxyprogesterone of perforation in the alkali-burned rabbit cornea: inhibition of collagenolytic activity. *Invest Ophthalmol Vis Sci* 1977;16:21-31.
10. Levinson RA, Paterson CA, Pfister RR. Ascorbic acid prevents corneal ulceration and perforation following experimental alkali burns. *Invest Ophthalmol* 1976;15:986-993.
11. Thoft RA. Indications for conjunctival transplantation. *Ophthalmology* (Rochester) 1982;89:335-339.
12. Paton D, Milauskas AT. Indications, surgical technique and results of thin conjunctival flaps on the cornea: a review of 122 consecutive cases. *Int Ophthalmol Clin* 1970;10:329-345.
13. Panda A, Mohan M, Gupta HK, Chawdhary S. Keratoplasty in alkali burned corneas. *Ind J Ophthalmol* 1984;32:441-446.
14. Abel R Jr, Binder PS, Polack FM, Kaufman HE. The results of penetrating keratoplasty after chemical burns. *Trans Am Acad Ophthalmol* 1975;79:584-595.
15. Dohlman CH, Boruchoff SA, Sullivan GL. A technique for the repair of perforated corneal ulcer. *Arch Ophthalmol* (Chicago) 1967;77:519-525.
16. Tragakis MP, Rosen J, Brown SI. Transplantation of the perforated cornea. *Am J Ophthalmol* 1974;78:518-522.
17. Kozarsky AM, Knight SH, Waring GO 3rd. Clinical results with a ceramic keratoprosthesis placed through the eyelid. *Ophthalmology* 1987;94:904-911.
18. Polack FM, Heimke G. Ceramic keratoprostheses. *Ophthalmology* (Rochester) 1980;87:693-698.
19. Bennett TO, Peyman GA, Rutgard J. Intracameral phosphate buffer in alkali burns. *Can J Ophthalmol* 1978;13:93-95.
20. McCulley JP, Whiting DW, Pettit MG, Lauber SE. Hydrofluoric acid burns of the eye. *J Occup Med* 1983;25:447-450.
21. Singh G, Foster CS. Epidermal growth factor in alkali-burned corneal epithelial healing. *Am J Ophthalmol* 1987;103:802-807.
22. Pfister RR, Friend J, Dohlman CH. The anterior segments of rabbits after alkali burns: metabolic and histologic alterations. *Arch Ophthalmol* 1971;86:189-193.
23. Korey M, Peyman GA, Berkowitz R. The effect of hypertonic ointments on corneal alkali burns. *Ann Ophthalmol* 1977;9:1383-1387.
24. Pfister RR, Paterson CA. Additional clinical and morphological observations on the favorable effect of ascorbate on experimental ocular alkali burns. *Invest Ophthalmol Vis Sci* 1977;16:478-487.
25. Pfister RR, Paterson CA, Hayes SA. Topical ascorbate decreases the incidence of corneal ulceration after experimental alkali burns. *Invest Ophthalmol Vis Sci* 1978;17:1019-1024.
26. Nirankari VS, Varma SD, Lakhanpal V, Richards RD. Superoxide radical scavenging agents in treatment of alkali burns. An experimental study. *Arch Ophthalmol* 1981;99:886-887.
27. Petroutsos G, Pouliquen Y. Effect of ascorbic acid on ulceration in alkali-burned corneas. *Ophthalmic Res* 1984;16:185-189.
28. Hirst LW, Smiddy WE, Stark WJ. Corneal perforations, changing methods of treatment 1960-1980. *Ophthalmology* (Rochester) 1982;89:630-635.
29. Croll M, Croll LJ. Egg membrane for chemical injuries of eye, new adjuvant treatment. *Am J Ophthalmol* 1952;35:1585-1586.
30. Belin MW, Hannush SB. Mucous membrane abnormalities. In: Abbot RI, ed. *Surgical intervention in corneal and external diseases*. Orlando, FL: Grune & Stratton, 1987;159-176.
31. Bazan HEP, Braquet P, Peddy STK, Bazan NG. Inhibition of the alkali burn-induced lipoxygenation of arachidonic acid in the rabbit cornea by a PAF antagonist. *J Ocul Pharmacol* 1987;3:357-365.
32. Bloom SM, Gittinger JW Jr, Kazarian EL. Management of corneal thermal burns. *Am J Ophthalmol* 1986;102:536.
33. Leibowitz HM, Berrospi AR. Initial treatment of descemetocele with hydrophilic contact lenses. *Ann Ophthalmol* 1975;1161-1166.
34. Bechara SJ, Kara-Jose N, Pettinati AH. Therapeutic use of contact lenses in alkali burns of the cornea. *Cornea* 1987;6:117-121.

35. Larsson S. Treatment of perforated corneal ulcer by autoplastic scleral transplantation. *Br J Ophthalmol* 1948;32:54-57.
36. Mandelbaum S, Udell IJ. Noninfected corneal perforations. In: Abbott RL, ed. *Surgical intervention in corneal and external diseases*. Orlando, FL: Grune & Stratton, 1987;87-106.
37. Cardona H, DeVoe AG. Prosthokeratoplasty. *Trans Am Acad Ophthalmol Otolaryngol* 1977;83:272-275.

Subject Index